# Manual of
# Ophthalmology

## Clinical Diagnosis and Treatment of Eye Disease

Etiology Symptoms Signs Differential Diagnosis Diagnosis Treatment

# Manual of Ophthalmology

## Clinical Diagnosis and Treatment of Eye Disease

⊘Etiology ⊘Symptoms ⊘Signs ⊘Differential Diagnosis ⊘Diagnosis ⊘Treatment

### HV Nema

*former* Professor and Head
Department of Ophthalmology
Institute of Medical Sciences
Banaras Hindu University
Varanasi, Uttar Pradesh

### Nitin Nema

Professor
Department of Ophthalmology
Sri Aurobindo Institute of Medical Sciences
Indore, Madhya Pradesh

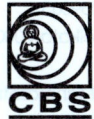

CBS

# CBS Publishers & Distributors Pvt Ltd

New Delhi • Bengaluru • Chennai • Kochi • Kolkata • Mumbai
Hyderabad • Nagpur • Patna • Pune • Vijayawada

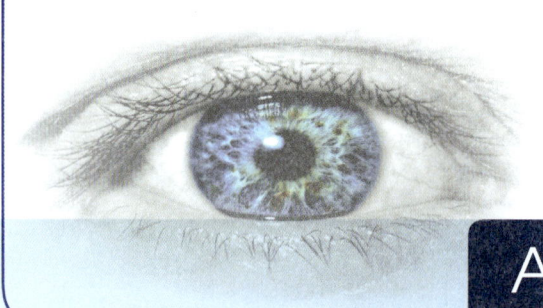

# Acknowledgments

We are grateful to Dr Prema Padmanabhan, Director, Sankara Nethralaya; Prof R Ramakrishnan, Aravind Eye Hospital, Tirunelveli; Prof Naresh Babu, Sr Consultant, Aravind Eye Hospital and Postgraduate Institute of Ophthalmology, Madurai; Prof Dhananjay Shukla, Senior Consultant, Aravind Eye Hospital and Postgraduate Institute of Ophthalmology; Dr SCL Chandravanshi, Assistant Professor, SS Medical College, Rewa; Dr Meena Chakrabarti, Chakrabarti Eye Care, Trivandrum; Dr Sushmita Kaushik, Associate Professor of Ophthalmology, Postgraduate Institute of Medical Education and Research, Chandigarh; Dr Rajul Parikh, Shreeji Hospital, Mumbai; and Dr Arun Bhargav, Retina Hospital, Indore; for their generous contribution of color photographs.

We thank Dr Pramod Sakhi, Department of Radiodiagnosis, for providing images.

Mr SK Jain (CMD), Mr Varun Jain (Director), Mr YN Arjuna (Senior VP, Publishing), CBS Publishers & Distributors, and their staff deserve our sincere thanks for their cooperation in the publication of the Manual.

**HV Nema**
**Nitin Nema**

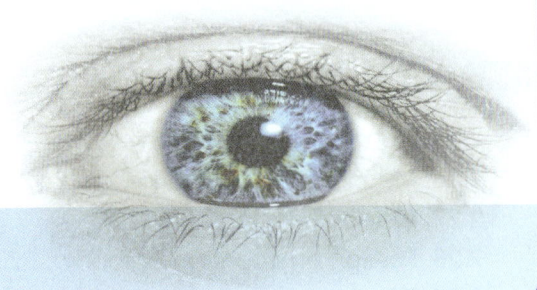

# Contents

## 6.  Glaucoma    105

## 7.  Cataract and Optics    128

## 12. Ocular Trauma                                        242

# Symptoms and Signs in Ophthalmology

## 1.1 SYMPTOMS AND THEIR CAUSES

It is essential to record the complaints of the patient before starting examination of the eye. All complaints, major or minor, should be recorded.

1. **Defective vision**
   - *Transient visual loss:* Causes of transient visual loss are migraine, bilateral vertebrobasilar insufficiency, papilledema, impending central retinal artery/vein occlusion, giant cell arteritis, ischemic optic neuropathy, glaucoma and ocular ischemic syndrome.
   - *Visual loss:* Visual loss may be sudden or gradual. It can be unilateral or bilateral and painless or painful.
   - *Sudden unilateral painless loss of vision:* It may occur in massive vitreous hemorrhage, retinal vascular occlusion, retinal detachment and dislocation of lens.
   - *Sudden bilateral painless loss of vision:* It may be found in patients with occipital lobe infarction, proliferative diabetic retinopathy, hypertensive retinopathy (grade IV) and posterior uveitis.
   - *Sudden painful loss of vision:* The sudden painful loss of vision is more frequent than painless loss of vision and it may be seen in acute angle-closure glaucoma, penetrating ocular injury, acute uveitis, ocular burns, central corneal ulcer and retrobulbar neuritis.
   - *Gradual painless impairment of vision in children:* It is due to refractive errors, developmental cataract, developmental/juvenile glaucoma, keratoconus and hereditary macular dystrophy.
   - *Gradual painless impairment of vision in old people:* It is common and is usually caused by cataract, glaucoma, corneal dystrophy, diabetic retinopathy (DR) and age-related macular degeneration (AMD).

2. **Night blindness**
   - Night blindness is often seen in the malnourished children of the third world countries.
   - Retinitis pigmentosa, advanced glaucoma, degenerative myopia, optic atrophy and congenital stationary night blindness are common causes of night blindness.
   - Iatrogenic night blindness may be seen following panretinal photocoagulation, very constricted pupil after the use of miotic therapy and chloroquine and quinine toxicity.

3. **Watering**
   - *Unilateral watering:* Common causes are corneal or conjunctival foreign

body (FB), corneal abrasion/ulcer, dacryocystitis, trichiasis, phlyctenular conjunctivitis, Bell's palsy and ectropion.

- *Bilateral watering:* Common causes include viral conjunctivitis, allergic conjunctivitis, trachoma, concretions and bilateral trichiasis/entropion.
- *Congenital or infantile watering* requires special attention as it may be caused by obstruction of nasolacrimal duct, congenital glaucoma, conjunctivitis and distichiasis.

4. **Discharge**
   - The discharge may be watery, mucopurulent, purulent, sanguineous and ropy.
   - Most viral conjunctivitis produces watery discharge.
   - Bacterial conjunctivitis gives mucopurulent or purulent discharge. *N. gonorrhoeae, Staphylococcus aureus* and *Streptococci* often cause purulent discharge.
   - Sanguineous discharge is found in herpes and traumatic conjunctivitis.
   - Ropy discharge is characteristic of vernal keratoconjunctivitis.

5. **Red eye:** The most common cause of red eye is conjunctivitis. Subconjunctival hemorrhage, exposure keratitis, corneal ulcer, episcleritis, scleritis, anterior uveitis, angle-closure glaucoma, dacrocystitis, orbital cellulitis, cavernous sinus thombosis drug reaction, and Stevens-Johnson (S-J) syndrome are other causes of red eye.

6. **Foreign body sensation:** Conjunctivitis, blepharitis, FB, superficial punctate keratitis (SPK), recurrent erosion of cornea, concretions, trichiasis, deposits on contact lens, post-trabeculectomy sutures, pterygium and dry eye disease can induce FB sensation.

7. **Burning:** Vernal keratoconjunctivitis, other types of allergic conjunctivitis, blepharitis, dry eye diseases, superior limbic keratoconjunctivitis, episcleritis and topical atropine, tropicamide, xylocaine, paracaine, fluorescein staining can lead to burning of eyes.

8. **Itching:** Causes of itchy eye are almost same as that of burning.

9. **Photophobia**
   - The most common cause of photophobia is corneal surface disorders like corneal abrasion, SPK and corneal ulcer.
   - Photophobia is often found in anterior uveitis, congenital glaucoma, conjunctivitis, mydriasis, aniridia and scleritis.
   - Systemic causes of photophobia are albinism, migraine, meningitis and trigeminal neuralgia.

10. **Swelling of eyelid**
    - Causes of inflammatory swelling of lid include hordeolum, blephroconjunctivitis, dacryocystitis, orbital cellulitis, agioneurotic edema, insect bite, herpes zoster ophthalmicus (HZO), dermatitis and trauma.
    - Noninflammatory conditions include chalazion, blepharochalasis, end-stage renal disorder, carotid-cavernous fistula (CCF), thyroid disorder and superior vena cava syndrome.

11. **Loss of eyelashes:** Eyelashes may be scanty or completely lost in blepharitis, leprosy, hypothyroidism, alopecia areata and postradiation.

12. **Inability of eyelids to close the eye:** Bell's palsy, marked proptosis, coma, burn and shortening of eyelid(s) during surgery may not allow proper closure of the eye.

13. **Twitching of eyelid**
    - Tic, FB in conjunctiva, blepharospasm, hemifacial spasm and albinism may induce twitching of lid.
    - It can also be induced in myasthenia gravis by tapping the lid (Cogan sign).

14. **Drooping of eyelid**
    - Drooping of lid or ptosis has varied etiology. It may be congenital or acquired.

- Depending on the cause of ptosis, it is often classified into five groups:

  (1) Myogenic, (2) aponeurotic, (3) neurogenic, (4) mechanical and (5) traumatic (*Refer* 9.1).

### 15. Proptosis

- Proptosis or bulging of eye may be unilateral or bilateral.
- Causes of unilateral proptosis include orbital cellulitis, retrobulbar hemorrhage, orbital cyst/tumor, orbital aneurysm, cavernous sinus thrombosis (early stage), mucocele of frontal sinus and orbital varix.
- Causes of bilateral proptosis are thyroid disorder (Graves' disease), congenital shallow orbits, late stage of cavernous sinus thrombosis, lymphoid tumors of the orbit and secondaries in orbits.

### 16. Double vision

- Double vision or diplopia can occur monocularly or binocularly.
- The causes of monocular diplopia include immature cataract, corneal opacity, additional iris hole (iridotomy/iridectomy), subluxated crystalline lens or intraocular lens (IOL) and retinal detachment.
- Binocular diplopia is more common; often found in paralytic strabismus following isolated III, IV and VI cranial nerves palsy.
- It is also seen in restrictive strabismus (thyroid ophthalmopathy, fracture floor of orbit, idiopathic orbital inflammation).
- Postoperative under or overcorrection of squint, retinal reattachment surgery, marked aniseikonia and ophthalmoplegia are other causes.

### 17. Jumping of objects

- Jumping of objects is a rare symptom. It may be associated with acquired nystagmus, internuclear ophthalmoplegia, ocular flutter and superior oblique myokymia.
- It may be found in myasthenia gravis and vestibular disorders.

### 18. Ocular pain

- Pain is often associated with refractive errors. Uncorrected or wrongly corrected refractive errors, ill-fitting spectacle glasses or decentered glasses, convergence insufficiency and spasm of accommodation are not uncommon causes of ocular pain.
- Patients with hordeolum internum, corneal abrasion, scleritis, anterior uveitis and optic neuritis usually suffer from mild to moderate pain in eye.
- Acute angle-closure glaucoma, HZO, secondary glaucoma, orbital cellulitis, acute dacryocystitis, acute dacryoadenitis, open-globe injury and migraine produce severe pain with headache and may need emergency treatment.

### 19. Headache

- It may be mild, moderate and severe.
- Mild headache can occur due to refractive errors, convergence deficiency, spasm of accommodation and anterior uveitis.
- Moderate to severe headache is associated with acute angle-closure glaucoma, secondary glaucoma, ocular ischemic syndrome and orbital cellulitis.
- Extraocular causes of headache include hypertension, raised intracranial pressure due to space occupying lesions or central nervous system (CNS) infection, intracranial hemorrhage, sinusitis, dental diseases, migraine, cervical spondylitis, giant cell arteritis and trigeminal neuralgia.

### 20. Cluster headache

- Etiology of cluster headache is not known.
- Use of alcohol and vasodilators and nitroglycerine are precipitating risk factors.

1

- Cluster headache is usually unilateral, extremely severe (boring or stabbing) and episodic in nature and shows remissions.
- It predominantly affects males and often awakens the patient from sleep.
- It is often associated with lacrimation, red eye, rhinorrhea, ptosis and Horner syndrome.

21. **Colored halos around light:** Patients with acute angle-closure glaucoma, corneal edema, corneal dystrophy, posterior polar cataract, purulent conjunctivitis, pigment dispersion syndrome and chloroquine or digitalis toxicity complain of color halos.

22. **Flashes of light:** Flashes of light may be seen in patients with posterior vitreous detachment (PVD), retinal detachment, neuroretinitis, lesions of the occipital lobe and migraine.

23. **Hallucinations**
    - Patients with bilateral patching, blindness, optic neuropathy and PVD may develop hallucinations.
    - Hallucinations are often found in lesions of parietotemporal lobes, Bonnet's syndrome and psychiatric patients.

24. **Floaters:** Floaters are caused by intermediate uveitis, vitreous hemorrhage, posterior uveitis, PVD, parasite in vitreous and migraine.

25. **Glare:** Patients with pseudophakia, post-LASIK (laser-assisted *in situ* keratomileusis), astigmatism, posterior polar cataract, PVD and dilated pupil often complain of glare.

26. **Distortion of vision**
    - Distortion of vision is commonly seen in macular diseases like central serous choroidopathy, macular edema, AMD and other causes of choroidal neovascular membrane (CNVM).
    - Less common causes include high astigmatism, ciliary spasm, cataract, corneal scar, keratoconus, postretinal detachment surgery, orbital fracture and hypotony.

## 1.2 CLINICAL SIGNS AND THEIR CAUSES

A thorough and systematic examination of eyes, elicitation of clinical signs and adequate knowledge of their differential diagnosis and causes are the basic prerequisite for the correct diagnosis of the eye disease. In certain conditions, assistance of neurophysician, pediatrician, pathologist and radiologist may be necessary.

1. **Face**
   - *Asymmetry of face:* It may be due to Bell's palsy, facial hemiatrophy or facial muscular dystrophy.
   - *Overaction of frontalis muscle:* The forehead may show excessive wrinkling, a sign of frontalis over action, to compensate the under action of levator, palpebrae, superioris in patients with partial ptosis.
   - *Loss of wrinkling of the forehead:* Complete loss of wrinkling on one half of the forehead denotes lower motor neuron facial palsy.
   - *The presence of pitted scars on one side of face:* It suggests an attack of HZO in the past.
   - *Scanty eyebrows:* The eyebrows may show scanty hair, especially in leprotic or myxedema patients.
   - *A face turn:* In horizontal incomitant strabismus, the face will turn in the direction of action of the paralyzed muscle to avoid diplopia.
   - *Head tilt:* Head tilt is adopted to avoid vertical diplopia in paralytic strabismus (vertical muscle palsy).
   - *Chin elevation or depression:* Chin elevation or depression is adopted to compensate the weakness of elevator or depressor muscles.
   - *Nystagmus:* When both eyes show rhythmic, repetitive oscillations, a sign which indicates that fixation reflex is not well-developed due to maldevelopment of eyes (congenital) or CNS and toxic

disorders. Nystagmus may be horizontal, vertical or torsional.

- **Nystagmoid jerks:** When the vision is impaired in infancy, the eyes often move arrhythmically and show searching movements.

## 2. Lids

- **Mongoloid obliquity of the palpebral aperture:** Normally, in the configuration of palpebral fissure, the level of medial and lateral canthi is more or less same, but in Mongolians the lateral canthus is at a higher level than the medial.

- **Antimongoloid obliquity of the palpebral aperture:** It is seen in Crouzon's disease wherein the outer canthus is at a considerably lower level than the medial.

- **Epicanthus:** A semilunar fold of skin runs over the inner canthus resulting in a pseudostrabismic appearance. It is usually congenital, bilateral and associated with ptosis. Epicanthus is a racial characteristic of Mongolians.

- **Telecanthus:** It is an abnormally increased intercanthal distance although the interpupillary distance remains normal. The condition is developmental and seen in Waardenburg syndrome.

- **Blepharophimosis:** The palpebral aperture may be all around narrow and is seen as a congenital anomaly.

- **Ptosis:** Ptosis is drooping of the upper lid. It is often seen as congenital anomaly or may be acquired due to trauma or CNS disorders (*Refer* 9.1 and 10.7).

- **Retraction of the upper lid:** Usually, the upper lid covers the upper one-sixth of the cornea. The upper limbus is visible due to contraction of the upper lid seen in thyrotoxicosis or sympathetic overactivity.

- **Distichiasis:** Distichiasis is a congenital anomaly of eyelashes marked by the presence of an additional posterior row of eyelashes which often cause irritation.

- **Trichiasis:** The eyelashes are directed forward and laterally. An inward misdirection of a solitary eyelash or a few eyelashes is known as trichiasis. It causes FB sensation and watering.

- **Entropion:** A complete in rolling of the upper or lower lid margin is called entropion, it is easy to diagnose (*Refer* 9.3).

- **Ectropion:** Ectropion is a mild sagging of the lower lid margin is commonly seen in old age. It induces annoying epiphora owing to the loss of contact of the lower punctum with the lacus lacrimalis (*Refer* 9.4).

- **Coloboma of lid:** A notch is found at the junction of medial-third and middle-third of the upper lid as a developmental defect associated with dermoid seen in Goldenhar syndrome.

- **Edema of the lid:** Edema of lid is common because of looseness of its skin. It may be caused by inflammatory conditions of lid, conjunctiva, lacrimal sac and orbit. Passive edema of lid may be found in cavernous sinus thrombosis, nephrotic syndrome, CCF, hypoproteinemia, etc.

- **Lid signs of Graves' disease**
  - Dalrymple sign: Unilateral or bilateral upper eyelid retraction is the most common (90%)
  - von Graefe: Upper eyelid lags on down gaze
  - Gifford sign: Eversion of upper eyelid is difficult
  - Stellwag sign: Infrequent and incomplete blinking
  - Kocher sign: Spasmatic retraction of upper lid during fixation
  - Rosenbach sign: On gentle closure or taping, tremors of eyelids may be evident

1

- Enroth sign: Fullness or edema of lower eyelid
- Pochin sign: Amplitude of blinking is reduced
- Boston sign: Jerky movements of upper lid on down gaze
- Jellinek sign: Abnormal pigmentation of upper lid
- Riesman sign: Bruit over eyelid.

3. **Conjunctiva**

The palpebral conjunctiva should be inspected for the presence of follicles, papillary hypertrophy, scarring, membrane, FB (especially in sulcus subtarsalis) and concretions. The upper fornix requires double eversion of the lid for detection of FB from the upper fornix. The distinction between the conjunctival and the ciliary injections should be made. Occasionally, both types of injections may coexist as seen in acute angle-closure glaucoma.

- *Follicles:* Follicles are found in trachoma, inclusion conjunctivitis, epidemic keratoconjunctivitis, M-A conjunctivitis, herpes, topical drug toxicity and benign folliculosis.
- *Papillary hypertrophy:* Papillary hypertrophy of conjunctiva is very common and seen almost all inflammatory conditions of conjunctiva; bacterial, viral or allergic.
- *Scarring:* Scarring is a characteristic feature of chronic trachoma. It is also seen in membranous conjunctivitis, oculocutaneous syndrome and ocular burns.
- *Membrane:* Presence of true or pseudo-membrane is an important sign of membranous conjunctivitis. The membranous conjunctivitis may be caused by *Streptococcus, Pneumococcus, Staphylococcus, Corynebacterium diphtheriae, Herpes,* adenovirus and acid burn.
- *Pterygium:* A wing-shaped encroachment of bulbar conjunctiva onto the cornea is known as pterygium. Dry, dusty and hot atmosphere cause microtrauma to the conjunctiva. Additionally, role of ultraviolet rays is also implicated.
- *Bitot spot:* A dry, lusterless, triangular spot (Bitot's spot) with the base toward the limbus is seen frequently in children with vitamin A deficiency.
- *Dryness of conjunctiva:* Excessive loss of goblet cells leads to dryness of conjunctiva. It is seen in chronic trachoma, Sjögren's syndrome, S-J syndrome, lagophthalmos, long-standing proptosis and cicatrical pemphigoid.
- *Subconjunctival hemorrhage:* Subconjunctival hemorrhage is common in children and found in acute hemorrhagic conjunctivitis, conjunctivitis caused by *Streptococcus pneumoniae* and *Haemophilus aegyptius (Koch-Weeks bacillus).* Trivial trauma often leads to small subconjunctival hemorrhage, but fracture of the base of skull leads to a large hemorrhage. Diabetes, hypertension, blood dyscrasias, scurvy and crush injuries are the other causes seen in adults.
- *Symblepharon:* Symblepharon is an adhesion of lid margin with bulbar conjunctiva or cornea (anterior). When obliteration of the upper or lower fornices occurs, it is known as posterior and a complete adhesion of lids with globe is called total symblepharon. Causes of symblepharon include chemical burn, membranous conjunctivitis, epidemic keratoconjunctivitis, cicatrical pemphigoid, S-J syndrome and trauma.
- *Pigmentation:* The conjunctiva may become yellow in jaundice, brown in Addison's disease and gray in ochronosis. Black discoloration occurs in precancerous melanosis, local use of mascara and adrenaline.

4. **Cornea**
   - *Microcornea:* A small cornea or *microcornea*, has a diameter of less than 10 mm. It is a developmental anomaly.
   - *Megalocornea:* An enlarged cornea with a diameter of more than 12.5 mm is known as megalocornea. Like microcornea, it is also a congenital anomaly and needs to be differentiated from *buphthalmos*.
   - *Keratoconus:* It is a localized conical bulge of the cornea mostly seen in young girls. It is a congenital anomaly of curvature of cornea.
   - *Keratoglobus:* The entire cornea appears globular (*keratoglobus*).
   - *Corneal abrasion:* Corneal abrasion is caused by trivial trauma resulting in a breach in the corneal epithelium that can be easily seen on fluorescein staining.
   - *Corneal edema:* Corneal edema is common and may be caused by ocular trauma, overwear of contact lens, keratitis, decompensated keratoconus, pseudophakic bullous keratopathy, corneal dystrophy, acute angle-closure glaucoma, congenital glaucoma and corneal graft rejection.
   - *Corneal opacification:*
     - The opacity in the cornea is found following birth trauma, interstitial keratitis, corneal ulcer and in congenital glaucoma and mucopolysaccharidosis.
     - Whorl-like corneal opacities may be found in Fabry disease and toxicity of chloroquine, amiodarone, phenothiazine and indomethacin.
   - *Corneal vascularization:* The vascularization of cornea may be superficial or deep or sometimes mixed. Causes of vascularization of cornea include trachoma, corneal ulcer, keratitis, ocular burns, herpes, sclerokeratitis, ill-fitting contact lens and ocular rosacea.
   - *Reduced corneal sensitivity:* The corneal sensation is reduced in herpes, leprosy, neuroparalytic keratitis, absolute glaucoma and cerebellopontine angle tumor.
   - *Enlarged corneal nerves:*
     - Corneal nerves may be enlarged and visible in neurofibromatosis, keratoconus, acanthamoeba keratitis and congenital glaucoma.
     - Multiple endocrine neoplasia, pheochromocytoma, mucosal neuroma and leprosy are systemic disorders wherein the nerves are enlarged.

5. **Anterior chamber**
   - *Shallow anterior chamber:* The anterior chamber is shallow in extremes of ages, angle-closure glaucoma, malignant glaucoma, postoperative wound leak and high hyperopia.
   - *Deep anterior chamber:* Anterior chamber is deep in high myopia, aphakia, posterior dislocation of lens, buphthalmos and keratoglobus.
   - *Irregular anterior chamber:* Anterior chamber is irregular in depth in iridiocyclitis, anterior synechia and anterior subluxation of the lens.
   - *Keratic precipitates:*
     - Keratic precipitates (KPs) are collection of inflammatory cells on the endothelium of the cornea. They may be fresh or old or macrophagic or lymphocytic.
     - Fresh KPs look white round shinning dots while old KPs appear as dull, with uneven margin and pigmented.
     - Macrophagic KPs are large and greasy (mutton-fat), a few in number and arranged in a triangular zone inferiorly. They are found in granulomatous uveitis.
     - Lymphocytic KPs are small, multiple and diffusely distributed and found in nongranulomatous uveitis.

- *Flare*
  - The presence of floating protein particles in the aqueous humor is called flare.
  - It may vary from faint to intense. Flare is moderate to intense in acute anterior uveitis while faint in chronic uveitis and acute angle-closure glaucoma.
- *Cells:* The aqueous may contain inflammatory cells in acute iridocyclitis.
- *Hypopyon:* Hypopyon is a collection of pus in the anterior chamber and seen in infective corneal ulcer, severe anterior uveitis, endophthalmitis, toxic IOL syndrome and Behçet syndrome.
- *Pseudohypopyon:* Tumor cells from retinoblastoma or malignant melanoma may migrate into the anterior chamber and produce *pseudohypopyon*. Pseudohypopyon may present a convex level of fluid in the chamber.
- *Hyphema*
  - The collection of blood in the anterior chamber is known as *hyphema*. It is caused by ocular trauma, intraocular surgery, herpes zoster and gonococcal iridocyclitis.
  - Fuchs' heterochromic iridocyclitis, use of anticoagulants, neovascularization of iris, intraocular neoplasm and blood dyscrasia are other causes.

6. **Iris**
   - *Heterochromia:* The two irides or a sector of one iris may be of different colors is known as *heterochromia*. It is found in chronic iridocyclitis, Fuchs' heterochromic iridocyclitis, Horner syndrome, Waardenburg syndrome, iris nevus, oculodermal melanosis, metastasis in iris and intraocular tumors.
   - *Neovascularization of iris:* It may develop in proliferative diabetic retinopathy, occlusion of the central/branch retinal vein or artery, longstanding uveitis, ocular ischemic syndrome, retinal detachment and melanoma of the iris.
   - *Nodules on iris:* Tuberculoma, leproma, gumma, FB granuloma, Koeppe's or Bussaca's nodules of sarcoidosis, melanoma, juvenile xanthogranuloma, Lisch nodule of neurofibromatosis may manifest as raised nodules on the iris.

7. **Intraocular pressure (IOP)**
   - *Increased IOP:* IOP is usually increased in acute angle-closure glaucoma, open-angle glaucoma, secondary glaucoma, retrobulbar hemorrhage, hyphema, intraocular tumors and suprachoroidal hemorrhage.
   - *Decreased IOP:* IOP is often decreased in penetrating ocular injury, retinal detachment, choroidal detachment, over-filtering trabeculectomy bleb, wound leak after intraocular surgery, traumatic shutdown of ciliary body, long-standing uveitis and dehydration.

8. **Lens**
   - *Cataract:* Opacity in the lens is called *cataract*. It can be developmental or acquired. Zonular cataract is the most common developmental cataract and senile cataract among the acquired cataracts.
   - *Luxated or subluxated lens:* (*Refer* 7.2)
   - *Iridescent particles in the lens:* Presence of iridescent particles in lens is uncommon and may be found in patients with myotonic dystrophy, hypothyroidism, hypocalcemia and complicated uveitic cataract.
   - *Anterior lenticonus:* It is a rare condition and is found in Alport syndrome.

9. **Choroid**
   - *Choroidal neovascularization:* Choroidal neovascularization is found in age-related macular degeneration, ocular histoplasmosis, choroidal rupture, choroidal neoplasm, high myopia, idiopathic polypoidal choroidal vasculo-

pathy, angioid streaks, drusen of optic disk.

- **Choroidal detachment:** (*Refer 5.23*).
- **Choroidal folds:** Choroidal folds may be found in orbital and choroidal tumors, posterior scleritis, marked hypotony, retinal detachment, papilledema, thyroid ophthalmopathy, pseudotumor orbit and trauma.
- **Malignant melanoma:** (*Refer 5.24*).

10. **Retina and vitreous**
    - **Cystoid macular edema (CME):** It may be found in host of condition like post-intraocular operation (Irvine-Gass syndrome), diabetic retinopathy, uveitis, central retinal vein occlusion (CRVO), branch retinal vein occlusion (BRVO), sarcoidosis, Eales' disease, Behçet syndrome, rhegmatogenous retinal detachment (RRD), AMD, idiopathic macular telangiectasia, etc.
    - **Macular hole**
      - The macular hole is characterized by a round-red spot with pin-headed yellow dots in the center of macula causing loss of vision.
      - It may be caused by trauma, CME, vitreomacular traction and epiretinal membrane.
      - Macular hole is classified in four stages: (i) impending hole with macular ring and yellow spots, (ii) a small macular hole, (iii) macular hole with cuff of subretinal fluid (SRF) and (iv) macular hole with SRF and complete PVD.
    - **Cherry-red spot at macula**
      - A striking cherry-red spot developed at the macula as the choriocapillaris shine against the ischemic white background of macular edema or deposits.
      - It is seen in the central retinal artery occlusion, commotio retinae, Tay-Sachs disease, Sandhoff disease, generalized gangliosidosis, Niemann-

Pick disease, sialidosis and galacto-sialidoses.

- **Bull's eye macula**
  - Bull's eye macula presents a characteristic ring of depigmentation surrounded by a ring of hyperpigmentation.
  - It is found in chloroquine toxicity, AMD, cone dystrophy, Stargardt disease and Batten's disease.

- **Cotton-wool spots**
  - Cotton-wool spots are white, ill-defined spots with fuzzy margins and found in the nerve fiber layer of retina.
  - They may be caused by an obstruction of axoplasmic flow and collection of its debris. Cotton-wool spots may be found in hypertension, diabetic retinopathy, CRVO, human immunodeficiency virus (HIV) retinopathy, giant cell arteritis, systemic lupus erythematosus (SLE), Wegener granulomatosis, retinal embolism and radiation retinopathy, etc.

- **Hard exudates:** Hard exudates are found in acute or chronic hypertension, diabetic retinopathy, renal retinopathy, retinal arterial microaneurysm and retinal telangiectasia.

- **Hollenhorst spot:** A bright yellowish cholesterol embolus at the bifurcation of retinal arteries seen in arteriosclerosis.

- **Drusen:** Idiopathic or may be seen in AMD.

- **Roth spots:** White-centered hemorrhages in retina may occur in DR, septic chorioretinitis, leukemia, SLE, pernicious anemia and sickle cell disease.

- **Retinal angiomas:** Retinal angiomas are not common. They may be seen in von Hippel's disease.

- **Retinal arterial macroaneurysm:** Retinal arterial macroaneurysm is seen at the bifurcation of artery or arteriovenous crossing and usually associated

**1**

with decreased vision and hemorrhages in almost all layers of retina and vitreous. It is caused by arteriosclerotic disease and hypertension.

- *Neovascularization of retina:* Neovascularization of retina may be central or peripheral. Neovascularization at the posterior pole is seen in DR and CRVO. Peripheral neovascularization is found in a number of conditions such as Eales' disease, BRVO, sarcoidosis, syphilis, chronic uveitis, diabetes, ocular ischemic syndrome, tumors, sickle cell and Coats' disease.

- *Epiretinal membrane:* Epiretinal membrane is also known as cellophane retinopathy, surface wrinkling retinopathy and macular pucker. It may be idiopathic or caused by retinal break, vitreous hemorrhage, ocular trauma, PVD, uveitis and following intraocular surgery, cryopexy and photocoagulation.

- *Retinal breaks or holes*
  - Breaks or holes in retina are not rare. They appear as round holes, horseshoe tear or tear and dialysis. Both horseshoe tear (with or without operculum) and dialysis are acute in onset and often caused by trauma.
  - Acute breaks may be associated with vitreous hemorrhage or PVD.
  - Chronic retinal breaks may remain asymptomatic and may be surrounded by pigments. A line of demarcation between detached and attached retina can be seen.
  - Aphakia, pseudophakia, high myopia, lattice degeneration, recent or old trauma and retinoschisis are risk factors for retinal breaks.

- *Retinoschisis:* (*Refer* 8.18)
- *Detachment of retina:* (*Refer* 8.20)
- *Sheathing of retinal veins:* Sheathing of retinal veins or periphlebitis retinae is commonly seen in Eales' disease, syphilis, sarcoidosis, multiple sclerosis

and sickle cell disease. It is also found in tuberculosis, viral and fungal retinitis, AIDS and Behçet disease.

- *Normal retina with marked loss of vision:* A complaint of decreased vision or gross visual loss with normal fundus poses a great challenge to a treating physician. Following conditions should be kept in mind while dealing with such patients: Amblyopia anisometropic, strabismus, toxic effect of drugs, tobacco, alcohol, retrobulbar optic neuritis, Leber hereditary optic neuropathy, cone dystrophy and psychiatric disorders.

- *Vitreous opacities*
  - Opacities in the vitreous are caused by the presence of blood, inflammatory exudates, parasites and tumor cells.
  - Occasionally, multiple small yellow and round bodies are suspended in the normal vitreous, they are known as asteroid hyalosis. These bodies are composed of calcium soaps of palmitate and stearate.
  - Some patients may see a shower of highly refractile small crystals in liquefied vitreous on ocular movements known as synchysis scintillans. The crystals are formed of cholesterol.

- *Blood in vitreous*
  - Blood in the vitreous often comes from retina. It may be localized or diffused.
  - Trauma, diabetes, retinal tear, hypertension, CRVO, Eales' disease blood dyscrasia, and retinovascular malformations are some of the causes of vitreous hemorrhage.
  - Long-standing vitreous hemorrhage may produce membrane formation and retinitis proliferans.

- *Posterior vitreous detachment* (*Refer* 8.30)

11. **Neuro-ophthalmology**
  - *Anisocoria*
    - The size of the two pupils is not equal in anisocoria; causes may be physiological, congenital and acquired.

- Physiological anisocoria is seen in about 15–20% of normal individuals. A difference of less than 0.5 mm may be found in the size of two pupils. This inequality remains in both light and dark.
- It is not rare to find that anisocoria may change sides.
- Causes of congenital anisocoria include heterochromia, coloboma of iris, ectopic pupil, polycoria and aniridia.
- Acquired anisocoria is caused by a host of conditions such as ocular trauma, intraocular surgery iritis, iris atrophy, tear of sphincter pupillae, unilateral instillation of miotic or mydriatic agent, palsy of third cranial nerve, Argyll Robertson pupil, Adie pupil, Horner syndrome, etc.

■ *Relative afferent pupillary defect (RAPD)*
- Normally, both pupils constrict equally to the swinging flashlight test.
- The degree of constriction depends on the brightness of light source; brighter the light, greater the constriction.
- In the presence of a unilateral or asymmetric optic nerve disease, the affected pupil shows reduced amplitude of constriction and accelerated dilatation (recovery) as compared with the contralateral eye (control).
- Other causes of RAPD are unilateral maculopathy, amblyopia and severe unilateral retinopathy.
- A contralateral RAPD is observed in lesions of optic tract, brachium of superior colliculus, dense unilateral cataract and complete ptosis. In latter two conditions, retina is dark adapted and thus shows greater stimulation to light.
- RAPD is not seen in bilateral optic neuropathy, which produces APD.

■ *Argyll Robertson pupil*
- Argyll Robertson pupil is caused by the syphilitic lesion of the tectum affecting the pupillary pathway.
- The pupils are small, irregular and show impaired light reaction but the reaction to convergence and accommodation is retained (light-near dissociation).
- They dilate poorly in dark and are asymmetrical.

■ *Adie's pupil*
- A tonic pupil of unknown etiology may be found in young women. Herpes simplex virus, varicella zoster, giant cell arteritis and orbital trauma are the causes.
- The pupil is irregular and shows a little or no reaction to light. A slow and tonic constriction is found on convergence followed by redilatation.
- Rarely, it may present involvement of both eyes with acute onset.

■ *Paradoxical pupillary reaction*
- It is an abnormal pupillary reaction characterized by dilatation of pupil in light and constriction in darkness.
- It may be seen in congenital stationary night blindness, optic nerve hypoplasia, congenital achromatopsia, Leber disease, Best disease and atypical retinitis pigmentosa.

■ *Miosis*
Miotic pupil is small and constricted, usually seen after the use of topical pilocarpine or systemic morphine. Pontine hemorrhage (pin-pointed pupil), Horner's syndrome and iridocyclitis can produce miosis.

■ *Mydriasis*
- Mydriatic pupil is dilated. Pupil is usually dilated after the use of topical mydriatic or cycloplegic drugs.
- Other causes of pupillary dilatation are acute congestive glaucoma (large

1

vertically oval pupil), absolute glaucoma, optic atrophy and the third nerve palsy (ophthalmoplegia interna).

■ *Horner syndrome:* (*Refer* 11.17)

■ *Leukocoria:* Leukocoria or white pupillary reflex may be seen in retinoblastoma, toxocariasis, cataract, retrolental fibroplasia, Coats' disease, persistent hyperplastic primary vitreous, retinal detachment, uveitis and coloboma of retina and choroid.

■ *Papilledema*
  • Papilledema is a noninflammatory swelling of optic disk head with obliteration of the cup and blurring of the disk margin. It is due to raised intracranial pressure. It may be unilateral or bilateral.
  • Causes of unilateral papilledema are central retinal vein occlusion, ischemic optic neuropathy, ocular hypotonia, orbital cellulitis, orbital venous thrombosis, meningioma of optic nerve sheath, carotid cavernous fistula, early thyroid ophthalmopathy, posterior fossa tumors, brain abscess, early cavernous sinus thrombosis, pseudotumor cerebri and Foster-Kennedy syndrome.
  • Bilateral papilledema may be seen in patients with midbrain tumors, parieto-occipital tumors, cerebellar tumor, aneurysms, cavernous sinus thrombosis, malignant hypertension, nephritis, toxemia of pregnancy, blood dyscrasias, giant cell arteritis and late thyroid ophthalmopathy.

■ *Optic neuritis*
  • Multiple sclerosis is the most common cause of optic neuritis.
  • Other causes include herpes, chickenpox, mumps, measles, tuberculosis, sarcoidosis, neurosyphilis, neuromyelitis and autoimmune vascular disorders.

■ *Optic atrophy:* The disk becomes pale and atrophic in optic atrophy. Glaucoma, occlusion of central retinal artery, optic neuropathy, optic neuritis, retinal degeneration, syphilis, drug toxicity (ethnambutol), radiation, compression of chiasma or optic tract by intracranial space occupying lesion and trauma can produce optic atrophy.

■ *Optic pit*
  • A small, gray or yellow, round depression is seen on the temporal part of optic disk. It is mostly congenital.
  • A pseudopit may be occasionally found in low tension glaucoma. Optic pit may be associated with serous macular detachment, shallow RD and retinoschisis.

■ *Visual field defect*
  • *Central scotoma:* Central scotoma is often found in optic neuritis, toxoplasma macular retinochoiditis, macular coloboma, occipital lobe lesion, macular hole, occlusion of cilioretinal artery and retinitis pigmentosa inversus.
  • *Paracentral scotoma:* Paracentral scotoma can be found in glaucoma and chloroquine toxicity.
  • Arcuate scotoma: Arcuate scotoma is more common field defect than central scotoma and is seen in glaucoma, ischemic optic neuropathy, optic neuritis and drusen of optic disk.
  • *Enlargement of blind spot:* Enlargement of blind spot is a feature of marked papilledema, optic disk drusen, high myopia with annular cresent, coloboma of optic nerve, opaque nerve fibers around the disk and multiple evanescent white dot syndrome.
  • *Concentric contraction of visual fields:* Retinitis pigmentosa, progressive glaucoma, long-standing papilledema, panretinal photocoagulation/cryopexy, bilateral infarction of

occipital lobe with sparing of macula and central retinal artery occlusion (CRAO) with sparing of cilioretinal artery cause concentric contraction of visual fields.

- *Homonymous hemianopia:* Stroke, neoplasm and aneurysm of parietal, temporal and occipital lobes often give homonymous hemianopia. It presents a typical field defect due to lesions of optic tract and lateral geniculate body.
- *Upper altitudinal quadrantanopia:* Lower BRVO or BRAO, ischemic optic neuropathy, optic neuritis and lesions of Meyer's loop in the temporal lobe produce upper altitudinal quadrantanopia.
- *Lower altitudinal defects:* Ischemic optic neuropathy, upper hemi-occlusion of retinal vein/artery, optic neuritis, glaucoma and lesions of Meyer's loop in the perietal lobe produce lower altitudinal quadrantanopia.
- *Bitemporal hemianopia:* Bitemporal hemianopia is caused by tumors of sella turcica, suprasellar aneurysm and chiasmal arachnoiditis. They press and destroy the nasal fibers of each retina in the chiasma.
- *Binasal hemianopia:* Binasal hemianopia is caused by enlargement of the third ventricle and atheromatous change and hardening of the carotids and/or posterior communicating arteries. They press and destroy the fibers of temporal halves of each retina.

## 12. Lacrimal apparatus

- *Watering*
  - Watering can occur due to obstruction in the tear drainage system by eyelashes and concretions (obstruct the punctum), stricture in the canaliculus and nasolacrimal duct and blockage of nasal opening of the duct by atrophic rhinitis and nasal polyp.

- Conjunctivitis, keratitis, dacryocystitis and dacryoadenitis cause profuse watering.
- *Dacryoadenitis:* Acute inflammation of lacrimal gland may occur in mumps, measles and infectious mononucleosis and chronic inflammation in sarcoidosis and tuberculosis.
- *Enlargement of lacrimal gland:* The lacrimal gland becomes enlarged in inflammatory and neoplastic conditions. Mixed cell tumor is common. Adenoid cystic carcinoma of lacrimal gland grows rapidly and is usually fetal. Both tumors cause proptosis and downward and inward dislodgment of the eyeball.
- *Enlargement of lacrimal sac:* The lacrimal sac is enlarged in dacryocystitis, mucocele and tumor of the sac.
- *Dry eye disease:* (*Refer* 9.9)

## 13. Orbit

- *Orbital cellulitis*
  - Orbital cellulitis is an inflammation of the orbit. An extension of infection from paranasal sinuses and teeth to the orbit is common.
  - Trauma, septic operation on the eyeball and facial erysipelas are considered as risk factors. Common organisms causing orbital cellulitis include *Streptococcus pyogenes, Streptococcus pneumoniae, Staphylococcus aureus, Pseudomonas aeruginosa, Aspergillus* and *Mucor.*

- *Proptosis*
  - Proptosis is a forward bulging of the eyeball with exposure of the lower limbus. It may be unilateral or bilateral.
  - Causes of unilateral proptosis include orbital cellulitis, tumors (meningioma, glioma, hemangioma, mixed-cell tumor of lacrimal gland, intraocular neoplasm), orbital cyst, orbital varix and early cavernous sinus thrombosis.
  - Bilateral proptosis is seen in systemic disorders like thyroid ophthalmopathy, lymphoma, lympho-

**1**

sarcoma, leukemia, late stage of cavernous sinus thrombosis, oxycephaly, Apert anomaly and Crouzon disease.

■ *Orbital tumors*

- Orbital tumors of childhood include dermoid, dermolipoma, teratoma, hemangioma, glioma of optic nerve, rhabdomyosarcoma, leukemia and neuroblastoma.

- Orbital tumors commonly seen in adults are meningioma, neurofibromatosis, neurofibroma, pleomorphic adenoma and malignant-mixed tumor of lacrimal gland.

- Carcinoma of lid or maxillary sinus, nasopharynx, breast or lungs, retinoblastoma cutaneous malignant melanoma may involve the orbit.

# Diagnostic Procedures in Ophthalmology

## 2.1 VISUAL ACUITY

### Visual Acuity Assessment in Adults

1. Testing of visual acuity is usually performed with the help of standard test types.
2. The Snellen test type and Bailey-Lovie chart (Fig. 2.1) are used for literate patients while E chart and C chart for illiterates.
3. Visual acuity can be measured in meters, feet, decimal or logarithm of minimum angle of resolution (logMAR).
4. In spite of 6/6 visual acuity, some individuals feel difficulties in their day-to-day visual functions.

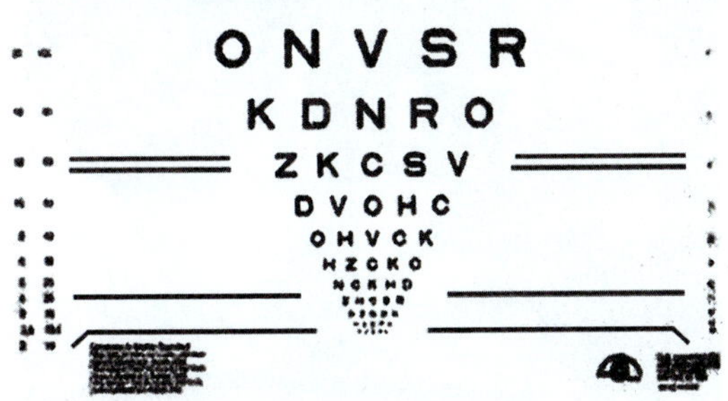

Fig. 2.1: Bailey-Lovie chart

5. Contrast sensitivity is considered a better measure of visual acuity and tested with the help of Pelli-Robson letter charts or CSV1000 charts of vector vision.
6. Near visual acuity is usually tested with the help of near vision charts. Jaeger type or Roman test types are often used. Rosenbaum pocket vision screener or Lebensohn chart may also be used.
7. Some mixed vision charts show music types, crosswords, tables, print types and playing cards.

### Visual Acuity Assessment in Infants and Children

1. Accurate assessment of visual acuity in infants is difficult. However, the infant's ability to fix and follow a moving object provides rough assessment.
2. Fixation develops at 4–8 weeks and by 6 months infant grasps objects. Central steady fixation indicates a vision of 6/60.
3. Induction of optokinetic nystagmus or involuntary pursuit movements with the help of a black and white strips drum are useful methods.
4. Preferential looking test and Teller acuity cards test are useful tests for estimating vision below the age of 18 months.
5. Miniature toys test, dot visual acuity test and coin test can measure the visual acuity in children between 1 and 3 years.

**2**

6. Visual acuity in children older than 3 years can be tested by Tumbling E test, HOTV test and Allen cards.

## 2.2 COLOR VISION TESTING

1. Various methods are available to assess the color vision in an individual. Color vision testing is essential before recruitment in certain jobs such as railway, navy, air force, etc.
2. Ishihara pseudoisochromatic plate test (Fig. 2.2) is commonly used to assess the color status of a patient. The test is based on the principle of color confusion. Other tests developed based on this principle include American optical company plates, Hardy-Rand-Rittler plates, Tritan plate and Dvorine booklet.
3. Some tests have been developed on the basis of color matching. They are Sloan achromatopsia test, Nagel's spectral matching test and Pickford-Nicolson anomaloscope.
4. Edridge-Green lantern, Farnsworth lantern test (Falant) and Homes-Wright lantern tests measure the proficiency of a person to recognize the color signals but do not grade the color vision defects.
5. Farnsworth-Munsell 100 hue test assesses the individual's ability to discriminate hues of color. It is an arrangement test consisting of 85 color chips of different hues. Patients with color deficiency make error in arranging the chips in each row in 2 minutes. Scores of knob/caps are plotted on a circular graph. The test can detect all types of color deficiencies.
6. Farnsworth D-15 test has only 15 color chips and is a more rapid than the 100 hue test.

## 2.3 SLIT-LAMP EXAMINATION

Slit-lamp examination (Fig. 2.3) is the most important procedure in diagnosing diseases

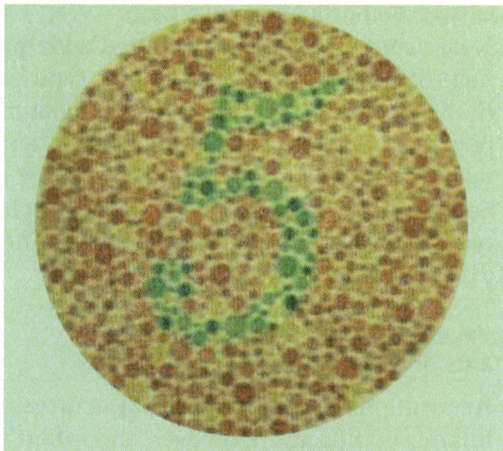
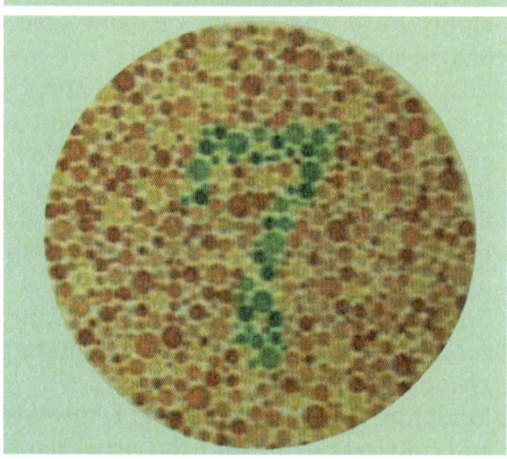

**Fig. 2.2:** Ishihara color vision plates

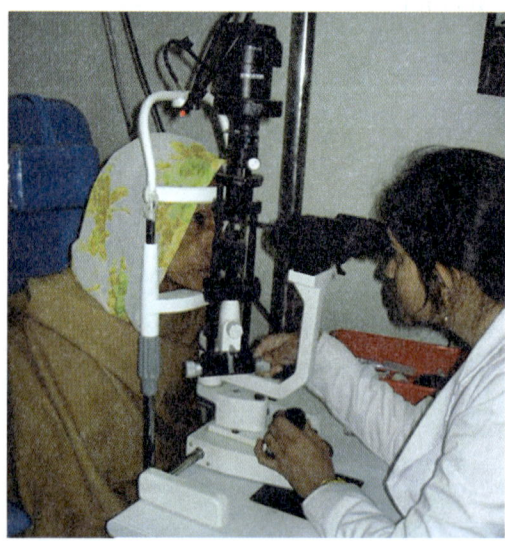

**Fig. 2.3:** Slit-lamp examination

of the anterior and posterior segments of the eye. It helps examination under magnification, bright light and stereopsis. The beam of the slit-lamp can be projected at any angle or moved while examining the ocular structure to locate the ocular pathology.

Various types of examinations are performed with the instrument.

### Direct Diffuse Illumination

1. It provides a wide field to examine the anterior surface of the cornea for scars, vascularization, tear debris and defects of eyelid margin.
2. Epithelial abrasion takes green stain with fluorescein dye and usually examined under cobalt blue filter.
3. Patients with keratoconjunctvitis sicca show pink stains of dead epithelial cells when stained with rose Bengal dye.
4. Direct diffuse illumination examination can distinguish a difference between conjuctival and ciliary/episcleral injections.

### Direct Focal Illumination

1. Direct focal illumination with a small slit and variable magnification is the most frequently used examination.
2. It is applied for localization of foreign body (FB) in layers of the cornea, keratic precipitates (KPs) at the back of cornea (Fig. 2.4),

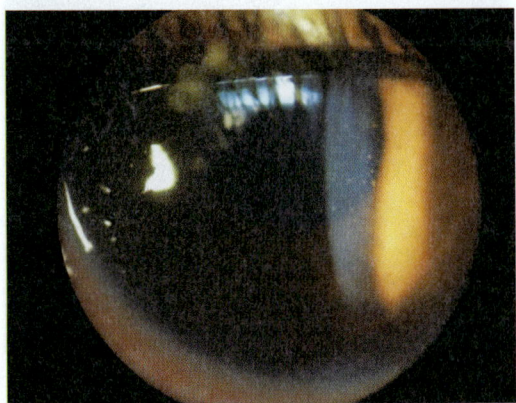

**Fig. 2.4:** Slit-lamp examination showing KPs

grading of flare and cells in the aqueous humor, nodules, neovascularization and FB on the iris and assessment of lens opacities.
3. Direct focal illumination can be used for grading the angle of the anterior chamber by Van Herick technique.

### Retroillumination

1. A small beam of light is reflected from iris to indirectly illuminate cornea to detect KPs, corneal epithelial or endothelial dystrophy.
2. The light from lens can easily show the atrophic defects in the iris.
3. Similarly, the light coming from the retina greatly helps in the diagnosis of posterior polar cataract or subcapsular posterior cataract.

### Sclerotic Scatter

A wide light beam is directed onto the limbus at a very low angle. It can detect small corneal opacities, FBs and edema of the cornea.

### Indirect Illumination

1. A sharp beam of light is focused on the cornea and the dark area just lateral or proximal to it is examined.
2. This examination can detect microcystic edema, corneal surface irregularity, infiltrates and opacities.
3. Slit-lamp examination is used in many diagnostic procedures such as specular reflection for viewing the endothelium of the cornea, contact lens fitting, applanation tonometry, gonioscopy and biomicroscopic fundus examination.

### 2.4 TONOMETRY

1. Tonometry is a method to measure the intraocular pressure (IOP) with the help of tonometer.
2. Both contact and noncontact tonometers are available for recording IOP.

**2**

3. Goldmann applanation is a contact tono-meter and is considered a gold standard for measuring IOP in the sitting posture.
4. Recently, it has been recognized that a variation in the central corneal thickness (CCT) would affect the accuracy of IOP measurements. A thin CCT would give a lower pressure while a thick CCT a higher.
5. A number of new tonometers have been introduced to measure IOP. Tonopen and pneumatonometer are widely used in ophthalmic clinics.
6. Tonopen is a hand-held tonometer and it works on principle of the Mackay-Marg tonometer. It contains a strain gauge that senses the force generated by the plunger of the tonometer to applanate the central cornea.
7. The probe of the pneumatic tonometer contains compressed air and sensor. A transducer converts pneumatic signals to electrical and amplifier and recorder of the tonometer amplify and provide the IOP reading respectively.

Pneumatic tonometer records fluctuations in the IOP due to cardiac cycle as well as ocular pulse amplitude. IOP shows diurnal variations. Corneal edema alters IOP. A low IOP is often recorded following keratorefractive surgery.

## 2.5 GONIOSCOPY

1. Visualization of the angle of the anterior chamber is known as gonioscopy.
2. The main purpose of gonioscopy is to detect developmental or acquired abnormalities in the angle of the anterior chamber.
3. Gonioscopy helps to classify glaucoma into open-angle and close-angle categories.
4. Gonioscopy is performed with the help of contact lenses. It is of two types:
   - *Direct gonioscopy:* It is performed with Koeppe lenses under microscope in infants and children. It provides a direct view of the angle in all quadrants allowing simultaneous comparison.
   - *Indirect gonioscopy:* It is performed with the help of lenses with mounted prisms. Common gonioscopes used are Goldmann, Zeiss and Posner four mirror.
5. In indirect gonioscopy, the visible angle (say lower) shows the picture of an opposite angle (the upper) due to reflecting prisms.
6. The landmark structures are iris root, ciliary body band, scleral spur, trabecular meshwork and Schwalbe's line (peripheral termination of the Descemet's membrane).
7. The width of angle recess between the iris and the surface of the trabeculum is of primary consideration in the classification of glaucoma.
   - *Classification*: Standard systems of grading system have been described by Shaffer and Speath.
     The Shaffer system grades the angle in following categories:
     - Grade 4: The angle is wide open and is 45° (Fig. 2.5).
     - Grade 3: The angle is more than 20° but less than 45° and angle closure does not occur.
     - Grade 2: The angle is 20° wide and angle closure is possible.
     - Grade 1: The angle is only 10° wide and angle closure is likely to develop.
     - Grade 0: The angle is already closed.

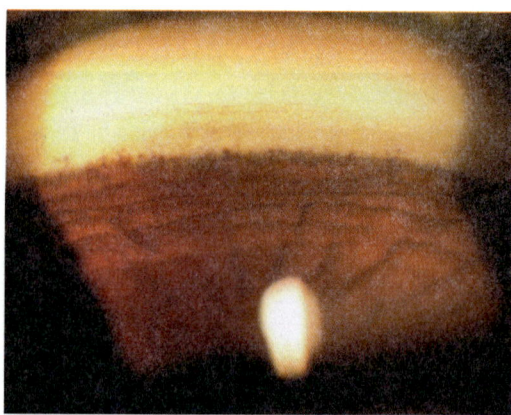

**Fig. 2.5:** Gonioscopy showing open angle of the anterior chamber. (*Courtesy:* Dr R Ramakrishanan, CMO, Aravind Eye Hospital, Tirunelveli)

The Speath's classification is more complete. It includes peripheral iris contour, location of insertion of iris root and effect of compression gonioscopy on the angle width.

- *Compression gonioscopy:* Compression gonioscopy is a technique in which an external pressure over the cornea using the Zeiss, Posner or Sussman four mirror lenses is exerted in patients with chronic angle-closure glaucoma. It helps to distinguish appositional angle-closure from synechial angle-closure glaucoma.

### 2.6 OPHTHALMOSCOPY

1. Ophthalmoscopy is an important tool for examination of the posterior segment of the eye.
2. Ophthalmoscopy is of three types: (1) direct, (2) indirect and (3) slit-lamp biomicroscopy.

#### Direct Ophthalmoscopy

1. Direct ophthalmoscopy is carried out after full dilatation of pupils with the help of a direct ophthalmoscope in a dark room.
2. It gives a magnification of about 15 times and a field of view of 6.5–10°.
3. Retinal blood vessels, optic disk, macula and peripheral retina in all quadrants should be critically screened.
4. The red-free filter in ophthalmoscope is used to study small hemorrhages, micro-aneurysms, retinal pigment epithelium (RPE) defects, nevus, choroidal melanoma, cup/disk ratio and drop out in retinal nerve fiber.

#### Indirect Ophthalmoscopy

1. Indirect ophthalmoscopy is the most commonly used procedure for the examination of retina.
2. A head-mounted binocular indirect ophthalmoscope is used in conjunction with a strong convex lens. The lens is placed in front of patient's eye to obtain a real, inverted and enlarged image of fundus between the lens and the observer.
3. Indirect ophthalmoscopy gives a small magnification depending on the power and position of lens.
4. Advantages of indirect ophthalmoscopy include binocular vision, stereopsis, a wide view of peripheral fundus (up to ora serrate), and fundus can be seen despite hazy media and high refractive error.

### Slit-lamp Biomicroscopy

1. Slit-lamp biomicroscopy is a very useful examination for studying the macular pathology.
2. It is performed after full dilatation of pupils with the help of slit-lamp and 78 or 90 lens (Fig. 2.6).
3. The technique presents a real, inverted and magnified image.
4. Hruby lens (–56.6 D planoconcave) mounted on slit-lamp can be used for visualization of central part of the fundus.
5. The method provides stereoscopic and a magnified view (virtual) of the central fundus.

### 2.7 VISUAL FIELDS

1. The orderly arrangement of nerve fibers in the visual pathway helps in precise

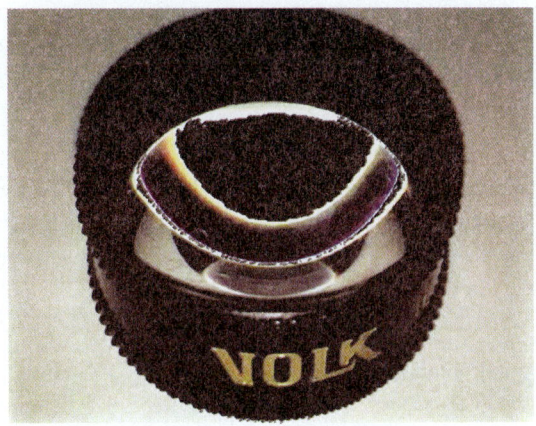

**Fig. 2.6:** 90 D lens for biomicroscopy

**2**

localization of lesions by charting visual fields (VFs). Humphrey (Fig. 2.7) and Octopus automated perimeters are widely used in the clinical practice. They have different range of suprathreshold and full strategies to screen VF loss.

2. Short-wavelength automated perimetry (SWAP) may detect the field defects earlier than Humphrey or Octopus.

3. Frequency-doubling technology (FDT) detects glaucomatous field defects in a very short time. The technique uses a sinusoidal contrast sensitivity as a stimulus and therefore likely to give false-positive results in patients with impaired contrast sensitivity.

4. VF record is not only helpful in the diagnosis of the diseases like open-angle-glaucoma, anterior ischemic optic neuropathy (AION) and pituitary adenoma but also provides information about the progress of the disease.

5. As true with almost all diagnostic procedures, VF defects should never be considered in isolation but should always be interpreted with overall clinical picture of the patient. Characteristic VF defects with their causes are summarized in Table 2.1.

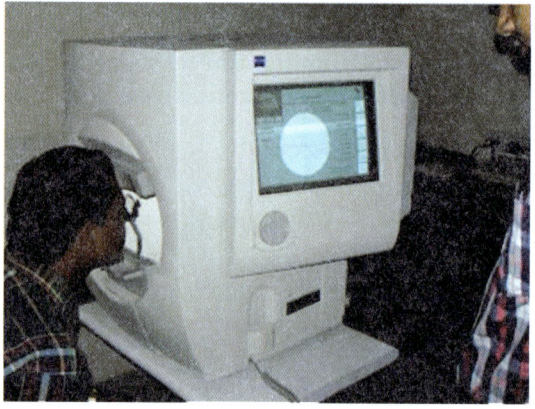

**Fig. 2.7:** Humphrey visual field analyser

**Table 2.1** Causes of typical VF defects in eye diseases

| Scotoma | Diseases |
|---|---|
| Paracentral | Early glaucoma |
| Altitudinal | AION, hemi-CRVO, glaucoma, chiasmal or occipital lobe lesions |
| Arcuate | Glaucoma, optic neuritis |
| Central or centrocecal | Optic neuritis, AION, macular disease, toxic amblyopia |
| Incongruous homonymous hemianopia | Lesions of optic radiation, LGB, temporal and parietal lobes |
| Congruous homonymous hemianopia | Occipital lobe lesions |
| Constriction of peripheral VF | Retinitis pigmentosa, long-standing glaucoma, papilledema, post-panretinal photocoagulation, CRAO with cilioretinal artery sparing, bilateral occipital lobes infarction with macular sparing |
| Enlargement of blind spot | Papilledema, glaucoma, drusen and coloboma of optic disk, high myopia, medulated nerve fibers of the disk |
| Binasal hemianopia | Enlargement of third ventricle, atheroma of the carotids or posterior communicating arteries |
| Bitemporal hemianopia | Chiasmatic lesions like pituitary adenoma, arachnoiditis, craniopharengioma, aneurysm |
| Pie in the sky/superior homonymous quadrantanopia | Temporal lobe tumor implicating Meyer's loop/lesion of optic radiation in temporal/temporoparietal lobe |
| Pie in the floor/inferior homonymous quadrantanopia | Lesion of superior fibers of optic radiation in parietal lobe |

## 2.8 PHOTOGRAPHY

1. The ophthalmic photography requires special skill to obtain high quality images which have direct influence on diagnosis, treatment and proper follow-up.
2. Ophthalmic photography helps in documentation of cases for retrospective clinical studies.
3. Digital photography has become an essential part of diagnostic procedures such as fundus fluorescein angiography (FFA), internal carotid artery angiography (ICAA), ultrasound biomicroscopy (UBM), optical coherence tomography (OCT), anterior segment optical coherence tomography (ASOCT), etc.
4. Fundus photography provides a wealth of information regarding the status of RPE, age-related macular degeneration (AMD), drug toxicity, macular dystrophy and choroidal tumors.
5. Wide angle photography is possible with the introduction of retcam (Fig. 2.8) which has a 3CCD chip. It provides easy screening of infants with retinopathy of prematurity.
6. With the advent of teleophthalmology images of the anterior and posterior segments of the eye are captured many miles away in rural areas, the quality must be near perfect to enable the treating ophthalmologist to make a correct diagnosis.

## 2.9 CORNEAL TOPOGRAPHY

1. Corneal topography is a noninvasive imaging technique for mapping the surface and curvature of the cornea.
2. It is performed by various methods such as Placido disk analysis, scanning slit beam and rasterstereography.
3. In Placido disk method, the images of the disk on the cornea are captured and analyzed by a computer. Color-coded maps are prepared depending on the power distribution (curvature) of the cornea.
4. The Orbscan II is a better technique wherein Placedo disk method is combined with scanning slit.
5. The corneal topography is very useful in diagnosis of subclinical keratoconus, corneal distrophies, marginal corneal degeneration.
6. Corneal topography helps in evaluating the suitability of patients for refractive surgery, IOL power calculation and fitting CLs.

## 2.10 SPECULAR MICROSCOPY

1. Specular microscope can examine and take photograph of the corneal endothelium *in vivo* (Fig. 2.9).
2. The cell count is about 2400 cells/mm$^2$.
3. Intraocular surgery should be avoided in case the cells are markedly reduced or they show extensive pleomorphism.

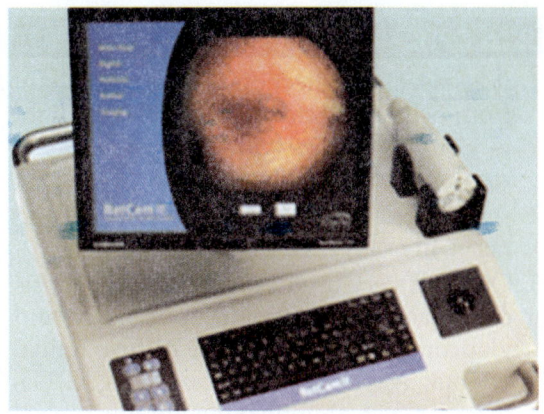

Fig. 2.8: Fundus camera: Retcam

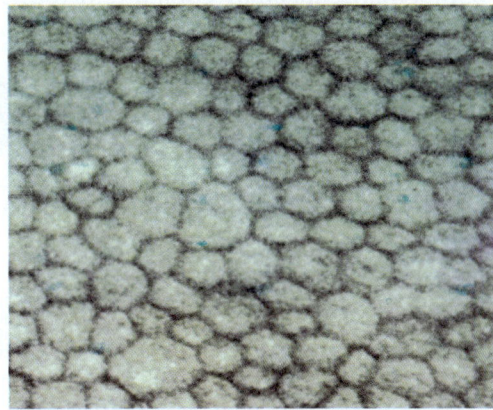

Fig. 2.9: Corneal endothelium on specular microscopy

**2**

## 2.11 CORNEAL PACHYMETRY

1. Corneal pachymetry measures corneal thickness. It is more in periphery (630–670 microns) than in center (520–560 microns). The superior cornea, in all the zones, is thicker than the inferior.
2. Ultrasonic pachymeter, or OCT can measure it.
3. CCT is often increased in corneal edema.
4. Corneal thickness can affect the reading of applanation tonometry.

## 2.12 CONFOCAL MICROSCOPY

1. Confocal microscopy presents a histological view of cornea *in vivo*. It images corneal endothelium and pathogens in the corneal layers.
2. Confocal microscopy can be done with the help of either confocal slit-scanning microscope or confocal laser-scanning microscope.
3. It can diagnose corneal dystropies more precisely.

## 2.13 CONFOCAL SCANNING LASER OPHTHALMOSCOPY

1. Confocal laser scanning microscope scans the cornea with high magnification.
2. HRT is used in the diagnosis of glaucoma, papilledema, macular edema and retinal and choroidal tumors.

## 2.14 ANTERIOR SEGMENT OPTICAL COHERENCE TOMOGRAPHY

1. ASOCT is an imaging technique that uses low coherence interferometry to axial resolution.
2. It uses a wavelength of 1310 nm.
3. ASOCT can measure corneal thickness, depth of the anterior chamber, angle of the anterior chamber (Fig. 2.10), thickness of laser-assisted *in situ* keratomileusis (LASIK) flap and residual stromal bed.

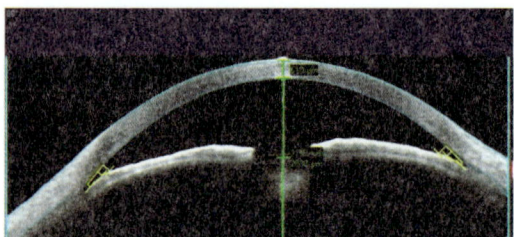

**Fig. 2.10:** Showing the closed-angle of the anterior chamber

4. It is particularly useful in implantation of anterior chamber IOLs and phakic IOLs, diagnosis of angle-closure glaucoma, and decentered IOLs.

## 2.15 PENTACAM

1. Pentacam is a comprehensive diagnostic tool that can imagine the anterior segment of the eye.
2. A Scheimpflung rotating camera is used to image all structures of the anterior segment of the eye.
3. It provides detail information regarding curvature and elevation of the posterior surface of the cornea, thickness of cornea (color-coded maps), depth of the anterior chamber, grading of the cataract, and IOL power calculation.
4. Pentacam also helps in planning refractive surgery and fitting of contact lenses.

## 2.16 OPTICAL COHERENCE TOMOGRAPHY

1. It is based on reflection of a coherent light from ocular structures. The reflected light is converted into images with high-resolution up to 3 microns.
2. A high reflectivity is noticed from RPE and nerve fiber layer.
3. OCT is a very useful tool for the diagnosis of diseases of retina and optic nerve and glaucoma. Diseases include diffuse retinal edema, AMD, macular hole (Fig. 2.11), macular cyst, epiretinal membrane, central serous choroidopathy, cystoid macular

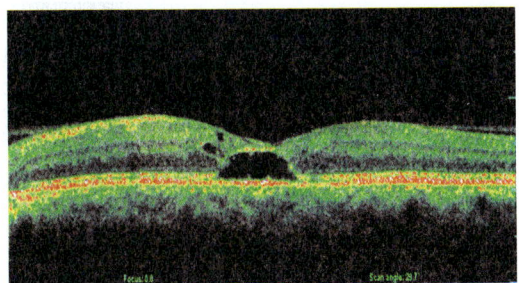

**Fig. 2.11:** Optical coherence tomography showing impending macular hole

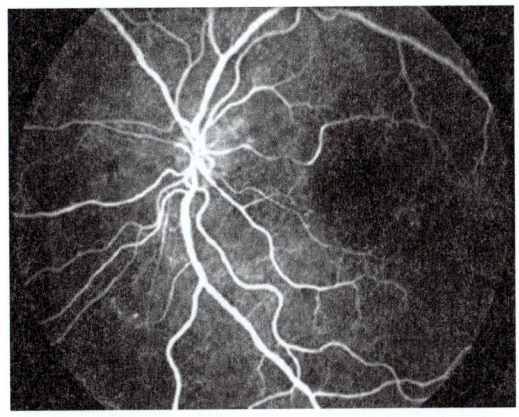

edema (CME), serous RPE detachment, drusen, retinal detachment, optic neuropathy, optic neuritis and papilledema.

4. Measurement of retinal nerve fiber thickness and optic disk cup, volume and rim characteristic may help in the early diagnosis of glaucoma.

### 2.17 FLUORESCEIN ANGIOGRAPHY

1. Fundus fluorescein angiography is of a useful diagnostic procedure for diseases of retina and optic nerve.
2. Serial photographs of fundus are taken after IV injection of 3 mL 25% sterile sodium fluorescein.
3. There are six phases in FFA:
   - Prearterial phase
   - Arterial phase
   - Arteriovenous phase
   - Venous phase
   - Recirculation phase
   - Late phase
4. The RPE and the endothelium of the retinal vessels act as barriers to fluorescein and thus the dye remains confined to the intravascular space.
5. Figure 2.12 shows an angiogram. The fluorescein in retinal disorders may either show hyperfluorescence or hypofluorescence.
6. Hyperfluorescence manifests in the form of leakage, pooling, staining, window defects, and autofluorescence.

7. Leakage is found in neovascularization of retina, proliferative diabetic retinopathy, AMD, papilledema, central serous choroidopathy and CME.
8. Pooling of fluorescein can be seen in REP detachment and central serous choroidopathy.
9. Staining may be found in retinal scar and drusen.
10. Window defects are seen in areas of RPE atrophy and laser scars.
11. Autofluorescence of optic nerve drusen can be recorded before the FFA.
12. Hypofluorescence occurs in central retinal vessel occlusion, and capillary nonperfusion. Retinal hemorrhages and pigmentation mask the fluorescein and lesions look hypofluorescent.

### 2.18 INDOCYANINE GREEN ANGIOGRAPHY

1. Indocyanine green angiography (ICGA) is an invaluable imaging technique used for studying the choroidal circulation and lesions. The indocyanine green is not absorbed by hemoglobin, melanin and exudates.
2. The ICG angiography shows much better choroidal circulation and subretinal vascularization than FA.
3. ICGA is used in the diagnosis of occult choroidal neovascularization (CNV),

**2**

recurrent CNV, AMD, polypoidal choroidal vasculopathy and serpiginous choroido-pathy.

## 2.19 A-SCAN ULTRASONOGRAPHY

1. A-scan ultrasonography is time-amplitude record of echoes. It uses 8–12 MHz ultrasound waves.
2. The ocular tissue can be calculated from the distance between echos position and thickness of individual.
3. A-scan can measure the axial length of the eyeball and power of IOL for implantation (Fig. 2.13).
4. A-scan is useful in the diagnosis of micro-phthalmos, nanophthalmos, congenital glaucoma, intraocular FB, intraocular and orbital tumors.
5. It can also measure the corneal thickness.
6. High spikes are obtained from cornea, lens and retina and low from aqueous and vitreous.

## 2.20 B-SCAN ULTRASONOGRAPHY

1. B-scan ultrasonography is a brightness-modulated scan which gives real-time, two-dimensional section of the eye.
2. It has a greater value in the examination of orbit than the A-scan. It provides a very rapid and convenient examination of intraocular structures even in opaque media.

3. B-scan ultrasonography is useful procedure for the diagnosis of retinal detachment (Fig. 2.14), choroidal detachment, optic nerve drusen, intraocular calcification, subluxation of lens, intraocular tumors, intraocular foreign body (IOFB), rupture of the globe and orbital diseases.
4. A combination of A and B ultrasonography can accurately localize IOFB.
5. Ultrasound can locate the FB even if it is lodged in the coats of eyeball.
6. Intraocular silicone oil and gas may distort the eye images, therefore, the patient's position should be upright during scanning.
7. A combination of B-scan ultrasonography with Duplex Doppler's technology is helpful in the diagnosis of vascular lesions like orbital varix, arteriovenous commu-nication, central retinal vascular occlusion, and ocular ischemic syndrome.

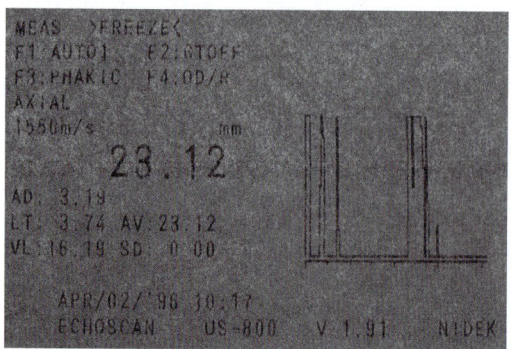

Fig. 2.13: A-scan

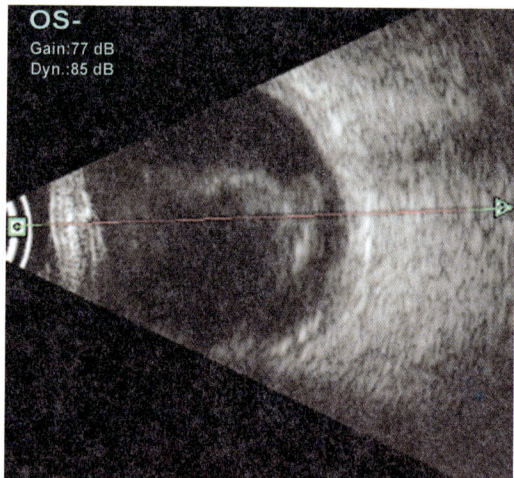

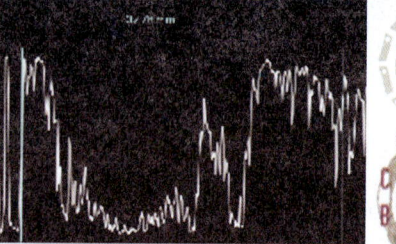

Fig. 2.14: B-scan showing retinal detachment

## 2.21 ULTRASOUND BIOMICROSCOPY

1. UBM requires high frequency ultasound (40–100 MH) for imaging of the anterior segment of the eyeball.
2. UBM is of immense help in the diagnosis of cysts and tumors of ciliary body, FB in the anterior chamber and prognosticating cases of keratoplasty.
3. UBM is an excellent technique for understanding the pathomechanisms of primary angle-closure glaucoma (Fig. 2.15).

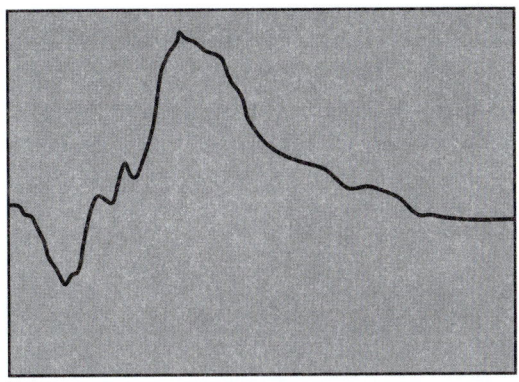

**Fig. 2.16:** Electroretinogram

## 2.22 ELECTRORETINOGRAPHY

1. Electroretinography records changes in the resting potential of the eye induced by to a flash of light (Fig. 2.16).
2. The ERG consists of three waves: Negative a-wave, a large positive b-wave, slight positive deflection c-wave.
3. Generally both photopic and scotopic ERGs are recorded. The b-wave response is normally about 150 mv or over; it arises from bipolar cells.
4. The b-wave remains subnormal in early pigmentary degeneration of retina and becomes extinguished in advanced RP, CRAO, total detachment of retina, etc.
5. Focal electroretinogram (FERG), multifocal ERG and pattern ERG are found useful in the diagnosis of maculopathies, glaucoma, retinal vascular disorders and retinal toxicity.

## 2.23 ELECTRO-OCULOGRAPHY

1. Changes in the resting potential during light and dark adapted retina (Fig. 2.17) are recorded in electro-oculography.
2. After placement of electrodes on lateral and medial canthi EOG is recorded 12 min in dark and 12 min in light.
3. Arden ratio is calculated by dividing the maximum height of light peak with minimum height of dark tracing multiplied by 100. Normally it is above 185.
4. Arden ratios below 100 and 125 are considered as flat and subnormal respectively. They may be found in myopia, RP, etc.

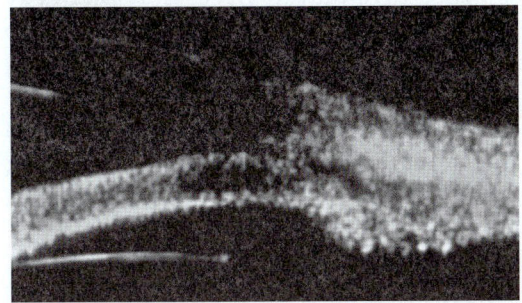

**Fig. 2.15:** Ultrasound biomicroscopy image showing the angle of the anterior chamber

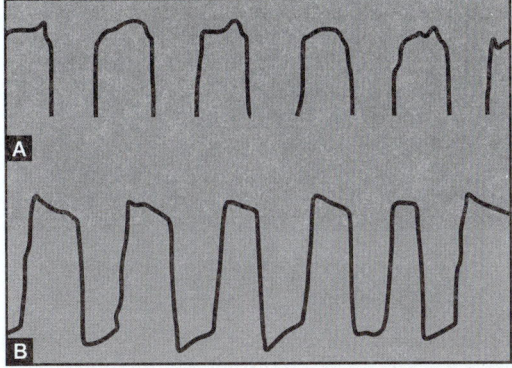

**Fig. 2.17:** Normal electro-oculogram—A: Dark adapted (for 15 minutes) and B: Light adapted (for 15 minutes)

## 2.24 VISUAL EVOKED POTENTIAL

1. Visual evoked potential or visual evoked response can be induced by a flash or patterned checkboard (Fig. 2.18).
2. Time of onset of response is a reliable sign. A delayed conduction time indicates retrobulbar neuritis.

## 2.25 COMPUTED TOMOGRAPHY

1. CT is a reliable technique for exploring diseases of eye, orbit and brain (Fig. 2.19).

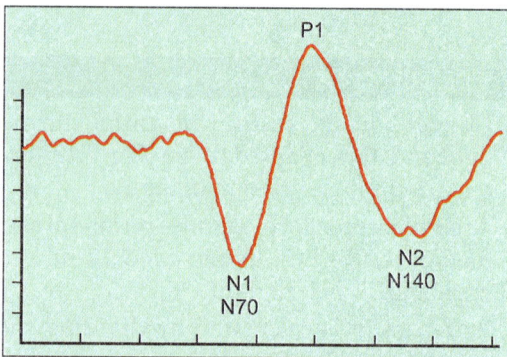

**Fig. 2.18:** Normal visual evoked potential

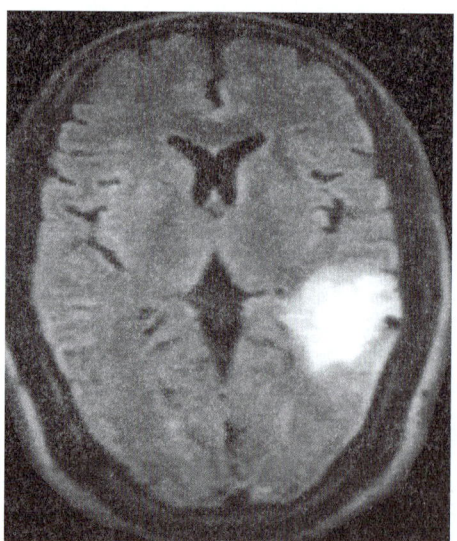

**Fig. 2.19:** CT scan showing small round hypodense lesion having eccentric nodule in left frontoparietal lobe (*Courtesy:* Dr (Prof) Pramod Sakhi/Dr Anup Gupta, Dept of Radiodiagnosis, Index Medical College, Indore)

2. It is an established procedure for localization of IOFB, diagnosing fractures of floor and walls of orbit, enlargement of extraocular muscles and tumors of the optic nerve.
3. In patients with suspected fracture of the orbit, both coronal and sagittal views should be taken; the muscle incarcination is best seen in coronal view.
4. A contrast study should be advised to find the vascular anomalies.

## 2.26 MAGNETIC RESONANCE IMAGING

1. Magnetic resonance imaging (MRI) is based on the ability of small number of protons within the body to absorb and emit radiowave energy when body is placed within a strong electromagnetic field. The emitted energy is analyzed by computer.
2. Differences in the density of protons differentiate one tissue from another.
3. Common pulse-sequence techniques used in MRI are T1- and T2-weighted images. T1 measures how fast tissue can become magnetized and T2 measures how fast it loses its magnetization.
4. It has techniques for fat suppression to diagnose optic neuritis and optic nerve sheath meningioma and cerebellopontine tumors (Fig. 2.20).
5. Intravenous gadolinium is used in augmented MRI in certain cases.
6. Fluid-attenuated inversion recovery (FLAIR) is used for lesions close to ventricular system, particularly plaques of multiple sclerosis.
7. Diffusion-weighted sequence (DWS) can identify acute cerebral infarction causing cortical visual impairment producing homonymous hemianopia.
8. MRI is free from the hazards of irradiation. It gives better resolution with three dimensional (3D) isotropic images for the diagnosis of lesions smaller than 2 mm.

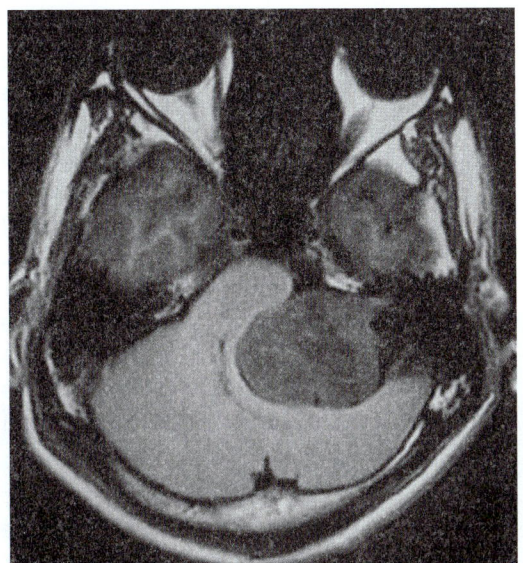

**Fig. 2.20:** MRI showing left cerebellopontine angle mass causing widening the left CP angle cistern and distortion of the fourth ventricle (*Courtesy:* Dr (Prof) Pramod Sakhi/ P. Shekhawatia, Radiodiagnosis, SAIMS, Indore)

9. MRI is contraindicated in patients suspected with magnetic metal (ferrous) FB and those using cardiac pacemaker, aneurysm clip, spinal or vagal nerve stimulators and straps, breast and penile implants. Contrast MRI should be avoided in renal insufficiency.

## 2.27 CEREBRAL ANGIOGRAPHY

1. Digital subtraction angiography (DSA) was a gold standard for imaging for extra and intracranial vasculature. Recently, it is replaced by less invasive CT angiography (CTA) and MR angiography (MRA).
2. In CTA, a contrast is injected in the antecubital vein followed by high-speed spiral CT scanning. During the procedure patient is moved and data are extracted.
3. In MRA, iodinated contrast material is not used and is free of ionizing radiation, time-of-flight imaging.
4. CTA provides superior image resolution, short examination time, and the procedure

can be performed even in patients with pacemaker and aneurysm clip.

5. Cerebral angiography is indicated in carotid stenosis or occlusion, intracranial aneurysm, arteriovenous malformation, hamartoma, carotid-cavernous fistula, and ocular ischemic syndrome.

## 2.28 POSITRON EMISSION TOMOGRAPHY

1. Positron emission tomography (PET) is used to measure cerebral blood flow and glucose consumption and metabolism of tissues.
2. PET imaging is useful in studying visual functions, visual pathway in amblyopia, neoplastic and metabolic diseases, recovery of stroke, and effects of drugs like neuro-protectants, and antidepressants or anti-dementia.

## 2.29 DIAGNOSTIC PROCEDURES FOR CONCOMITANT STRABISMUS

1. A concomitant strabismus has an onset in early childhood and characterized by absence of limitation of ocular motility and diplopia and a constant angle of deviation (no deviation in latent squint) in all directions of gaze.
2. The strabismus may be convergent or divergent. Each can be subdivided into latent, intermittent and manifest.
3. Vertical and pattern strabismus may also be seen.
4. Protocol for the diagnosis of incomitant strabismus includes examination of motor and sensory status.

### Motor Status

1. History of age of onset, mode of onset, family history, glasses, surgery, etc.
2. Head posture
3. Monocular and binocular movements
4. Vision and refraction

5. Dilated funduscopy to exclude organic lesions
6. Type of deviation
7. Cover test to unmask latent squint
8. Cover-uncover test confirms type of deviation, latent nystagmus and visual dominance.
9. Measurement of ocular deviation: The deviation can be measured by following methods:
   ▪ Hirschberg corneal reflex test (light reflex on the pupillary border 15°, mid-surface of iris 30° and limbus 45°) is the most popular test.
   ▪ Prism bar cover test measures the amount of deviation in prism diopters.
   ▪ Krimsky corneal reflex test measures the deviation by placing prisms of increasing strength in front of the fixing eye so as to bring the light reflex in the center of the deviating eye.
   ▪ Synoptophore is a very useful instrument for the measurement of horizontal and vertical deviations as well as torsion.
   ▪ Horizontal and vertical vergences should be measured by prisms or synoptophore. If vergence amplitudes are large, the patient remains symptom-free.

## Sensory Status

Sensory status of the patient can be evaluated by examination of binocularity, suppression, retinal correspondence, amblyopia and stereopsis.
▪ Binocularity can be tested by dissociation of eyes.
▪ Suppression indicates an active inhibition of images originating from the retina of squinting eye to avoid confusion. Binocularity and suppression can be detected by red-green glasses, Bagolini striated glasses, two Maddox rods test, after image test and synoptophore.
▪ Retinal correspondence is considered normal (NRC) when patient has bifoveal

fixation and retinal points nasal to the fovea in one eye correspond to the retinal points temporal to the fovea in the fellow eye. A correspondence between fovea of one eye and extrafoveal point in the contralateral eye is called anomalous retinal correspondence (ARC). In NRC, the objective and subjective angles of deviation are equal. ARC may be harmonious or unharmonious. If subjective angle is zero but objective angle is equal to the angle of deviation, it is termed harmonious ARC. Unharmonious ARC presents a greater objective angle than subjective angle of deviation on synoptophore.

The objective angle of deviation can be measured by prism bar cover test or synoptophore and subjective angle by Worth four dot test, Bagolini striated glasses after-image test or synoptophore.

▪ Amblyopia is an unilateral or bilateral decrease of visual functions. Strabismic, anisometropic and vision deprivation amblyopia are common. Worth four dot test and synoptophore can detect amblyopia.
▪ Stereopsis is the ability of eyes to appreciate depth perception. Stereoacuity can be assessed by synoptophore, Randot stereotest and Lang's two-pencil test.

## 2.30 DIAGNOSTIC PROCEDURES FOR INCOMITANT STRABISMUS

1. An incomitant strabismus may be congenital or acquired.
2. The acquired incomitant strabismus is characterized by a limitation of action of paralyzed muscle in the direction of action and often associated with diplopia.
3. The strabismus may be convergent, divergent or vertical.
4. Protocol for the diagnosis of incomitant strabismus includes following examinations.

- History of onset, congenital or acquired, diplopia, nausea, vertigo, systemic illness, head trauma and surgery.
- Compensatory face turn, head tilt and chin elevation or depression.
- Examine the ocular motility, see the direction of restriction of ocular movements, measure deviations in different directions of gaze. Saccades should also be tested; slow saccades suggest reduced muscle strength.
- Corneal light reflex test helps to determine approximate degree of deviation.
- In incomitant strabismus, the secondary deviation (normal eye under cover and squinting eye is fixing) is always greater than primary deviation (deviation of squinting eye when normal eye is fixing) due to Hering's law of equal innervation of muscles.
- Cover test should be performed after correction of head posture and deviation is measured with prism cover test in all 6 cardinal positions of gaze.
- Synoptophore can also be used for measurement of the deviation.
- False projection or orientation occurs as a result of increased innervational impulse to the paralyzed extraocular muscle. Therefore, the patient overshoots the object when asked to locate it after the closure of the sound eye.
- Diplopia is maximal in the area in which the muscle action is limited. Diplopia charting can provide information about involvement of horizontal or vertical muscle. Vertical separation with crossed images suggests vertical rectus muscles involvement.
- Maddox double rod test can determine the degree of torsion.
- Foveal position on funduscopy may diagnose and qualify torsion.
- Long-standing paralyzed muscles undergo secondary changes such as contracture of the direct antagonist, overaction of the contralateral synergist and inhibitional palsy of the contralateral antagonist muscle.
- Hess or Lee screen test is based on Hering's law. It provides information about paralyzed muscle as well as secondary changes in other muscles.
- Forced duction test is performed to differentiate between paralytic strabismus and restrictive strabismus. Force generation test and saccadic velocity may also be used for this purpose.
- Examination of CNS may help in determining the etiology of incomitant strabismus.
- In doubtful cases, electromyography, CT and MRI of orbit and brain are recommended.

## 2.31 DIAGNOSTIC PROCEDURES FOR DRY EYE DISEASE

1. Dry eye disease can be diagnosed during ophthalmic practice with relative ease provided the clinician has a high index of suspicion.
2. Patients with history of blepharitis, trachoma, S-J syndrome, lagophthalmos, proptosis, frequent use of eyedrops with preservatives and chemical or radiation injury are prone for dry eye.
3. Systemic disorders like arthritis, sarcoidosis, rosacea, atopic dermatitis, lymphoma and chronic viral infection can aggravate dry eye.
4. Use of antihistaminic drugs, beta-blockers, diuretics and antidepressants may exacerbate symptoms of dry eye.
5. Smoking, air-conditioning, low humidity, dry atmosphere and working long hours on systems are known to cause dry eye.

Diagnostic procedure for dry eye disease is usually based on the following points:
- Ocular surface disease index (OSDI) questionnaires may help in the diagnosis of the dry eye.

2

- Tear meniscus height is reduced.
- Tear breakup: Put a drop of fluorescein and examined the eye on slit lamp. Ask the patient to blink. The time taken between the last blink and development of first dry spot on the cornea is known as tear breakup time (Fig. 2.21). The normal breakup time ranges between 15 and 35 seconds. A time of less than 10 seconds or less indicates dry eye.
- Schirmer test: The aqueous production is measured with the help of a 5 × 35 mm Whatman paper strip. About 5 mm of the bent strip is kept in the lower fornix and wetting of the strip from the bent part is measured after 5 min. A secretion of less than 5 mm suggests dry eye.
- Rose Bengal staining: It detects damaged and dead epithelial cells. A staining of bulbar conjunctiva is diagnostic of keratoconjunctivitis sicca.
- Fluorescein staining: It may show diffuse staining of cornea with filaments in the dry eye.
- Lissamine green B: It detects dead or degenerated cells and causes less irritation than rose Bengal.
- Fluorescein clearance test: The dye is instilled in the conjunctiva and the color of the lower tear meniscus is compared with the standardized scale.
- Tear film osmolarity: It has great sensitivity and specificity and considered a gold standard test for the diagnosis of dry eye disease.
- Tear ferning: Ferning pattern of conjunctival scraping under microscope is a quantitative test for mucin deficiency.
- Conjunctival impression cytology: It allows the evaluation of conjunctival epithelium and goblet cells of the ocular surface. A decrease in the density of goblet cells and metaplastic change in the epithelium indicate mucous deficiency and tear film instability.
- Lysozyme and lactoferrin assays: Lysozyme and lactoferrin concentrations are low in dry eyes.
- Serum autoantibodies: Antibodies (anti-Ro or anti-La) have been detected in Sjögren's syndrome.

## 2.32 DIAGNOSTIC PROCEDURES FOR INFECTIOUS KERATITIS

1. Infectious keratitis is caused by bacteria, fungi, parasite and viruses.
2. Different protocols are usually followed for diagnosis of these etiological agents.
3. Basic investigative procedures include characteristic clinical picture, examination of smear, culture on specific media and sensitivity test, corneal biopsy, immunology and molecular biology based tests.

- Corneal scrapings for smear should be collected by using platinum spatula or disposable blade after topical anesthesia. The collected material is spread over a small area on glass slides. The smears are fixed with KOH and stained with Gram for light microscopy (Fig. 2.22). Smear stained with calcoflur white or acridine need fluorescent microscopic examination.
- Organisms identified during smear examination provide basis for provisional diagnosis. Gram-positive bacteria, fungi and *Acanthamoeba* can be easily recognized by Gram staining. Fungal hyphe

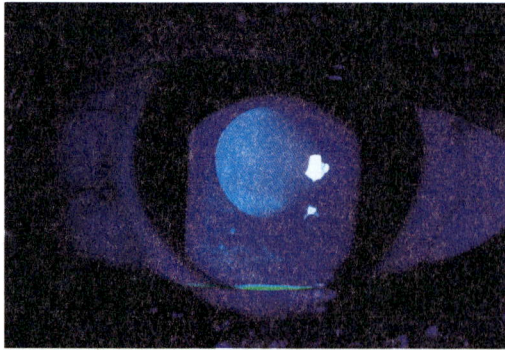

**Fig. 2.21:** Measurement of tear break-up time (BUT)

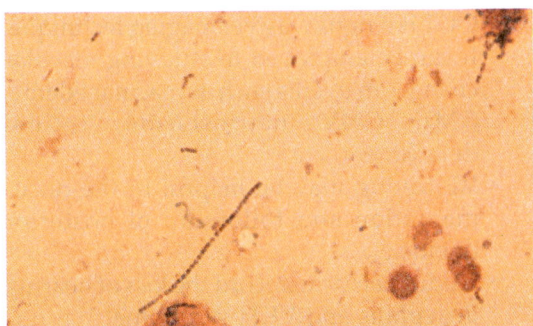

Fig. 2.22: Conjunctival scraping showing Streptococci (*Courtesy:* PK Mukherjee and Bandhopadyay, Bacterial infection. Eye in Systemic Disorders. HV Nema et al, editors, New Delhi, Wiley, 2015)

and cysts of *Acanthamoeba* show staining but not their walls.

- Isolation of organism in culture confirms the diagnosis. Antibiotic susceptibility of organism *in vitro* provides rational guidelines for the treatment.
- Polymerase chain reaction (PCR) on corneal scraping is highly sensitive test. If test is not performed meticulously, false-positive results can occur.
- Diagnosis of viral keratitis requires a more strict protocol than bacterial.
- Corneal material should be collected and transported in a viral transport medium for PCR, culture and histopathology.
- Examination of smears of corneal scraping are stained with Giemsa, Papanicolaou and hematoxylin and eosin (H & E) stains may show multinucleated giant cells, intranuclear or intracytoplasmic inclusions and lymphocytes.
- Viral antigen can be detected in corneal scraping collected in buffer fluid by enzyme-linked immunosorbent assay (ELISA).
- Virus isolation is possible by tissue culture method. HeLa, Vero, HEp-2 and MRC-5 cell lines are used for culture.
- PCR technique is widely employed for the detection of viral DNA.

## 2.33 DIAGNOSTIC PROCEDURES FOR UVEITIS AND ENDOPHTHALMITIS

1. There is a significant advancement in the clinical diagnosis of uveitis.
2. In spite of advances, the etiology of only 50% cases may be established.
3. The workup for the diagnosis of uveitis can be summarized as follows:
   - History of present and past illness and associated systemic disease.
   - Clinical evidence based on slit-lamp and fundus examinations
   - The list of investigations for uveitis is huge. However, ordering of all investigations is not practical but only a tailored approach to obtain maximal information from minimal tests should be followed.
   - Basic investigations like white blood cells (WBC) count, erythrocyte sedimentation rate (ESR) and C-reactive protein may provide clue for the association of uveitis with systemic diseases.
   - Rh factor, antinuclear antibodies, antineutrophilic cytoplasmic test, etc. are indicated if connective diseases are suspected.
   - Human leucocyte antigens are found to be associated with some uveitic entities.
   - Serology is helpful in syphilis.
   - ELISA for toxoplasmosis, toxocariasis, leptospirosis, Lyme disease, HIV, etc. is recommended.
   - Aqueous can be obtained from paracentesis (tap). It is very useful for the diagnosis of anterior uveitis and also endophthalmitis, toxoplasmosis, intraocular tumors and Behçet disease.
   - Vitreous tap or diagnostic vitrectomy is indicated in endophthalmitis, cytomegalovirus (CMV) retinitis, intraocular neoplasms, toxoplasmosis, Behçet's disease, sympathetic ophthalmitis, etc.
   - Biopsy
     • Iris or ciliary body biopsy for the diagnosis of granuloma, cyst and tumors is preferred.

**2**

- Retinochoroidal biopsy for tuberculoma, tumors, etc.
- Conjunctival or lacrimal gland biopsy for the diagnosis of sarcoidosis (Fig. 2.23), tuberculosis and coccidioidomycosis.
- Mucosal biopsy for Behçet's disease
- Lymph node biopsy for tuberculosis and sarcoidosis.
- Arterial biopsy for giant cell arteritis.
- FFA is indicated in birdshot retinochoroidopathy, geographic helicoid peripapillary choroiditis, acute posterior multifocal placoid pigment epitheliopathy, sympathetic ophthalmia, etc.
- ICGA allows imaging of choroidal and retinal circulation and helps in the diagnosis of Behçet's disease, sarcoidosis, tuberculosis, Vogt-Koyanagi-Harada (VKH) syndrome, birdshot retinochoroidopathy, etc.
- Ultrasound can diagnose inflammatory thickening of choroidal and scleral thickening. It is helpful in locating granuloma cyst, abscess and scolex of cysticercosis.
- UBM can identify intermediate uveitis and distinguish between inflammation and metastatic tumors of ciliary body.

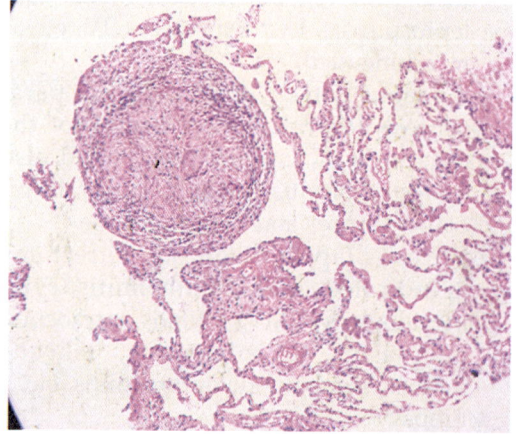

**Fig. 2.23:** Histopathology of biopsy shows noncaseating granuloma of sarcoidosis. (*Courtesy:* Dr OP Sharma, Keck School of Medicine, Los Angeles)

- OCT is a noninvasive imaging technique. It can be employed in studying macular changes in uveitis such as macular edema, CME, CNV, neurosensory retinal detachment, etc.
- VF testing may be helpful in the documentation and follow-up of posterior uveitis.
- Audiometry can record the loss of hearing in syphilis and VKH syndrome.
- Skin test: Mantoux test is advised in tuberculosis.
- Radiological investigations are often advised to study the associated joint inflammation with uveitis. Chest X-rays are indicated in tuberculosis and sarcoidosis. Complicated cases may need CT or MRI.
- PCR is a reliable test for the diagnosis of bacterial endophthalmitis. It is often employed for the confirmation of tuberculous uveitis, Eales' disease and toxoplasmosis.

## 2.34 LOCALIZATION OF INTRAOCULAR FOREIGN BODY

1. The incidence of IOFB has markedly increased with the industrialization.
2. IOFBs may be of two types: Metallic or nonmetallic and metallic is further divided into magnetic and nonmagnetic.
3. Diagnosis or localization of IOFBs is of immense importance from the point of view of their management (Fig. 2.24).
4. The IOFB can be diagnosed by adopting following approach:
   - History of injury provides important clues about FBs. IOFBs are mostly metallic in industrial setup while they are organic in rural area.
   - Slit-lamp examination can localize the FB in the anterior chamber as well as provide definitive evidence of entrance of FB by finding track of FB in cornea, lens or vitreous and iris hole. An embedded FB in the iris and lens may be found.

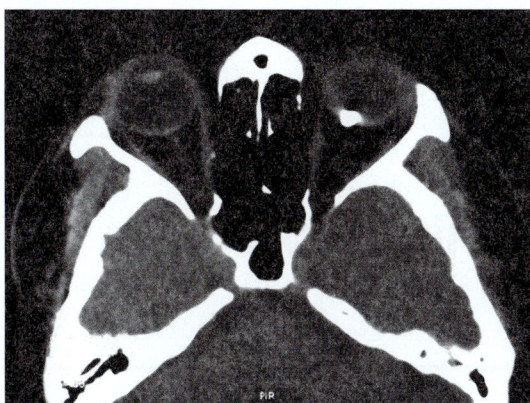

**Fig. 2.24:** CT showing IOFB in the left eye

- Gonioscopy can identify FB in the angle of the anterior chamber. FB in the ciliary area may not be visible; UBM may localize it.
- Fundus examination with indirect ophthalmoscope with scleral indentation may find a FB on the retina provided media are clear. Vitreous or retinal hemorrhage is common. Identification of old IOFB becomes difficult when it undergoes capsulation. FB cannot be detected if it causes double perforation.

- Berman and Roper-Hall localizers to diagnose IOFB are no more in use with the availability of more precise tests.
- A combined B-scan and A-scan ultrasonography is capable of detecting metallic as well as nonmetallic IOFBs. Metallic FBs produce bright signals on B-scan and highly reflective echoes on A-scan. Small IOFB trapped in the vitreous hemorrhage may be missed.
- UBM can identify IOFB lodged in the ciliary body area.
- CT scan is the most established method for the localization of IOFB. It has replaced old radiological methods with marker.
- MRI is employed in locating wooden IOFBs not easily detected by CT scan. It is contraindicated in metallic IOFB because the applied magnetic field may move the IOFB and damage the intraocular structures.
- Intraoperative localization of IOFBs should be attempted if IOFB is associated with endophthalmitis or encapsulated or attached to the eye wall following double perforation.

# Diseases of Conjunctiva

### Etiology

1. Mucopurulent conjunctivitis (Fig. 3.1) is caused by *Staphylococcus aureus, Koch-Weeks bacillus, Pneumococcus Streptococcus, Haemophilus influenzae* and *H. aegypitus.*
2. *Haemophilus* infects children more than adults.

### Symptoms

Acute onset of redness, foreign body sensation, grittiness, initial watering followed by mucopurulent discharge, difficulty in opening the eyes in the morning, ocular discomfort or mild pain and photophobia are common.

### Signs

1. Mild edema of lids, mucopurulent discharge at the medial canthus or matted eyelashes and chemosis of conjunctiva.

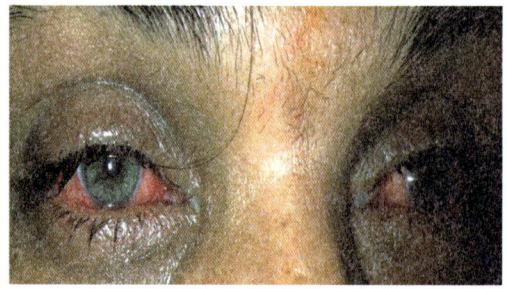

**Fig. 3.1:** Mucopurulent conjunctivitis

2. Conjunctival injection, diffuse papillary hypertrophy of the upper palpebral conjunctiva and petechial hemorrhages in bulbar conjunctiva (pneumococcal conjunctivitis) may be found.
3. Cornea is usually not involved, some cases show superficial punctate erosions in the cornea.

### Diagnosis

1. History of recent epidemic or recurrent conjunctivitis.
2. Culture and sensitivity test.

### Treatment

1. Mild infection shows spontaneous resolution.
2. Recent cases are managed by gatifloxacin drops (0.3%, 4 times a day for 1 week) or moxifloxacin (0.5%, 3 times a day for 7 days).
3. Patients with dacryocystitis need systemic antibiotics.

### Etiology

1. Acute purulent conjunctivitis of adults (Fig. 3.2) is caused by *N. gonorrhoeae* as well as other organisms such as *S. aureus S. pneumoniae, S. haemolyticus* and *Chlamydia* responsible for ophthalmia neonatorum.

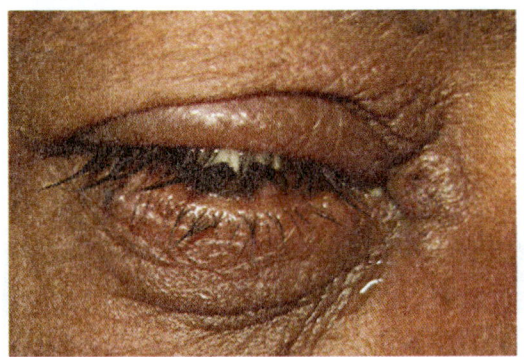

**Fig. 3.2:** Purulent conjunctivitis (*Courtesy:* Dr SCL Chandravansi, SS Medical College, Rewa)

2. It is associated with urethritis and arthritis.
3. The infection is transmitted from genitals to the eye. Males are more affected.

## Symptoms

Gritty sensation, photophobia, profuse purulent discharge, blurring of vision, pain in the eye are common.

## Signs

1. The eye is tender and painful.
2. The upper lid has brawny edema and eyelashes are matted.
3. The conjunctiva is intensely hyperemic, chemotic and edematous with velvety appearance.
4. Occasionally, pseudomembrane develops over the conjunctiva.
5. The cornea is hazy with central gray area of infiltrations and marginal ulcers.
6. Iridocyclitis may develop early.
7. The patient is febrile and preauricular lymph nodes are enlarged.
8. Rarely, septicemia may also be found.

## Diagnosis

1. Immediate Gram-staining of the smear should be done.
2. Conjunctival swab must be sent for culture and sensitivity test.

## Treatment

1. Repeated irrigation and intensive therapy with penicillin drops (10000 units/ml half hourly), gentamicin or ciprofloxacin (0.3%) eye drop 2 hourly and erythromycin 1% eye ointment at bedtime often bring improvement. The therapy should be continued for 2–3 weeks.
2. Topical atropine is applied to prevent uveitis.
3. Analgesics are helpful in ameliorating the general symptoms.
4. A single dose of ceftriaxone 1 g IM is very effective.
5. Severe infection needs treatment with ceftriaxone 1 g IV twice a day for 3–4 days.

## 3.3 ACUTE MEMBRANOUS CONJUNCTIVITIS

### Etiology

1. The membranous conjunctivitis (Fig. 3.3) was earlier known as diphtheritic conjunctivitis since *Corynebacterium diphtheriae* causes membrane formation.
2. It is seen in unimmunized children.
3. *Streptococcus hemolyticus, Streptococcus pneumoniae, Neisseria gonorrhoeae, Staphylococcus aureus, H. aegyptius, E. coli, adenoviruses* and *herpes simplex virus* also cause membranous conjunctivitis.

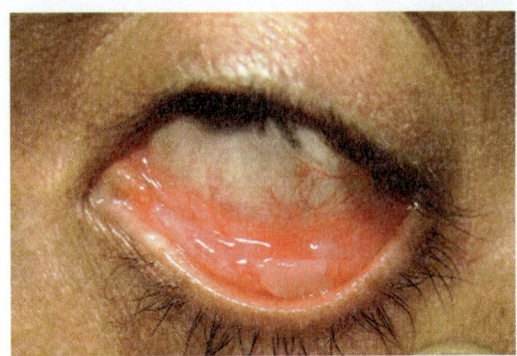

**Fig. 3.3:** Membranous conjunctivitis (*Courtesy:* Dr SCL Chandravansi, SS Medical College, Rewa)

## Symptoms

Mucopurulent discharge, foreign body sensation, matting of eyelashes, mild pain and constitutional symptoms like fever, malaise and sore throat are common.

## Signs

1. Swelling of the conjunctiva and lids, a white pseudomembrane on the palpebral conjunctiva and regional lymphadenopathy may be seen in the mild form of conjunctivitis.
2. In severe form, the patient is acutely ill. Pain is often severe. The lids are swollen, red and tense.
3. In the acute phase, the conjunctiva is markedly chemosed and infiltrated with exudates that may impair corneal transparency. A true membrane is found on palpebral conjunctiva and rarely on the bulbar conjunctiva. The regional lymphadenopathy is often present. The diphtheritic conjunctivitis may be associated with a membrane covering the throat and nasal mucosa.
4. During acute phase sloughing of conjunctiva is common.
5. During healing, adhesions develop between the raw areas on the palpebral and the bulbar conjunctiva resulting in symblepharon, and entropion.

## Diagnosis

Bacterial culture establishes the diagnosis.

## Treatment

1. Proper immunization in infancy is essential.
2. Initially, every case of membranous conjunctivitis is treated as diphtherial.
3. Anti-diphtheritic serum (ADS) and penicillin drops are used topically several times in a day.
4. Atropine sulfate (1%) applied.
5. ADS (10,000 units) and crystalline penicillin (5 lacs unit) are given 12 hourly.

6. Use contact shell. Amniotic membrane transplantation may prevent symblepharon formation.
7. The nondiphtheritic conjunctivitis requires treatment with topical and systemic antibiotic.

## 3.4 HERPES SIMPLEX VIRUS CONJUNCTIVITIS

### Etiology

Acute conjunctivitis is also caused by herpes simplex virus (HSV).

### Signs

HSV1 causes unilateral blepharoconjunctivitis, vesicles on the lids, conjunctival papillary hypertrophy and follicular conjunctivitis and dendritic lesion on the cornea.

### Treatment

It is a self-limiting disease. Topical acyclovir (3%) or ganciclovir gel (0.05%), 5 times a day is effective in controlling the infection. (*Refer* 4.8).

## 3.5 ACUTE ADENOVIRUS CONJUNCTIVITIS

Adenoviruses can produce acute follicular conjunctivitis. It is a very contagious virus often transmitted through tonometers, contaminated towels and respiratory secretion.

### Pharyngoconjunctival Fever

#### Etiology

PCF primarily affects children and appears in an epidemic form. It is caused by adenovirus serotypes 3, 4 and 7.

#### Symptoms

Symptoms are foreign body sensation, itching, watering, redness, sore throat and fever.

#### Signs

1. Acute follicular conjunctivitis, chemosis, pseudomembrane and conjunctival hemorrhages.

2. Punctate epithelial keratitis, subepithelial and stromal infiltrates are corneal signs of the disease.
3. Systemic manifestations include pharyngitis, fever and preauricular lymphadenopathy.

### Treatment

1. The conjunctivitis is self-limiting.
2. There is no specific treatment except preservative-free artificial tears.
3. Topical antibiotics should be used to control secondary bacterial infection and topical steroids may be used for keratitis.

### Epidemic Keratoconjunctivitis

### Etiology

EKC is due to adenovirus serotypes 3, 7, 8 and 19. It spreads through infected ophthalmic instruments.

### Symptoms

Foreign body sensation, itching, scanty discharge, redness and photophobia.

### Signs

1. Follicles and/or membrane on the palpebral conjunctiva are common.
2. Petechial hemorrhages or sub-conjunctival hemorrhages on bulbar conjunctiva.
3. Diffuse punctate epithelial infiltrates are the earliest corneal lesion and later discrete anterior stromal infiltrates (coined-shaped opacities) appear which may cause visual disturbances.
4. Preauricular lymphadenopathy.

### Diagnosis

1. History of epidemic
2. Clinical features especially coin-shaped opacities in the cornea
3. Recovery of the virus in cell culture.

### Treatment

1. The cleaning and sterilization of all instruments that touch the patient's eye must be done for preventing the spread of epidemic.
2. Use of antibiotics can control secondary infections.
3. Topical corticosteroids benefit patients with conjunctival membrane or photophobia.

## 3.6 ACUTE HEMORRHAGIC CONJUNCTIVITIS

### Etiology

1. Acute hemorrhagic conjunctivitis is caused by coxsackie virus and enterovirus 70 of picornavirus group.
2. It is contagious and spreads by hand-to-eye contact.

### Symptoms

Red eye, watery discharge, blurring of vision and ocular discomfort are common.

### Signs

1. It has sudden onset marked by mixed papillary and follicular hyperplasia. Multiple hemorrhages in the bulbar (Fig. 3.4) and the tarsal conjunctiva are seen. Preauricular lymph glands are enlarged.
2. Edema of eyelids and chemosis of the conjunctiva are often present and occasionally, punctate keratopathy may be seen.

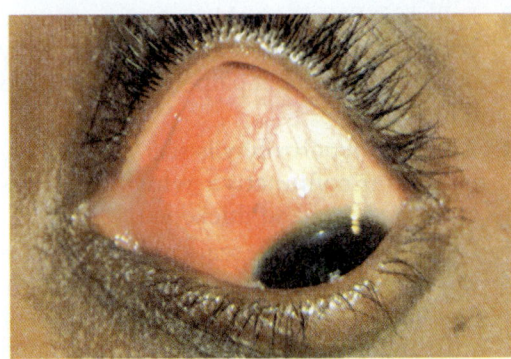

**Fig. 3.4:** Hemorrhagic conjunctivitis (*Courtesy:* Dr SCL Chandravansi, SS Medical College, Rewa)

3

## Treatment

1. It has a self-limiting course.
2. Topical antibiotics may be used to prevent bacterial and cross-infection
3. Rarely, myelitis may develop that needs proper treatment.

## 3.7 TRACHOMA

### Etiology

1. Trachoma is caused by *Chlamydia trachomatis*.
2. Fourteen serotypes of *Chlamydia* are recognized and designated by the letters A, B, Ba, C, D, Da, E, F, G, H, I, Ia, J and K. Serotypes A–C are responsible for trachoma.

### Symptoms

1. Trachoma in pure form is a symptom free disease which undergoes spontaneous cure in patients with good personal hygiene.
2. Gritty sensation, mucopus discharge, red eye, photophobia and ocular discomfort are common symptoms of trachoma of acute onset.

### Signs

1. Trachoma is common in children in endemic areas and has an insidious onset and often complicated by bacterial conjunctivitis.
2. Trachoma in adults has an acute onset.
3. Follicle is the classical lesion of trachoma. Follicles are multiple and preferentially appear on the upper palpebral conjunctiva (Fig. 3.5).
4. Papillary hypertrophy is seen on both the palpebral conjunctiva which becomes congested, red and thickened.
5. Localized or diffuse scars are seen on the upper palpebral conjunctiva (Fig. 3.6). Majority of scars look star-shaped. Linear scarring in the sulcus subtarsalis is known as Arlt's line.
6. Cornea is almost always involved.

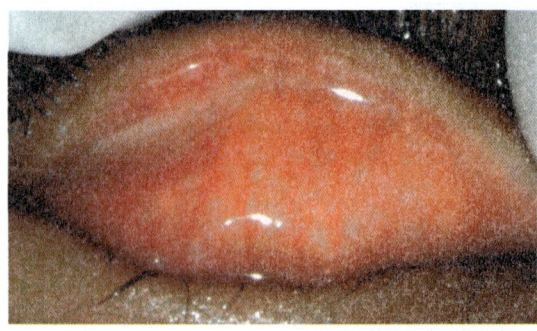

**Fig. 3.5:** Follicular trachoma *(Courtesy:* HV Nema, Nitin Nema. Textbook of Ophthalmology, New Delhi, Jaypee-Highlights, 2012)

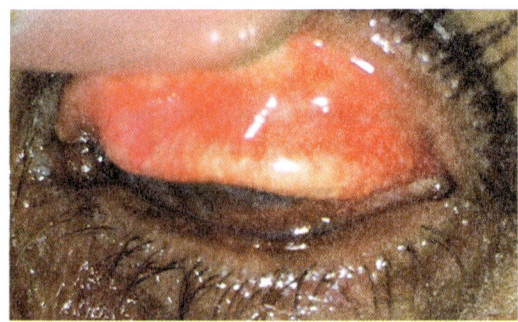

**Fig. 3.6:** Cicatricial trachoma

7. Small punctate epithelial erosions over the upper half of the cornea can be demonstrated by fluorescein stain.
8. Subepithelial infiltration in the upper-third of cornea is usually associated with vascularization, called pannus.
9. Typical follicles (Herbert's follicles) develop on the limbus; they leave round pits known as Herbert's pits at the limbus (Fig. 3.7).
10. Trichiasis, entropion, ectropion, dry eye and corneal opacity are common sequelae of trachoma.

### Classification

1. MacCallan had divided the course of trachoma into four stages: Stage 1: Incipient trachoma, Stage 2: Manifest trachoma, Stage 3: Healing trachoma and Stage 4: Healed trachoma.

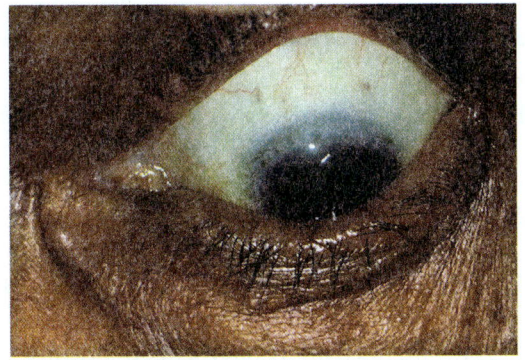

**Fig. 3.7:** Herbert's pits

2. The World Health Organization (WHO) Expert Committee on trachoma had adopted it but later simplified the classification (Table 3.1).

## Diagnosis

1. The clinical diagnosis of trachoma requires the presence of at least two of the following signs: Follicles or Herbert's pits, epithelial or subepithelial keratitis, pannus and cicatrization.
2. The diagnosis can be confirmed by laboratory tests such as: (i) demonstration of the inclusion bodies in conjunctival scrapings (ii) isolation of the virus, (iii) demonstration of trachoma antibodies by microimmunofluorescence technique and (iv) PCR.

## Treatment

1. All cases of active trachoma should be treated. Azithromycin is the drug of choice. It is given in a single dose of 20 mg/kg body weight in children and a single oral dose of 1–1.5 g in adults.
2. Topical ciprofloxacin (0.3%) or ofloxacin (0.3%) eye drop 4 times a day and application of 1% erythromycin or tetracycline ointment at bedtime for 6 weeks control the infection in most cases.
3. To combat trachomatous blindness, the WHO has developed the SAFE strategy. It is an acronym for:
   **S**urgery for trichiasis
   **A**ntibiotic treatment of active infection
   **F**acial cleanliness
   **E**nvironmental improvement

## 3.8 INCLUSION CONJUNCTIVITIS

### Etiology

1. Inclusion conjunctivitis (IC) is caused by D to K *Chlamydia trachomatis*.
2. IC manifests in two forms: Papillary form and follicular form. Acute papillary IC is seen in newborn while follicular IC occurs in children/adult after taking bath in swimming pool. Hence known as swimming pool conjunctivitis.
3. The infection appears to come from mild urethritis.

| Table 3.1 WHO simplified system of classification of trachoma | | |
|---|---|---|
| **Simplified system** | **Signs** | **Implication** |
| TF | Trachomatous inflammation: Follicular | The presence of 5 or more follicles in the upper tarsal conjunctiva |
| TI | Trachomatous inflammation: Intense | Pronounced inflammatory thickening of the upper tarsal conjunctiva that obscures more than half the normal deep tarsal vessels. |
| TS | Trachomatous scarring | The presence of scarring in the tarsal conjunctiva |
| TT | Trachomatous trichiasis | At least, one eyelash rubbing on the eyeball |
| CO | Corneal opacity | Easily visible corneal opacity over the pupil |

In this system, TF and TI represent active trachoma

**3**

## Symptoms

Symptoms are watering, discharge, red eye, FB sensation and discomfort.

## Signs

1. The disease has an acute onset.
2. Signs include acute follicular hypertrophy of the lower palpebral conjunctiva (Fig. 3.8). Papillary hyperplasia and mild superficial punctate keratitis are also seen.
3. Micropannus may be found.
4. Preauricular lymph nodes are enlarged.

## Diagnosis

1. Predominantly involves the lower palpebral conjunctiva and cicatrization of follicles and vascularization of the cornea are absent or minimal.
2. Laboratory tests of trachoma.

## Treatment

1. A single dose of azithromycin 1 g oral is effective in controlling the infection.
2. Topical erythromycin (1% drops or ointment, 3 times in a day for 3 weeks) is also effective.

## 3.9 VERNAL KERATOCONJUNCTIVITIS

### Etiology

1. In vernal keratoconjunctivitis (VKC) immunoglobulin (IgE) and cell mediated immune mechanism play some role.
2. The mechanism involves both type I and type IV hypersensitivity reactions.
3. VKC affects children in the age group of 5–15 years, often boys more than girls.
4. The patients usually have a history of atopy in the family.
5. It shows exacerbations and remissions with change of weather.

### Symptoms

Intense itching, foreign body sensation, burning, watering, photophobia and white ropy discharge.

### Signs

1. VKC manifests in two forms: (1) palpebral and (2) limbal or bulbar.
2. The *palpebral form* is relatively more common than the limbal.
3. The upper palpebral conjunctiva shows the presence of papillae. They may take giant size (Fig. 3.9).

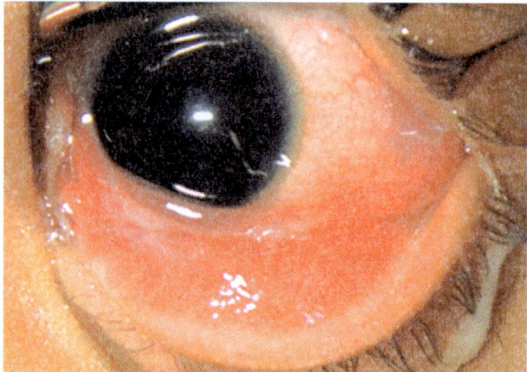

**Fig. 3.8:** Inclusion conjunctivitis (*Courtesy:* Dr SCL Chandravansi, SS Medical College, Rewa)

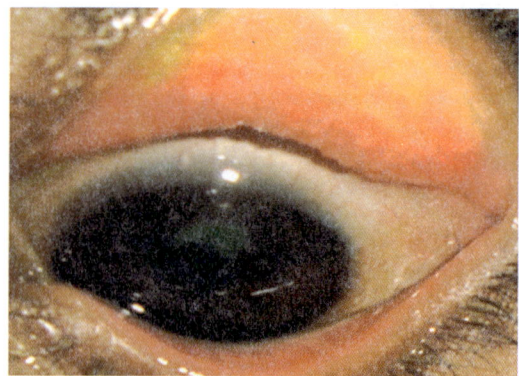

**Fig. 3.9:** Palpebral VKC with shield ulcer (*Courtesy:* Dr SCL Chandravansi, SS Medical College, Rewa)

4. Papillae have polygonal shape with flat-tops and tufts of capillaries and look like cobblestone. They impart bluish white color due to hyaline degeneration. The papillae may also seen in the lower palpebral conjunctiva.

5. A fibrinous pseudomembrane (Maxwell-Lyons sign) may sometimes be found.

6. The *limbal* or *bulbar form* is less common and seen in black races.

7. The characteristic lesion is a wall of gelatinous thickening at limbus (Fig. 3.10).

8. A few white, superficial dots or nodules (*Horner-Trantas' spots*) mainly composed of degenerated eosinophils are present at the limbus.

9. In some cases, both palpebral and limbal forms of VKC may be seen.

10. Vernal keratopathy or corneal lesions of vernal conjunctivitis are superficial punctate keratitis, epithelial erosions, noninfectious oval ulcers (shield ulcers), pseudogerontoxon and peripheral corneal vascularization.

11. VKC may be associated with keratoconus.

## Diagnosis

Smears of conjunctiva show the presence of eosinophilic granules in great numbers.

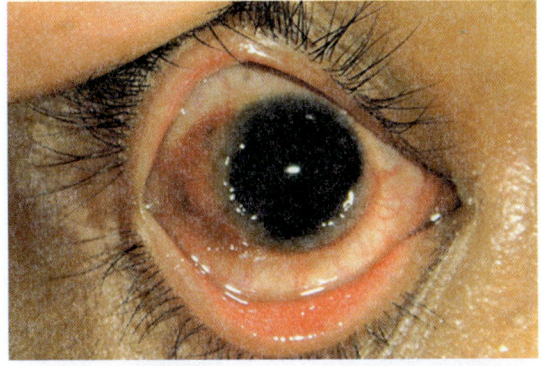

**Fig. 3.10:** Limbal vernal conjunctivitis (*Courtesy:* Dr SCL Chandravansi, SS Medical College, Rewa)

## Treatment

The treatment of VKC varies depending on the severity of the disease:

1. Mild to moderate VKC:
   - *Mast cell stabilizers.* They include cromolyn, ketorolac tromethamine, ketotifen, epinastine, azelastine and lodoxamide tromethamine.
   - Olopatidine has double actions: Mast cell stabilizing and antihistaminic.
   - Lodoxamide tromethamine (0.1% solution 4 times daily).

2. Severe VKC:
   - *Topical corticosteroids* are often needed. Prednisolone eye drops may be used 2–3 times a day and gradually tapered because steroid may raise the IOP.
   - Some cases may need fluorometholone (1%) therapy.

3. Refractory VKC:
   - An immunosuppressive agent cyclosporine topically (0.05–2%) may be used. It inhibits chemotaxis and is found effective in the management of shield ulcers.
   - Tacrolimus ointment (0.03–1%) is recommended in patients if VKC is associated with atopic dermatitis.
   - Use of acetylcysteine can check the early plaque formation. However, thick plaques are removed by phototherapeutic keratectomy.
   - Photophobia in VKC can be prevented by wearing dark glasses.

## 3.10 ATOPIC KERATOCONJUNCTIVITIS

### Etiology

1. Atopic keratoconjunctivitis (AKC) may be seen in patients with atopic dermatitis especially eczema.

2. It is a type-I hypersensitivity response that releases of histamine, prostaglandins and leukotrienes.

**3**

3. Patients with AKC are susceptible to herpes simplex keratitis and *Staphylococcus blepharitis*.

## Symptoms

Symptoms are severe itching and burning of eyes, watering and photophobia.

## Signs

1. AKC is a bilateral symmetrical disease characterized by milky edema of conjunctiva and presence of medium-sized papillae on upper and lower palpebral conjunctiva. Occasionally, giant papillae are seen.
2. Later, subepithelial fibrosis and conjunctival scarring develop.
3. The skin of the eyelids is red, macerated, fissured and inflamed.
4. Punctate erosions, plaque formation, ulcer and secondary infection may be found in the cornea.
5. Later, cornea becomes opaque and vascularized due to limbal stem-cell dysfunction
6. Occasionally, posterior and anterior lens opacities may be found.
7. A scaly dermatitis involving lids, face and neck may be seen.
8. VKC and keratoconus may be associated in a small percentage of patients with AKC.

## Treatment

1. Drugs used in the treatment of VKC are effective in AKC.
2. In severe cases, oral cyclosporine or tacrolimus should be used.
3. Additionally, concurrent infection with herpes or Staphylococcus must be treated.
4. AKC needs a prolonged treatment.

## 3.11 PHLYCTENULAR CONJUNCTIVITIS

### Etiology

1. Phlyctenular conjunctivitis is a (type IV, cell-mediated) response to endogenous microorganisms and their proteins.

2. Phlyctenulosis may develop after *Staphylococcal blepharitis*. It is commonly seen in malnourished children.

## Symptoms

Red eye, mild discomfort, irritation, photophobia and mucopurulent discharge are common.

## Signs

1. The most characteristic lesion of phlyctenulosis is a *phlycten* or *phlyctens* (blebs).
2. Small round, single or multiple, gray phlyctens appear at or near the limbus (Fig. 3.11).
3. Phlyctens may also involve the cornea or sclera. They may undergo ulceration.
4. Corneal phlycten is usually associated with subepithelial cellular infiltration and wedge-shaped vascularization.
5. Later, overlying epithelium ulcerates and a shallow fascicular ulcer develops.
6. The ulcer heals by scarring. The limbal scar undergoes nodular degeneration, Salzmann nodular dystrophy.
7. Regional lymph glands are enlarged.

## Differential Diagnosis

1. Inflamed pinguecula
2. Infected filtering bleb
3. Limbal foreign body
4. Nodular scleritis
5. Ocular rosacea.

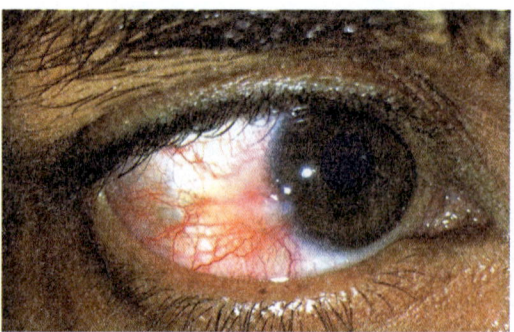

**Fig. 3.11:** Phlyctenular conjunctivitis

## Diagnosis

Diagnosis is based on clinical features.

## Treatment

1. Frequent instillation of antibiotic-steroid eye drops is very effective.
2. Cycloplegic should be applied if cornea is involved.
3. Associated secondary infection should be treated with erythromycin (200 mg twice a day) or doxycycline (100 mg, once a day) for 1–2 weeks.
4. The general health should be improved.

## 3.12 GIANT PAPILLARY CONJUNCTIVITIS

### Etiology

Giant papillary conjunctivitis is caused by mechanical irritation of tarsal conjunctiva by spoiled contact lens (hydrophilic lenses), ocular prosthesis, filtering bleb and left-over corneal sutures.

### Symptoms

Patients complain of itching, foreign body or gritty sensation, redness, watering, mucous discharge, photophobia and intolerance to contact lens (CL) or ocular prosthesis.

### Signs

1. Giant papillae are seen on the upper palpebral conjunctiva. They are polygonal and look like cobblestones (Fig. 3.12).

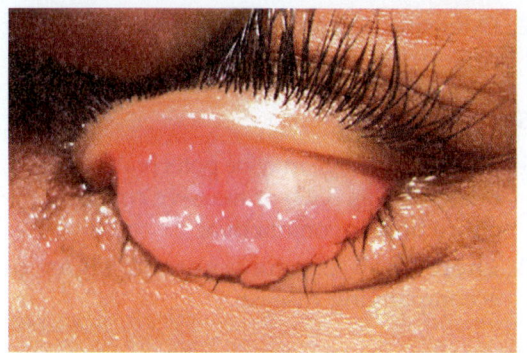

**Fig. 3.12:** Giant papillary conjunctivitis (*Courtesy:* Dr SCL Chandravansi, SS Medical College, Rewa)

2. Focal scarring may be found.
3. Deposit of mucous on CL or prosthesis.
4. Corneal complications are rarely seen.

## Treatment

1. Discontinue CL or prosthesis wear for a short period.
2. Thoroughly clean CLs with CL solution.
3. Old and spoiled CLs and prosthesis should be replaced.
4. Reduce the CLs wear time.
5. Use of topical mast cell stabilizer and corticosteroid drops for a short period is effective in severe cases.

## 3.13 PARINAUD OCULOGLANDULAR SYNDROME

### Etiology

1. Parinaud oculoglandular syndrome (POS) is caused by *Bartonella hensalae* (cat-scratch disease).
2. Tularemia, tuberculosis, syphilis, mumps, sarcoidosis, sporotrichosis and fungal infection can also cause the disease.

### Symptoms

1. Irritation, foreign body sensation, red eye and mucopurulent discharge are common.
2. Fever, headache and anorexia are constitutional symptoms.

### Signs

1. POS may manifest as follicular conjunctivitis or granulomatous nodule on the palpebral conjunctiva.
2. Occasionally, it may cause optic atrophy.
3. Regional lymph glands are enlarged.
4. Rarely, the disease may cause encephalitis and hepatitis.

### Diagnosis

1. Cat-scratch skin test and serology
2. Conjunctival culture may help

3. Excision biopsy of nodule
4. X-ray chest to rule out sarcoidosis and tuberculosis.

## Treatment

1. Azithromycin in high doses (500 mg 4 times a day) is effective in cat-scratch disease.
2. Systemic tobramycin (5 mg/kg/day, 8 hourly) combined with topical gentamicin drops can improve the patients with tularemia.

## 3.14 TOXIC CONJUNCTIVITIS

### Etiology

1. Toxic conjunctivits is caued by ophthalmic medications or accompanying preservatives.
2. Preservatives like benzalkonium chloride and thiomersal may cause toxic reaction.
3. Atropine, miotics, timolol, antivirals, etc. may induce follicular conjunctivitis.
4. Prostaglandin analog and brimonidine are known to cause adverse reaction.

### Symptoms

Irritation, foreign body sensation, burning, watering, redness, swelling of lids and ocular discomfort may occur.

### Signs

1. Chronic follicular conjunctivitis or papillary hyperplasia may occur.
2. Follicles are mostly seen on the inferior tarsal conjunctiva and in the fornix.
3. Edema and flushing of lids may be seen.
4. In severe reaction, face is usually involved.
5. Occasionally, a progressive scarring may develop in the conjunctiva.

### Differential Diagnosis

- Allergic conjunctivitis
- Infective conjunctivitis.

## Diagnosis

1. History of use of topical drug.
2. Stoppage of the drug relieves clinical features.

## Treatment

- The medication must be immediately discontinued.
- Withdrawal of drug is followed by normalization of condition.
- Use of preservative-free lubricant drops provides relief.

## 3.15 SUBCONJUNCTIVAL HEMORRHAGE

### Etiology

1. Subconjunctival hemorrhage or ecchymosis is caused by acute hemorrhagic conjunctivitis.
2. Hemorrhages in conjunctiva may be seen in whooping cough, blood dyscrasias, scurvy, diabetes, arteriosclerosis and hypertension.
3. Subconjunctival hemorrhages are common following crush injuries and fracture of the base of skull (appears after 8–12 hours).
4. Children and aged people are more prone to subconjunctival hemorrhages.

### Symptoms

1. Patient is symptom free or may complain of red eye.
2. Extensive hemorrhage covering the bulbar conjunctiva may cause anxiety.

### Signs

1. The hemorrhage may be petechial, sectorial, bilateral (Fig. 3.13) or massive covering the entire bulbar conjunctiva.
2. There may or may not be signs of accompanying disease.

### Treatment

1. Try to stop bleeding by cold compresses.

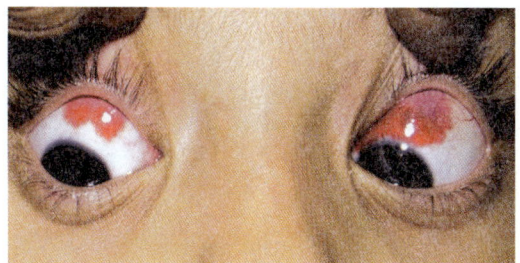

**Fig. 3.13:** Bilateral subconjunctival hemorrhage

2. Small subconjunctival hemorrhage resolves in 2 weeks time without any treatment.

## 3.16 XEROSIS

Xerosis is a dry lusterless condition of the conjunctiva which manifests in two forms: (1) parenchymatous xerosis and (2) epithelial xerosis.

### Etiology

1. Parenchymatous xerosis is usually caused by trachoma, membranous conjunctivitis, ocular cicatricial pemphigoid, chemical burns, and lagophthalmos.
2. Epithelial xerosis or xerophthalmia is caused by an inadequate intake of vitamin A or a defective absorption from the gut.

### Symptoms

1. Night blindness is the earliest symptom of xerophthalmia.
2. If cornea is involved, photophobia, watering and visual impairment develop.

### Signs

Almost all signs of xerosis are included in the WHO classification of xerophthalmia:

- *XN—Night blindness.*
- *X1A—Conjunctival xerosis.*
- *X1B—Bitot's spot.*
- *X2—Corneal xerosis.*
- *X3A—Corneal ulceration or keratomalacia* affecting less than one-third of the corneal surface.

- *X3B—Corneal ulceration or keratomalacia* affecting more than one-third of the corneal surface.
- *XS—Corneal scars* of different densities appear after healing of ulcers. They impair the visual acuity.
- *XF—Xerophthalmic fundus*

Bitot's spot is a characteristic dry lusterless triangular spot with base toward limbus and apex toward outer canthus. It is often bilateral and temporal (Fig. 3.14)

Cornea becomes lusterless, insensitive and its surface becomes pebbly. It is not rare to find a dry plaque on it.

Keratomalacia is an advanced stage of xerophthalmia wherein cornea melts and a large ulcer is formed. Perforation of ulcer or thick corneal scarring results in blindness.

Presence of multiple scattered yellow dots in the periphery of retina is a characteristic appearance of the xerophthalmic fundus.

### Diagnosis

1. Diagnosis is based on clinical picture
2. Serum vitamin A level.

### Treatment

1. Adequate treatment of chronic conjunctival diseases (known to cause scarring) and use of protective devices to prevent chemical burns can prevent parenchymatous xerosis.

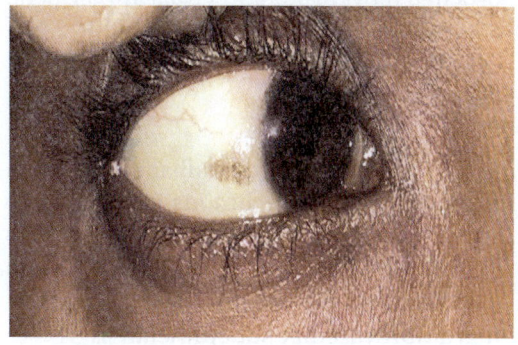

**Fig. 3.14:** Bitot's spot

2. Ocular chemical burn should be treated aggressively. Frequent use of preservative-free tear substitutes and grafting are often needed.
3. Administration of prophylactic vitamin A (50000–100000 IU, 6 monthly) and breast feeding prevent epithelial xerosis in infants.
4. The daily requirement of vitamin A for a child is 3,000–4,000 IU.
5. Proper treatment of worm infestations is necessary.
6. Methyl cellulose or lubricating eye drops are used locally several times in a day.
7. If secondary infection is feared, topical antibiotic is added.
8. Children with corneal ulcers (X3A and X3B) need energetic treatment in order to avoid corneal blindness.

## 3.17 PTERYGIUM

### Etiology

1. Pterygium is a growth disorder induced by UV rays damaging the limbal stem cells.
2. There is overexpression of p53 protein, vimentin, and overproduction of transforming growth factor (TGF) beta 1 resulting in cellular migration.
3. Incidence of pterygium is high in people living in hot, dry, dusty and windy climate.

### Symptoms

1. Symptoms include mild irritation, redness, dry eye, cosmetic disfigurement, restriction of ocular movements and visual impairment.
2. Contact lens wearers with pterygium often develop discomfort.

### Signs

1. A wing-shaped fold of bulbar conjunctiva encroaches over the limbus and onto the superficial cornea in the horizontal axis (3–9 o'clock position) in the interpalpebral aperture (Fig. 3.15).
2. It is a fibrovascular subepithelial ingrowth usually seen nasally.

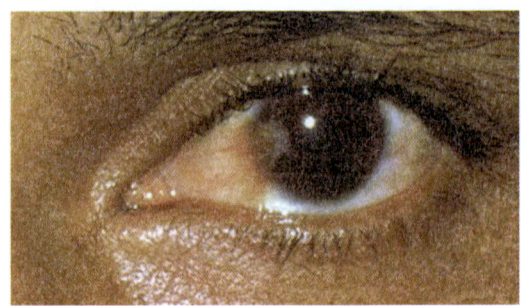

**Fig. 3.15:** Pterygium

3. The pterygium consists of 4 parts: (1) A cap consists of infiltrates on the apex, (2) head is the apex, (3) neck is the limbal part and (4) body is formed by bulbar part.
4. An iron line or Stocker's line may be seen in the epithelium anterior to the apex.
5. A progressive pterygium is always thick, fleshy and vascular. It may extend to the pupillary area and cause severe visual impairment.
6. Pterygium induces high degree of astigmatism as a result of flattening of the cornea.
7. When pterygium stops growing, it looks pale and thin and known as regressive pterygium.
8. Superficial keratitis and thinning of the cornea may be found.

### Differential Diagnosis

- *Pseudopterygium:* A fold of conjunctiva gets attached to the peripheral cornea following corneal ulceration
- *Pinguecula:* It does not encroach on to the cornea.

### Diagnosis

1. Slit-lamp examination can establish the diagnosis
2. Refraction reveals presence of astigmatism
3. Biopsy.

### Treatment

1. Fleshy pterygium should be treated with topical corticosteroid drops (prednisolone

1%, 2–3 times a day for 10–15 days). However, IOP should be monitored for the possibility of steroid-induced glaucoma.

2. Pterygium requires excision with conjunctival autograft.

3. Amniotic membrane graft is used if there is an extensive damage to the conjunctiva.

4. To prevent the recurrence, intraoperative mitomycin C (0–2%) may be applied.

5. Superficial keratectomy or lamellar graft may be needed for improving the visual acuity if pterygium causes a corneal scar.

## 3.18 CICATRICIAL PEMPHIGOID

### Etiology

1. Cicatricial pemphigoid is a bilateral chronic disease of autoimmune etiology with dysregulation of T-lymphocytes.

2. It affects adults and shows remissions and exacerbations.

### Symptoms

The patient may present with ocular discomfort, dryness, foreign body sensation, redness, itching, photophobia, lacrimation, pain and diminution of vision.

### Signs

1. In the initial stage, reactive conjunctivitis with vesicles and bullae are seen.

2. Later rupture of vesicles/bullae forms ulcers and gradually symblepharon may develop stretching between bulbar conjunctiva/cornea and lid margin. It causes limitation of ocular movements.

3. Shortening or obliteration of the lower fornix is common.

4. The eye becomes dry.

5. Trichiasis, entropion, SPK and corneal ulcer are found.

6. Skin and mucous membrane of oral cavity, genitals and esophagus are often involved. Vesicles appear on mucous membrane and rupture of vesicles causes scarring and stricture.

### Differential Diagnosis

1. Membranous conjunctivitis
2. Chemical burns
3. Pemphigus
4. Stevens-Johnson syndrome.

### Diagnosis

1. Diagnosis is mostly clinical.

2. Conjunctival biopsy for direct or indirect immunofluorescence test for antibodies is helpful.

### Treatment

1. Medical
   - One or two hourly instillation of preservative-free artificial tears
   - Topical antibiotic ointment at bedtime
   - Oral doxycycline (100–200 mg) daily for 3 weeks for blepharitis.
   - Systemic prednisolone 60 mg, daily may control acute exacerbations.
   - Immunosuppressive agents: Methotrexate, mycophenolate mofetil, cyclophosphamide, etc. are effective.

2. Surgical
   - Occlusion of puncta for dry eye
   - Correction of trichiasis, entropion and symblepharon (reconstruction of fornices and cutting of bands).

## 3.19 STEVENS-JOHNSON SYNDROME

### Etiology

1. Stevens-Johnson syndrome (SJS) or erythema multiforme is a delayed type of hypersensitivity reaction against various agents.

2. *Mycoplasma pnuemoniae* is the most common cause in children.

3. Herpes, vaccinia, mumps, *M. tuberculosis*, etc. are other microbes which play important role in the etiology of SJS.

**3**

4. Adverse reactions to some drugs like sulfonamides, penicillin, tetracycline, barbiturates, nonsteroidal anti-inflammatory drugs (NSAIDs) are also implicated.

## Symptoms

1. Dryness, foreign body sensation, redness, itching, photophobia, lacrimation, pain and diminution of vision are ocular symptoms.
2. Headache, fever, malaise, nausea and vomiting are general symptoms.

## Signs

1. Initially, crust formation on the skin of eyelids and acute papillary conjunctivitis appear.
2. Membrane or pseudomembrane may form on the conjunctiva.
3. Heavy scarring of conjunctiva causes obliteration of fornices.
4. Trichiasis, entropion and symblepharon often develop due to cicatrization
5. Loss of goblet cells results in dry eye. Severe meibomitis is present.
6. Keratinization of the tarsal conjunctiva and the cornea appear.
7. Corneal facets, corneal vascularization and stromal ulcers are not uncommon.
8. Erythematous papular eruptions appear on soles, palms and hands.
9. The classical dermatological lesions of SJS are target or "bull's eye spots". Each spot shows a central area of erythema surrounded by a zone of normal-looking skin and again followed by an erythematous ring.
10. Mucous membrane of nose, mouth, anus, vagina and conjunctiva is often involved. Vesicles and bullae develop and soon rupture followed by scarring.

## Diagnosis

1. History of fever or an acute side effect of a drug.
2. Characteristic lesions in the skin and simultaneous involvement of mucous membrane.

## Treatment

1. Frequent use of lubricants
2. Topical cycloplegic, antibiotic and steroid drops
3. Bandage CLs
4. Amniotic membrane and stem cell grafts
5. Tarsorrhaphy and plastic repair
6. Lamellar or penetrating keratoplasty
7. Keratoprosthesis.

## 3.20 CYST AND BENIGN TUMORS OF CONJUNCTIVA

### Epibulbar Dermoid

Epibulbar dermoid is a congenital white or yellow, oval cyst seen at limbus (Fig. 3.16). It may cover partly the conjunctiva and partly the cornea. The dermoid grows slowly and is composed of epidermoid epithelium and fibrous tissue containing hair follicles and sebaceous glands. It may be associated with upper eyelid coloboma. Excision of dermoid followed by keratoplasty is the treatment of choice.

Dermolipoma is a yellowish-white, fibrofatty, solid, subconjunctival benign tumor. It is usually found in the suprotemporal region. It often extends posteriorly in the orbit. Dermolipoma, like dermoid, may be associated with Goldenhar syndrome.

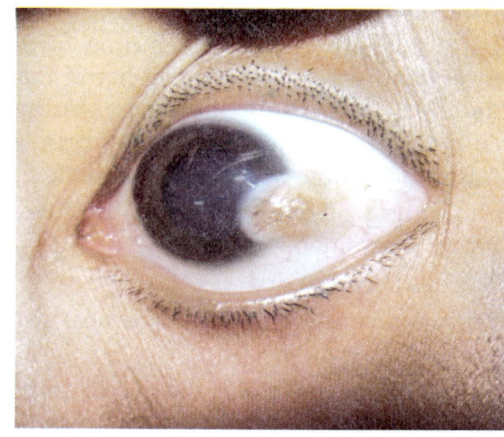

Fig. 3.16: Epibulbar dermoid at limbus

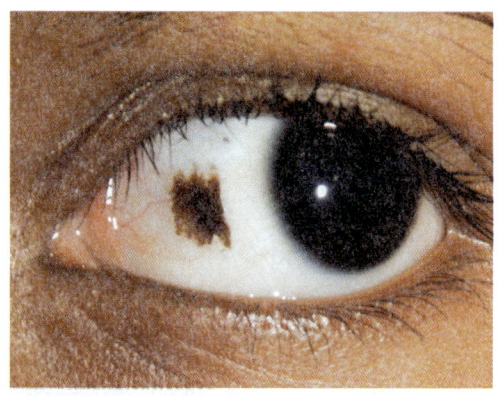

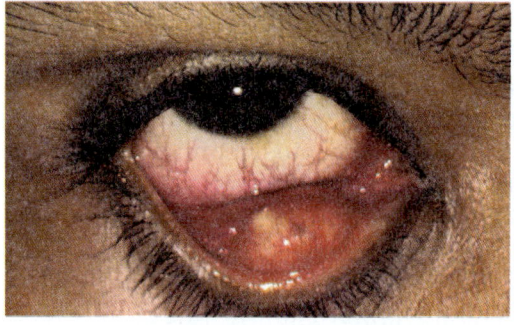

Fig. 3.18: Conjunctival granuloma

Fig. 3.17: Conjunctival nevus

## Nevus

Nevus or congenital mole is frequently seen on the bulbar conjunctiva (Fig. 3.17). It may grow at puberty. It appears as brownish or black flat small growth. It contains pigmented nevus cells. The nevus does not require excision lest malignant changes develop.

## Papilloma

Papilloma is a benign polypoid or sesile tumor of the conjunctiva caused by human papilloma virus. It may be single or multiple often seen in the fornix or at the canthus. Most papillomas undergo spontaneous resolution. Cimetidine (150 mg twice a day orally) is an effective treatment.

Papilloma found in elderly patients is nonviral in origin. It is usually found near limbus. It may appear like cock's comb type of tuberculosis. It should be excised completely because it has a tendency to become malignant.

## Granuloma

Granuloma of the conjunctiva usually develops on the palpebral conjunctiva. The tumor should be excised. Granuloma may be found after strabismus surgery and extrusion of chalazion (Fig. 3.18), sarcoidosis and tuberculosis. Granuloma presents as a rapidly growing, reddish, fleshy and vascularized mass. Later, it may appear as a huge growth. Majority of granulomas need surgical removal while sarcoid granuloma responds to systemic corticosteroids therapy.

## 3.21 MALIGNANT TUMORS OF CONJUNCTIVA

### Squamous Cell Carcinoma

Squamous cell carcinoma or epithelioma is a malignant growth of the conjunctiva seen in old age. It is characterized by a vascular gelatinous mass at lid margin or limbus (Fig. 3.19). The epithelioma can invade the cornea or the eye. In the event of intraocular spread, enucleation should be performed.

### Intraepithelial Neoplasia

Intraepithelial neoplasia (Bowen's disease) is a rare epibulbar tumor. It involves conjunctiva as well as cornea. A free excision is the treatment of choice.

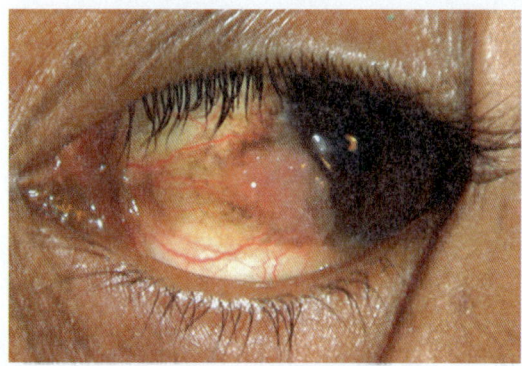

Fig. 3.19: Squamous cell carcinoma (*Courtesy:* Dr SCL Chandravansi, SS Medical College, Rewa)

3

## Basal Cell Carcinoma

Basal cell carcinoma is a locally malignant tumor. The tumor frequently involves the lower lid and plica semilunaris. Surgical excision is the most common mode of treatment. It may be followed by radiotherapy.

## Lymphoid Tumor

Salmon-colored slightly raised and oval-shaped tumor appears in the bulbar conjunctiva. The growth can take a horizontal or cresent shape in the fornix. The diagnosis requires biopsy and immunohistochemical studies. The lesion should be completely excised.

## Kaposi Sarcoma

Kaposi sarcoma is a bright-red subconjunctival nodule found in patients of AIDS. It is a slow growing nontender malignant tumor. It may resolve with highly active antiretroviral therapy (HAART) or may need excision.

## Malignant Melanoma

Malignant melanoma may arise *de novo* or from a prexisting nevus in the conjunctiva. It involves limbus. Melanoma appears as a dark-brown nodular mass which is heavily vascularized. Intraocular and intraorbital spread can occur. Metastases can also occur elsewhere in the body, commonly in liver. Exenteration of orbit is often needed.

# Diseases of Cornea and Sclera

## Etiology

1. Superficial punctate keratitis (SPK) is caused by virus, adenovirus and chlamydia. Dry eye, trauma and blepharitis may predispose it.
2. Drugs like antivirals, atropine, gentamicin, or their preservatives and ultraviolet (UV) burn can also induce the disease.
3. Both corneal dystrophy and corneal degenerations (band-shaped and Salzmann nodular degeneration) may present with SPK.

## Symptoms

1. Photophobia, foreign body sensation, watering, ocular discomfort and mild pain are common symptoms.
2. Vision may or may not be affected.

## Signs

1. Multiple, small, pin-head size, round lesions in the epithelium and superficial stroma of the cornea appear.
2. Lesions of SPK take fluorescein stain.
3. Depending on the etiology of SPK, clinical signs vary.

## Diagnosis

1. Slit-lamp examination after staining of cornea with fluorescein confirms the diagnosis.

2. Degenerated or devitalized cells stain better with Rose Bengal than fluorescein.
3. If diffuse staining of the entire cornea and conjunctiva occurs, an early bacterial/viral/toxic keratitis should be suspected.
4. Superior limbal staining of infiltrations suggests trachoma/vernal keratoconjunctivitis (VKC)/superior limbic keratoconjunctivitis (SLK), staphylococcal infection/trichiasis or contact lens (CL) overwear.
5. Paracentral or central stained dendrites point to herpes and linear stains to mechanical injury.
6. Horizontal staining of the inferior cornea in the interpalpebral area is a sign of exposure keratitis.

## Treatment

1. If CL is causing SPK, discontinue its use.
2. Use of toxic drugs should be stopped.
3. Dark glasses may relieve annoying photophobia.
4. Patients with exposure keratitis need tarsorrhaphy.
5. Trichiasis and ectropion should be corrected surgically.
6. Generally, SPK responds to frequent use of preservative-free tear lubricant.
7. Topical acyclovir (3%) is beneficial in herpes simplex infections.

8. Topical antibiotics are needed to treat infective cases. If multiple SPK coalesce to form an epithelial defect or corneal ulcer, use of antibiotic and cycloplegic is recommended.

## 4.2 THYGESON'S SUPERFICIAL PUNCTATE KERATITIS

### Etiology

1. Thygeson's SPK is a bilateral, asymmetrical, and coarse epithelial keratopathy of unknown etiology.
2. More often a viral infection is implicated.
3. The response to corticosteroids suggests that it may be an immune mediated disease.

### Symptoms

Foreign body sensation, ocular discomfort, watering and photophobia are common symptoms.

### Signs

1. Multiple coarse, round opacities in the cornea.
2. Corneal lesions stain with fluorescein.
3. It has a chronic course.
4. Exacerbations and remissions are common.

### Diagnosis

1. Slit-lamp examination
2. Stain with fluorescein and rose Bengal dyes.

### Treatment

1. Use preservative free artificial tears.
2. Topical fluorometholone (0.1%) provides relief. Resistant cases may need bandage contact lens.

## 4.3 SUPERIOR LIMBIC KERATOCONJUNCTIVITIS

### Etiology

1. The etiology of superior limbic keratitis is not known. It affects more females than males.

2. It occurs more frequently in patients with hypothyroidism.

### Symptoms

Ocular discomfort, watering and irritation may occur.

### Signs

1. Marked papillary hyperplasia is seen at the upper limbus as well as in the upper palpebral conjunctiva.
2. Blood vessels are dilated over the superior limbus and bulbar conjunctiva (Fig. 4.1).
3. Superficial punctate corneal lesions take fluorescein stain.
4. Keratinization of superior limbus and conjunctiva may be seen.

### Treatment

1. Preservative-free artificial tears and corticosteroid drops may provide relief.
2. BCL may be helpful in relieving symptoms.
3. Application of 1% silver nitrate on the upper tarsal conjunctiva or recession of 2 mm strip of upper limbal conjunctiva is recommended if other measures fail.

## 4.4 FILAMENTARY KERATITIS

### Etiology

Filamentary keratitis is seen in kerato-conjunctivitis sicca SPK, HSK, bullous

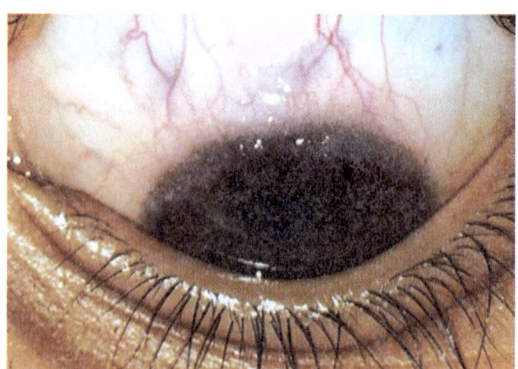

**Fig. 4.1:** Superior limbic keratitis

keratopathy, radiation keratopathy and prolonged eye patching.

## Symptoms

Foreign body sensation, dryness, photophobia and mild to severe pain especially on closure of lids or ocular movements.

## Signs

1. The filament is composed of a mucus core enveloped by the corneal epithelium.
2. One end of the filament moves freely while the other remains attached to the epithelium. Pain occurs due to stretching of filament during ocular movements.
3. Slit-lamp examination after fluorescein staining reveals epithelial erosions and filaments (Fig. 4.2).

## Treatment

1. The cause of the condition should be treated.
2. Use of hourly or 2 hourly preservative-free tear substitute provides relief in dry eye disease.
3. Instillation of hypertonic saline (5%) 5 times a day and debridement of filaments relieve pain.
4. The use of topical acetylcysteine (10–20%) benefits the patient as it is a mucolytic agent.
5. High water content CL (Perma lens) is also helpful.

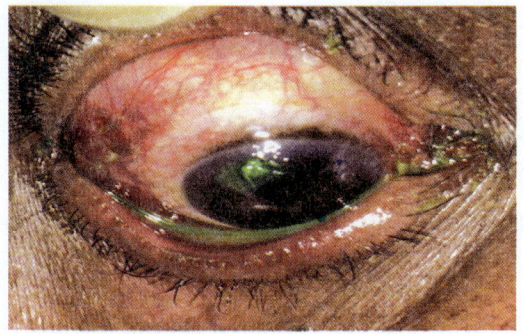

**Fig. 4.2:** Filamentary keratitis

## 4.5 RECURRENT CORNEAL EROSIONS

### Etiology

1. Recurrent corneal erosions are nonspecific lesions caused by an old fingernail or paper-cut injury which may heal rapidly.
2. After some interval symptoms recur as a result of imperfect healing of basement membrane.
3. It can also occur in epithelial basement membrane dystrophy, stromal dystrophy, corneal degeneration (Salzmann nodular and band keratopathy) and after cataract surgery, penetrating keratoplasty (PKP) and keratorefractive procedures.
4. Increased levels of metalloproteinase-2 and 9 in tears may cause loose adhesion between the corneal epithelium and basement membrane.

### Symptoms

1. Recurrent corneal erosions cause intense pain and the patient is awakened by it in the early morning.
2. Photophobia, foreign body sensation, irritation, watering and redness are other symptoms.

### Signs

1. In minor episodes, no ulcers or abnormalities may be found in the cornea.
2. Severe episodes may reveal an ovoid or triangular ulcer with attached filament of detached epithelium in the lower part of the cornea after fluorescein staining.
3. The loose corneal epithelium may be heaped at the margin of the ulcer and hinder its healing.
4. Epithelial defect after healing may recur in a short time.
5. Retroillumination can demonstrate loose attachment of epithelium with the underlying Bowman membrane during an attack.
6. Both eyes may show corneal dystrophy or degeneration.

4

## Treatment

1. Frequent use of lubricants and bandage contact lens relieve the symptoms.
2. Apply lubricant and antibiotic ointment and patch the eye in the acute phase.
3. Administration of doxycycline and use of topical low concentration corticosteroids are effective.
4. Multiple stromal punctures of the cornea is recommended.
5. Superficial keratectomy or excimer laser ablation may prevent the corneal erosions.

## 4.6 BACTERIAL CORNEAL ULCER

### Etiology

1. Corneal ulcers are caused by *S. aureus, Pseudomonas, S. pneumoniae, S. hemolyticus, Haemophilus spp.* and *Moraxella spp.*
2. Some risk factors disturb the integrity of the corneal epithelium. They include trauma, frequent use of steroids, prolonged wear of contact lens, poor general health and persistent chronic dacrocystitis.
3. Except *N. gonorrheae* and *C. diphtheriae* no other bacteria can invade the intact corneal epithelium.
4. The epithelium at the margins of the ulcer swells with infiltration of inflammatory cells. Enzymes released by neutrophils and corneal metalloproteinases exacerbate necrosis.
5. Bacterial toxins may diffuse in the anterior chamber and cause iritis.

### Symptoms

Pain, redness, lacrimation, photophobia, blepharospasm and impairment of vision.

### Signs

1. The corneal ulcer starts as a gray or white localized infiltrate.
2. Fluorescein staining (Fig. 4.3) shows a discontinuity of the corneal surface.

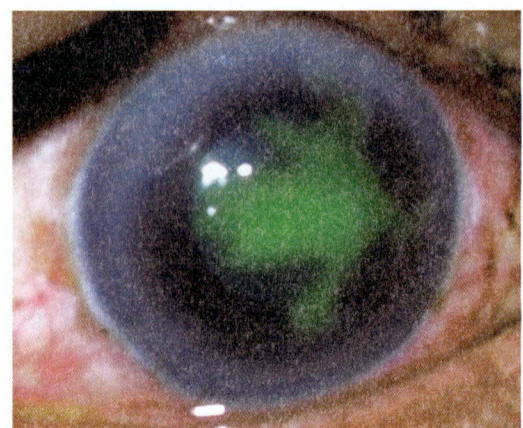

**Fig. 4.3:** Superficial corneal ulcer showing fluorescein staining

3. The ulcer may take any shape, oval or irregular shape. The margin of the ulcer is usually overhanging with sloping edges.
4. There is a marked ciliary injection.
5. Generally, superficial blood vessels invade the margin of the ulcer. Sometimes, a fleshy growth may cover it.
6. In some cases, the entire corneal stroma becomes necrotic and exposes the Descemet's membrane which may bulge *descemetocele*.
7. The ulcer may perforate causing iris prolapse which on healing forms *adherent leucoma*.
8. If perforation of ulcer is in the central area, a *corneal fistula* develops.
9. Other complications of perforation of corneal ulcer include collapse of the anterior chamber, anterior capsular cataract, extrusion of the lens from the eye, prolapse of the vitreous and intraocular hemorrhage and anterior staphyloma.

### Hypopyon Corneal Ulcer

#### Etiology

1. *S. pneumoniae, S. hemolyticus, S. gonorrhoeae* and *Proteus vulgaris* are common pyogenic organisms capable of producing the ulcer.
2. *Pseudomonas pyocyanea* causes a rapidly sloughing hypopyon corneal ulcer.

3. Old, debilitated and malnourished individuals are prone to develop hypopyon ulcer. Presence of concurrent chronic dacryocystitis and history of injury by organic matters (leaf, twigs, coal particles) or finger-nail are considered as high-risk patients.

### Pneumococcal Corneal Ulcer

1. A typical pneumococcal ulcer begins as a central disk-shaped ulcer with infiltrating edges.
2. The cornea becomes hazy and edematous.
3. The toxins induce violent iridocyclitis associated with *hypopyon* (Fig. 4.4) if the hypopyon remains sterile. The Descemet's membrane is intact.
4. The ulcer spreads on the edge of infiltration which looks as a yellowish crescent anterior to the Descemet's membrane. The double infiltration renders the cornea weak.
5. The corneal stroma becomes necrotic and breaks down.
6. The intraocular pressure (IOP) is often elevated.

### Staphylococcal Corneal Ulcer

1. Staphylococcal corneal ulcer is seen in compromised cornea.

2. The stromal ulcer appears gray white with sharp border associated with corneal edema.
3. A chronic ulcer spreads in the deeper layers of cornea and forms an abscess and causes perforation.

### Streptococcal Corneal Ulcer

1. Streptococcal infection can produce a mild to severe reaction in the cornea.
2. *S. viridance* induces an indolent reaction or crystalline keratopathy.
3. *Streptococcus haemolyticus* gives purulent infiltrates associated with severe anterior chamber reaction and hypopyon.

### Pseudomonas Corneal Ulcer

1. Pseudomonas causes a rapidly progressive ulcer in the cornea with greenish discharge.
2. It presents a diffuse epithelial and stromal infiltration.
3. The ulcer progresses and involves the entire width and depth of the cornea.
4. It is usually associated with severe anterior chamber reaction and hypopyon (Fig. 4.5).
5. Pseudomonas strains produce exotoxin A that melts the cornea leading to perforation.

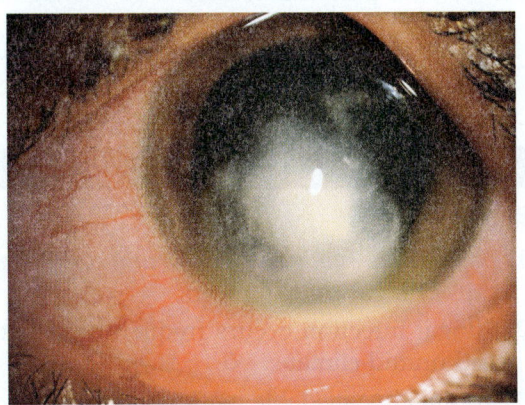

Fig. 4.4: Bacterial corneal ulcer with hypopyon (*Courtesy:* Dr Prema Padhamanabhan, Sankara Nethralaya, Chennai)

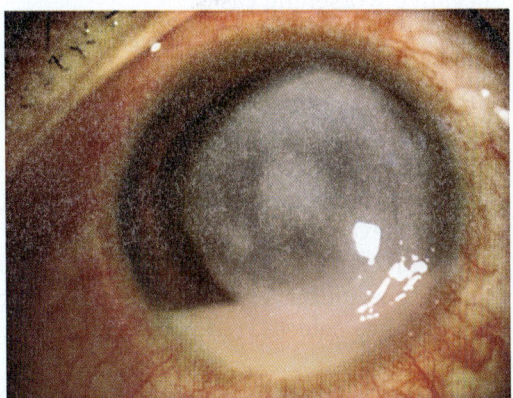

Fig. 4.5: Pseudomonas corneal ulcer (*Courtesy:* Dr Prema Padhamanabhan, Sankara Nethralaya, Chennai)

4

## Marginal Corneal Ulcer

1. Marginal corneal ulcers are caused by *Staphylococcus aureus*, *Morax-Axenfeld diplobacilli* and *Haemophilus aegyptius*.
2. Marginal ulcers are seen in old age and patients may be suffering from staphylococcal blepharitis.
3. The marginal corneal ulcer is oval in shape and often involves the inferior half of the cornea.
4. It may occur as a shallow infiltrated crescent with vascularization.
5. It has a chronic indolent course and occasionally forms a deep marginal gutter.

### Differential Diagnosis

1. Hypersensitivity-mediated marginal corneal ulcer: It is caused by a reaction to staphylococcal exotoxin resulting in the deposition of antigen–antibody complex in the periphery of the cornea with lymphocytic infiltration. Culture is negative and the ulcer responds to topical steroid drops.
2. Mooren ulcer.

### Diagnosis

1. Smear and culture examinations should be carried out before starting the treatment.
2. Corneal biopsy may be needed in culture-negative worsening cases.

### Treatment of Corneal Ulcers

1. Prophylaxis includes wearing protective glasses and treatment of trichiasis.
2. Systemic analgesics and anti-inflammatory agents (diclofenac sodium, ibuprofen, etc.) relieve pain.
3. The infection is controlled by the topical use of specific bactericidal or bacteriostatic antibiotics selected after the sensitivity test.
4. Gram-positive cocci are treated with cefazolin (100 mg/mL), ciprofloxacin, moxifloxacin or gatifloxacin.

5. Gram-negative cocci with ceftriaxone or ceftazidime (50 mg/mL), levofloxacin, or moxifloxacin.
6. Gram-positive bacillus are sensitive to tobramycin (14 mg/mL), gentamicin (14 mg/mL), vancomycin or penicillin G (100,000 U/mL).
7. Gram-negative bacilli are sensitive to moxifloxacin, tobramycin or ceftazidime (50 mg/mL). Oxytetracycline is effective against Moraxella.
8. In severe infection, fortified antibiotics freshly prepared from their injectable preparations are used.
9. Subconjunctival and intravenous (IV) injections of antibiotics are recommended in nonhealing ulcers with deep infiltrates.
10. Homatropine (2%) eye drop or atropine sulfate (1% drop or ointment) is used twice a day.
11. The eye with corneal thinning is protected by collagen shield. It may also be used for a high concentration of drug delivery purpose.
12. Reduction of IOP with oral acetazolamide and/or IV mannitol can prevent perforation of the cornea.
13. BCL and conjunctival flapping can also help in prevention of perforation.
14. Corneal perforation should be managed by penetrating therapeutic keratoplasty, cynoacrylate glue and collagen plug or shield.

## 4.7 FUNGAL CORNEAL ULCER

### Etiology

1. *Aspergillus fumigatus*, *Fusarium*, *Candida* cause fungal corneal ulcers.
2. Fungal infection occurs frequently in hot and humid climate.
3. Trauma by vegetable matter, CL wear, dry eye and herpes infection are considered as risk factors.

## Symptoms

1. Red eye, discharge, photophobia, impairment of vision and pain are common.
2. Pain is relatively less as compared to alarming signs.

## Signs

1. Progressive gray or grayish-white infiltrates with feathery extensions in the stroma are characteristic signs (Fig. 4.6).
2. Epithelium over the infiltrates ulcerates.
3. Ciliary injection is marked.
4. Small round satellite lesions surround the ulcer.
5. A dense white plaque appears on the corneal endothelium.
6. A severe anterior chamber reaction with nonsterile hypopyon is seen.
7. A white immune ring *(Wesseley ring)* is seen in the midperiphery of the cornea.
8. A corneal abscess often develops in fulminating corneal ulcer.

## Diagnosis

1. Smear with KOH or calcoflour white helps in detecting the fungus.
2. Gram-stain can diagnose *Candida*.
3. Culture on the Sabouraud's dextrose agar medium on room temperature may yield the offending fungus in 7–15 days.

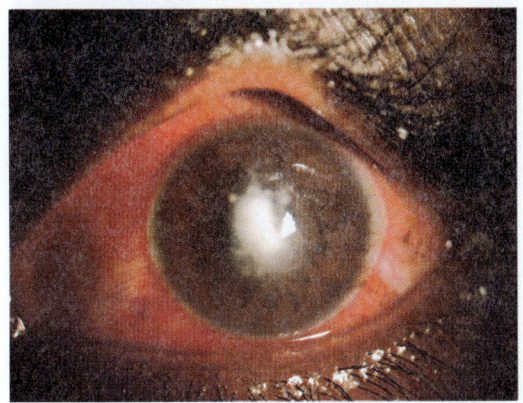

**Fig. 4.6:** Fungal corneal ulcer with satellites (*Courtesy:* Dr. Prema Padhamanabhan, Sankara Nethralaya, Chennai)

## Treatment

1. Fungus ulcer requires speedy and aggressive treatment.
2. Topical natamycin (5%) is used for the treatment of ulcer caused by filamentous fungi.
3. Amphotericin B (0.15%) and voriconazole (1%) eye drops are effective against a wide range of fungi.
4. Oral fluconazole (100–200 mg, 4 times a day), ketaconazole (200–400 mg, 2 times a day) or voriconazole (200 mg twice daily) are administered for deep fungal corneal ulcer.
5. Topical cycloplegic is used in all cases.

## Surgical Therapy

1. Debridement removes the necrotic tissue and increases the action of antifungal drugs.
2. Non-healing ulcer may need conjunctival flapping.
3. Therapeutic PKP not only removes the infected tissue but also saves the eye.

## 4.8 HERPES SIMPLEX KERATITIS

### Etiology

1. Herpes keratitis is caused by herpes simplex virus (HSV). It has two strains: (i) HSV-1 and (ii) HSV-2
2. HSV-1 affects mouth, lips and eyes
3. HSV-2 affects the anogenital region
4. The HSV infection manifests in two forms: (1) primary and (2) recurrent:
   - *Primary herpetic infection:*
     - Primary herpetic infection is seen in nonimmune subjects and remains subclinical in about 50% of patients.
     - Skin, eye, oral cavity and central nervous system (CNS) may be involved in neonatal herpes. The disease may be potentially devastating.
     - Primary herpes may cause fever, malaise and preauricular lymphadenopathy.

4

**4**

- It can cause ophthalmia neonatorum, follicular conjunctivitis and corneal dendrites.
- Lesions heal without causing any complications.
- Primary herpes remains dormant for many years.
    - *Recurrent infection:* Reactivation of the virus may occur due to trivial trauma, attack of flu, and involves the eye often unilaterally.

## Symptoms

Symptoms include watering, pain, red eye, photophobia, reduced visual acuity, vesicular rash near the angle of mouth and eyelid.

## Signs

1. The most characteristic lesion of herpes in the corneal epithelium is *dendritic keratitis* or *ulcer* (Fig. 4.7). It is a thin, linear branching ulcer with club-shaped terminal bulbs at the end of each branch. The center of the ulcer takes fluorescein stain.
2. The epithelium at the edge of the ulcer is often heaped up and stains well with Rose Bengal.
3. The dendritic ulcer can spread and forms a *geographical ulcer.* The geographical corneal ulcer is due to rapid viral replication.
4. The corneal sensitivity is always reduced.

5. Recurrent corneal erosions may occur due to persistent defect in the basement membrane. The lesion is known as *trophic* or *metaherpetic keratitis.*
6. Herpes can produce both nonnecrotizing and necrotizing lesions in the corneal stroma.
7. The nonnecrotizing lesion is called *disciform keratitis;* a hypersensitivity response of stroma.
8. The classical features of disciform keratitis are disk-shaped edema of stroma, a ring of infiltrates (Wesseley ring) (Fig. 4.8), folds in the Descemet's membrane and a mild anterior uveitis with lymphocytic keratic precipitates (KPs).
9. *Stromal necrotizing keratitis* (Fig. 4.9) is caused by destruction of corneal stroma and presents a yellowish-white necrotic appearance. It is associated with ciliary injection, corneal vascularization, hypopyon, anterior uveitis and secondary glaucoma.

## Differential Diagnosis

1. Herpes zosters ophthalmicus (HZO) presents dendrites without terminal bulbs and they do not stain with fluorescein.

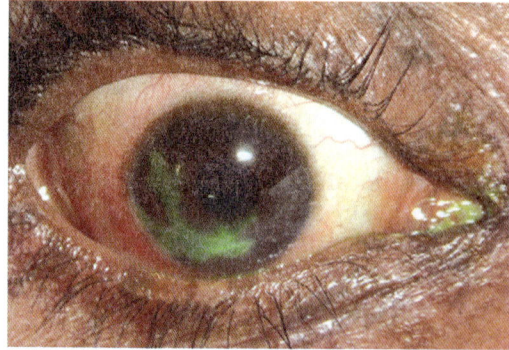

**Fig. 4.7:** Herpetic corneal ulcer (*Courtesy:* Dr SCL Chandravansi, SS Medical College, Rewa)

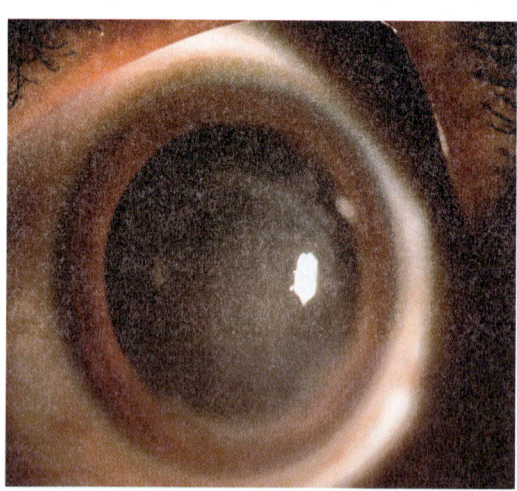

**Fig. 4.8:** Stromal herpetic immune keratitis (*Courtesy:* Dr. Prema Padhamanabhan, Sankara Nethralaya, Chennai)

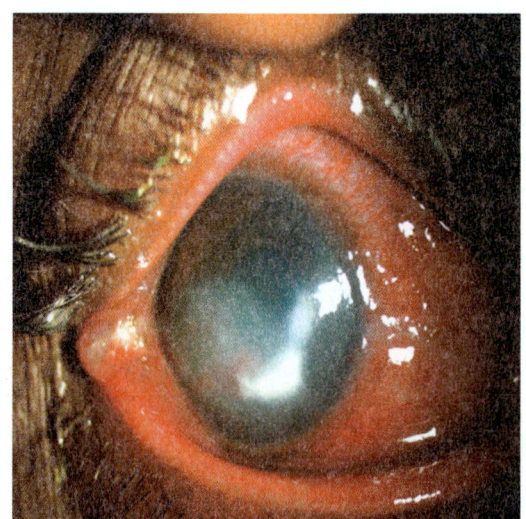

**Fig. 4.9:** Necrotizing HSV keratitis (*Courtesy:* Dr. Prema Padhamanabhan, Sankara Nethralaya, Chennai)

2. Recurrent cornea erosions may also present dendrites during the process of healing. If they are associated with lattice dystrophy, a geographic ulcer may be formed.
3. Acanthamoeba keratitis causes severe pain out of proportion to signs and raised epithelial lesions. The patient may give history of use of CL.

### Diagnosis

1. Corneal scrapings show multinucleated giant cells and intranuclear inclusions.
2. Virus isolation
3. Polymerase chain reaction is a sensitive test for the diagnosis of herpetic infection in tear sample.

### Treatment

1. Ganciclovir gel (0.15%), vidarabine (3% ointment 5 times a day) and trifluoro-thymidine (1% drops 9 times a day) are quite effective for the epithelial lesions.
2. Resistant cases require both topical and oral acyclovir 800 mg 5 times a day for 2 weeks and debridement.

3. Besides the antiviral agents, topical cyclo-plegic drugs are always recommended for the management of HSK.
4. According to Herpetic Eye Disease Study topical corticosteroids prednisolone (1%) used initially 2 hourly and then tapered and oral acyclovir should be given in patients with disciform and necrotizing stromal keratitis.
5. Administration of oral acyclovir may not prevent the recurrence of the disease.
6. Valaciclovir has greater bioavailability than acyclovir and is beneficial in herpetic uveitis.
7. Famciclovir (500 mg, 3 times a day for 7–10 days) is also effective.
8. Oral corticosteroids may be needed to save the eye from necrotizing stromal disease. The dose should be gradually tapered.
9. Tectonic PKP is indicated in impending corneal perforation.
10. Patients with stromal scarring may need PKP for visual improvement.
11. Eyelid lesions are treated by acyclovir ointment or ganciclovir (0.15%) gel, 5 times per day.

### 4.9 HERPES ZOSTER OPHTHALMICUS

#### Etiology

1. HZO is caused by varicella zoster virus.
2. The virus remains dormant in gasserian ganglion.
3. It gets activated at a later age causing HZO involving the supraorbital, supratrochlear and infratrochlear branches and frequently the nasal branch of trigeminal nerve.
4. The occurrence of HZO is frequently found in patients with acquired immune deficiency syndrome, malignancy, debilita-ting disease.

#### Symptoms

1. Severe neuralgic pain on one side of the forehead and scalp associated with fever, nausea, vomiting and malaise.

2. The pain often diminishes after the appearance of vesicles.

3. Other symptoms include watering, photophobia, red eye, ocular discomfort, swelling of lids, inability to open the eye or blepharospasm.

### Signs

1. Multiple vesicular eruptions occur on one side of forehead in the distribution of the supraorbital, supratrochlear, infratrochlear and nasal branches of trigeminal nerve (Fig. 4.10).

2. The eye is usually involved if the vesicles appear on the tip and side of the nose (*Hutchinson's rule*).

3. The corneal lesion may be a small infiltrate to a big vesicle. Later, the vesicle ulcerates.

4. Other corneal lesions are superficial punctate keratitis, microdendrites and nummular keratitis.

5. The dendrites of HZO are small and are without central ulceration and terminal bulbs.

6. HZO can cause disciform keratitis, interstitial keratitis and scleritis.

7. Anterior iridocyclitis, secondary glaucoma, sector iris atrophy, focal choroiditis, occlusive retinal vasculitis, anterior segment ischemia, retinal detachment, optic neuritis, extraocular muscle palsy and Bell's palsy are other manifestations of HZO.

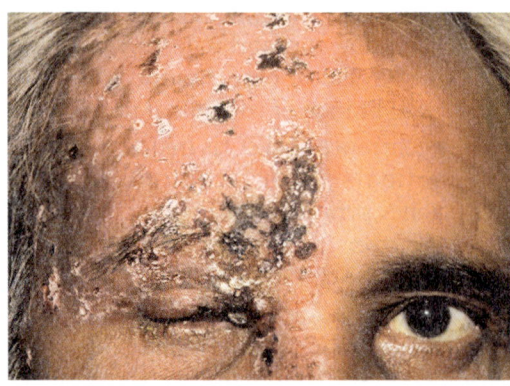

**Fig. 4.10:** Herpes zoster ophthalmicus

8. Postherpetic neuralgia is a painful condition that may persist for many years.

### Diagnosis

1. Characteristic unilateral eruption of vesicles

2. Demonstration of giant cells and inclusion bodies in scrapings

3. Polymerase chain reaction (PCR) test.

### Treatment

1. Early initiation of antiviral therapy decreases the occurrence of postherpetic neuralgia and uveitis.

2. Topical antivirals are not effective.

3. Oral famciclovir (500 mg, 3 times a day), valacyclovir (1 g, 3 times a day) or acyclovir (800 mg, 5 times a day) for 7–10 days should be administered.

4. Immunocompromized patients should be given IV acyclovir.

5. Oral corticosteroids may prevent pain and crust formation in vesicles.

6. Symptoms of SPK and pseudodendrites are relieved with the use of preservative-free artificial tears.

7. Keratitis and keratouveitis are treated with topical cycloplegic and corticosteroids.

8. Neurotrophic keratopathy needs BCL or tarsorrhaphy.

9. Small corneal perforation is sealed with tissue adhesive but large perforations needs therapeutic keratoplasty.

10. Antibiotic-corticosteroid or acyclovir cream should be applied to vesicles on forehead.

11. Capsaicin cream decrease postherpetic neuralgic pain; amitriptyline and pregabalin may be needed for severe pain.

### 4.10 VACCINIA KERATITIS

### Etiology

Vaccinia keratitis may be caused in laboratory workers dealing with poxvirus or in babies by autoinoculation from an arm pustule within 3 weeks of smallpox vaccination.

## Symptoms

1. Lacrimation, itching, redness, photophobia and pain may occur.
2. Patient may suffer from fever and rash.

## Signs

1. Vesicles develop on the lid due to contact with poxvirus. They progress to pustules formation.
2. It may be associated with edema of eyelid and ulcerative conjunctivitis.
3. Corneal lesions include SPK, superficial dendritic or geographical ulceration and corneal edema.
4. Anterior uveitis and secondary glaucoma may develop.

## Diagnosis

1. History of vaccination
2. Virus culture
3. PCR
4. Restriction endonuclease analysis.

## Treatment

1. Ganciclovir (0.15%) gel or vidarabine (3%) ointment 5 times a day are effective.
2. Topical and systemic vaccinia immuno-globulins (6,000 U/kg IV) may help in the resolution of lesion.
3. Topical homatropine or atropine is often used.

## 4.11 ACANTHAMOEBA KERATITIS

### Etiology

1. It is caused by protozoan, *Acanthamoeba*.
2. The protozoan may adhere to the CL or may be found in CL solution, bath-tub and tap water.
3. Use of CL and substandard CL solution for cleaning, swimming in ponds and trauma are risk factors.

## Symptoms

Severe ocular pain (out of proportion to signs), foggy vision and watering.

## Signs

1. Pseudodendrites and dendritiform infiltrates are the early manifestations of Acanthamoeba keratitis.
2. Epithelial erosions may occur.
3. Stray infiltrates appear in the corneal stroma which form a ring ulcer (Fig. 4.11).
4. Radial keratoneuritis causes visibility of the corneal nerves.
5. The ulcer may be associated with anterior uveitis and hypopyon.
6. It may suppurate and form corneal abscess and perforation of the cornea may occur.
7. Nodular or diffuse scleritis may be found.
8. Corneal neovascularization is minimal.

## Diagnosis

1. Corneal scrapings should be examined after staining with calcoflur white.
2. Confocal microscopy for cysts of *Acanthamoeba*.
3. A corneal tissue biopsy can confirm the diagnosis.
4. PCR test.

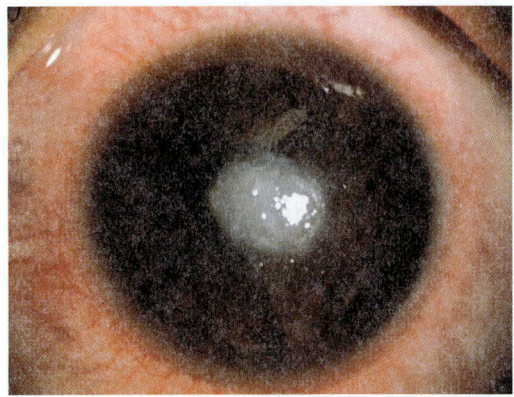

Fig. 4.11: Acanthamoeba keratitis (*Courtesy:* Dr Prema Padhamanabhan, Sankara Nethralaya, Chennai)

4

4

## Treatment

1. Use of daily disposable CL and proper cleaning and disinfection of CLs can prevent the occurrence of *Acanthamoeba keratitis* in CL wearers.
2. Hydrogen peroxide and chlorhexidine solution may be used for cleaning.
3. *Acanthamoeba keratitis* has no satisfactory treatment.
4. Propamidine isethionate (0.1%, 1–2 hourly intervals), polyhexamethylene biguanide (PHMB), 0.02% or chlorhexidine (0.02%) eye drop hourly for 1 week, then taper over 2–3 months and dibromopropamidine (0.15%) ointment at night time have been tried.
5. Topical miconazole (1%) and clotrimazole (1%) may be effective.
6. Ketaconazole (200–400 mg, once or twice a day) or itraconazole (a loading dose of 300–450 mg followed by 150 mg a day) is also effective.
7. Topical cycloplegic is used 2–3 times a day.
8. The disease is chronic and requires a prolonged treatment.
9. Some patients may need PKP for improving vision.

## 4.12 SYPHILITIC INTERSTITIAL KERATITIS

### Etiology

1. Syphilitic interstitial keratitis (IK) is an inflammation of the stroma of the cornea. It is secondary to primary anterior uveitis; which may be triggered by a trivial trauma.
2. It is seen in children with congenital syphilis.
3. *Treponema pallidum* infection can occur through transplacental route.
4. IK affects children in 5–15 years of age group and it is usually bilateral.

### Symptoms

Watering, photophobia, decreased vision, pain and blepharospasm are symptoms of the acute stage of IK. However, poor vision is the only symptom of the chronic stage.

### Signs

1. Acute stage of IK
   - Cloudiness of the cornea due to edema of deeper layers is the main sign.
   - A dense bilateral infiltration of inflammatory cells in the stroma causes folds in the Descemet's membrane.
   - Presence of anterior uveitis may be masked by corneal clouding.
   - Over a period of time, the corneal lamellae undergo necrosis.
   - Blood vessels from the limbus grow in a brush-like manner in a sector of the cornea.
   - The vascularized area looks dull pinkish-red or like "salmon patch" due to overlying corneal edema.
   - Besides ciliary injection, conjunctival vessels are congested and there may be heaping of conjunctiva at the limbus.
2. Chronic stage of IK
   - Healing starts by proliferation of corneal fibroblasts.
   - Gradually the necrotized stromal area is converted into a vascularized scar.
   - The disease shows regression; the corneal edema disappears and the corneal vessels start obliterating.
   - However, ghost vessels remain throughout the life as fine lines.
   - Chorioretinal scars and salt-and-pepper fundus in children are seen on funduscopy.
   - Frontal prominence, depressed bridge of nose, deafness, mental retardation and Hutchinson's teeth may be present as stigmata of the congenital syphilis.

### Differential Diagnosis

IK can also occur in acquired syphilis, tuberculosis, sarcoidosis HZO, leprosy, trachoma, Lyme disease, mumps, brucellosis, trypanosomiasis, onchocerciasis and malaria.

## Diagnosis

1. Rapid reagent test and Venereal Disease Research Laboratory (VDRL) test.
2. Fluorescent treponemal antibody absorption (FTA-ABS) test
3. Microhemagglutination-treponema pallidum (MHA-TP) test.

## Treatment

1. Topical prednisolone (1% eye drops 2 hourly) and cycloplegics (atropine 1%, 2–3 times per day) are used to treat anterior uveitis.
2. Nonresponding cases are treated with subconjunctival or sub-tenon injections of corticosteroids.
3. Systemic corticosteroids should always be combined with antisyphilitic therapy like benzathine penicillin (50,000 U/kg IM once) and procaine penicillin (10,000 U/kg IM daily for 10 days).
4. Children with penicillin allergy should be treated with erythromycin and children more than 8 years of age with doxycycline.
5. The treatment should not be terminated abruptly, otherwise recurrence may occur.
6. PKP can restore vision in patients with dense corneal opacities.

## 4.13 NEUROTROPHIC KERATOPATHY

### Etiology

1. Neurotrophic keratopathy is caused by damage to the trigeminal nerve.
2. The sensory nerve damage causes hydration and exfoliation of the corneal epithelial cells.
3. The nerve can be damaged in the following conditions:
   - Infection from HSV and varicella zoster virus.
   - Surgical ablation of trigeminal ganglia for trigeminal neuralgia, stroke, aneurysm,

acoustic neuroma, multiple sclerosis (MS) and leprosy.
   - Refractive surgery, chemical burns, abuse of local anesthesia and, rarely, Riley-Day syndrome.

## Symptoms

The patient may remain symptom-free or complain of red eye, foreign body sensation initially, and later decreased vision.

## Signs

1. There is a complete loss of corneal sensation with ciliary injection.
2. The corneal epithelium appears slightly opaque and edematous.
3. Persistent epithelial defect develops showing fluorescein stain.
4. The ulcer looks gray with heaped-up epithelial borders.
5. The enlargement of epithelial defect is accompanied by stromal edema, cellular infiltration and vascularization.
6. The ulcer may perforate following secondary infection.

## Diagnosis

1. History of present or past infection or surgical intervention on the cornea
2. Loss of corneal sensation
3. Computed tomography (CT) scan or magnetic resonance imaging (MRI) can confirm the central nervous system (CNS) lesions.

## Treatment

1. Frequent instillations of preservative-free artificial tears or autologous serum.
2. Topical antibiotic drops/ointment and atropine ointment
3. Mild cases get relief by botulinum toxin injection; as it induces ptosis and protects the eye.
4. Protection of the eye either by patching or bandage CL.

5. Tarsorrhaphy.

6. Some cases may need amniotic membrane graft.

## 4.14 EXPOSURE KERATOPATHY

### Etiology

1. Exposure keratitis is caused by incomplete closure of the palpebral aperture.

2. Causes of exposure keratopathy include Bell's palsy, marked proptosis, ectropion, eyelid scarring, burns, cicatricial pemphigoid, facial eczema, overcorrection of ptosis, coma, Parkinsonism and floppy eyelid syndrome.

### Symptoms

The patient may present with foreign body sensation, irritation, redness, lacrimation, dry eye and reduced vision.

### Signs

1. There is incomplete closure of the eyelids and frequency of blinking is reduced.

2. Initially, punctate epithelial changes are seen in the lower half of cornea.

3. Soon epithelial breakdown occurs (Fig. 4.12).

4. Other changes include SPK, corneal erosion, nocturnal lagophthalmos, lid deformities and poor Bell's phenomenon.

5. Later, opaque, dry and ulcerated horizontal bands may be seen in the lower one-third of the cornea.

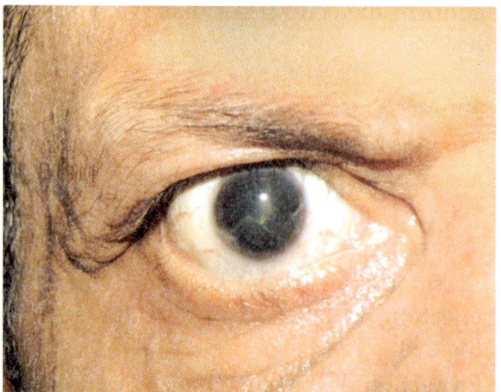

**Fig. 4.12:** Exposure keratopathy

6. Secondary infection may supervene and cause melting and perforation of cornea.

### Diagnosis

1. History of seventh nerve palsy or ptosis surgery

2. Evaluation of Bell's phenomenon and extent of corneal exposure after eyelid closure.

3. Assess corneal sensation

4. Investigate for dry eye disease

5. Examine for systemic disorders like Parkinsonism, thyroid or CNS disease.

### Treatment

1. Frequent use of preservative-free tear substitutes in daytime and eye ointment at night may relieve symptoms.

2. If corneal ulcer develops, it should be treated with antibiotic ointment and cycloplegic drops and the eye is protected by a patch or BCL.

3. Partial tarsorrhaphy is often needed in majority of cases.

4. Lid deformity must be corrected early.

## 4.15 ROSACEA KERATITIS

### Etiology

1. The etiology of rosacea is unknown.

2. It is an idiopathic chronic dermatosis that affects the exposed skin.

3. Environmental changes, beverages and certain food may precipitate the disease.

### Symptoms

The patient complains of irritation, foreign body sensation, burning and mild redness of the eyes.

### Signs

1. A chronic recalcitrant keratitis is not uncommon.

2. Rosacea keratitis is usually associated with acne of face, blepharitis, telangiectasia

of lid margins, recurrent chalazia and phlyctenulosis.

3. The conjunctival vessels are dilated.
4. The cornea is vascularized in the periphery.
5. The ulcers leave irregular corneal facets.
6. Map-dot subepithelial opacities, corneal erosion, vascularization and thinning may be found.
7. Iritis and perforation of cornea may occur.
8. Typical skin lesions is butterfly-like erythema of cheeks.
9. Besides skin lesions, rhinophyma develops late in the disease.

## Diagnosis

Presence of telangiectasia on lid margin, meibomitis and corneal lesions associated with butterfly-like erythema of cheeks facilitates clinical diagnosis.

## Treatment

1. The treatment is unsatisfactory.
2. The keratitis should be treated.
3. Prolonged use of systemic tetracyline or doxycycline gives beneficial results. Oral tetracycline 1 g is administered for 1 month followed by 250 mg daily for 6 months.
4. Topical cycloplegic and antibiotics are needed for the ulcerative lesion of the cornea.
5. Chronic ocular rosacea can be managed by cyclosporine (0.05%) drops.

## 4.16 BAND-SHAPED KERATOPATHY

### Etiology

1. Band-shaped keratopathy may be found in chronic anterior uveitis in children, juvenile idiopathic arthritis, Paget disease, gout, repeated trauma, postretinal detachment surgery and vitamin D intoxication.
2. Advanced age, hereditary and metabolic disorders are risk factors.

### Symptoms

Irritation, watering, foreign body sensation, disfigurement of eye (white band of opacities) and decreased vision.

### Signs

1. Band-shaped keratopathy starts in the peripheral cornea in the interpalpebral area.
2. A clear corneal zone remains between the band and the limbus (lucid interval).
3. Gradually, it involves the central cornea and calcium salts are deposited in the Bowman's membrane and anterior stroma of the cornea.
4. The band or calcareous plaque is not uniformly opaque but shows small holes and crypts (Fig. 4.13).
5. Later, the lesion becomes nodular and raised and overlying epithelium ulcerates causing pain and discomfort.
6. Additionally, signs of accompanying disease may be found.

### Diagnosis

1. Characteristic clinical picture
2. Biopsy reveals calcium salts deposit.

### Treatment

1. Mild cases of band keratopathy can be managed by preservative-free artificial tears 6 times a day and a bland ointment in the night.

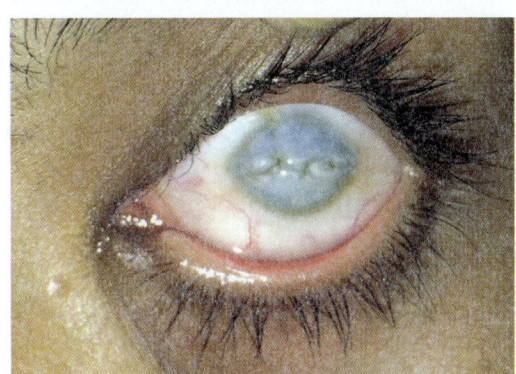

Fig. 4.13: Band-shaped keratopathy

2. Use of BCL may relieve symptoms.
3. The choice of treatment of band-shaped keratopathy is chelation:
   - Scrape the corneal epithelium containing calcium
   - Apply 0.01 M solution of ethylene diamine tetra-acetic acid (EDTA) with cotton-tipped bud and gently rub it to remove calcium.
   - Irrigate the eye with normal saline and apply antibiotic ointment and cycloplegic drop and patch the eye.
4. Excimer laser keratectomy (phototherapeutic keratectomy) can be helpful in improving the vision.
5. Recurrence may occur following surgical removal.

## 4.17 MOOREN CORNEAL ULCER

### Etiology

1. The etiology of Mooren ulcer is not known. It is presumed to be an idiopathic disease.
2. It is considered type III hypersensitivity reaction because it has some similarities to peripheral ulcerative keratitis.
3. The ulcer affects males more than females and manifests bilaterally in approximately one-third of cases.
4. Trauma, surgery, herpes and other causes of marginal corneal ulcer and worm infestation are considered as risk factors.

### Symptoms

1. Severe pain, watering, photophobia and blurred vision.
2. The pain is always out of proportion to the presenting signs.

### Signs

1. A crescent-shaped indolent ulcer develops at the periphery of the cornea and progresses.

2. The growing edge of Mooren's ulcer lies in corneal stroma and is marked by cellular infiltration and vascularization. The ulcer has overhanging edge.
3. It advances in the direction of its infiltrated edge which may take fluorescein stain due to epithelial defect.
4. A low-grade iritis is seen.
5. The ulcer progresses slowly with ultimate loss of entire corneal stroma leaving behind thinned vascular cornea.
6. Trivial trauma and secondary bacterial infection can cause perforation.
7. Vision may be lost due to vascularization and scarring of the cornea.

### Diagnosis

1. Typical clinical picture with indolent course
2. Exclude other causes of peripheral ulcerative keratitis
3. Estimation of serum immune complexes.

### Treatment

1. Mooren ulcer has no effective treatment.
2. Topical cycloplegic, antibiotic, steroids, acetylcysteine and cyclosporine are used without much success.
3. Excision of the conjunctiva adjacent to the growing edge of the ulcer with application of cyanoacrylate glue and soft CL and administration of topical steroids and systemic immunosuppressants showed encouraging results.
4. Systemic tetracycline should be given to check the collagenolytic activity.
5. Bilateral progressive Mooren ulcer needs treatment with systemic immunosuppressants like methotrexate, cyclophosphamide, azathioprine (1–1.5 mg/kg body weight/day for 4–6 weeks) or cyclosporine.
6. Lamellar keratoplasty or PKP often fails, but in the event of perforation, tectonic graft should be given.

## 4.18 APHAKIC/PSEUDOPHAKIC BULLOUS KERATOPATHY

### Etiology

Aphakic/pseudophakic bullous keratopathy is caused by intraocular surgery in patients with corneal endothelial dysfunction (Fuchs corneal dystrophy, complicated cataract and compromised cornea).

### Symptoms

Foreign body sensation, pain, watering, decreased vision, photophobia and red eye are common complaints.

### Signs

1. Initially, mild to moderate corneal edema develops following cataract surgery (Fig. 4.14).
2. The corneal haze increases and bullae appear in the epithelium associated with folds in the Descemet membrane.
3. The rupture of bullae results in severe ocular pain.
4. Over a period of time, subepithelial fibrosis may develop which prevents bullae formation. It reduces the ocular pain but decreases the vision markedly.

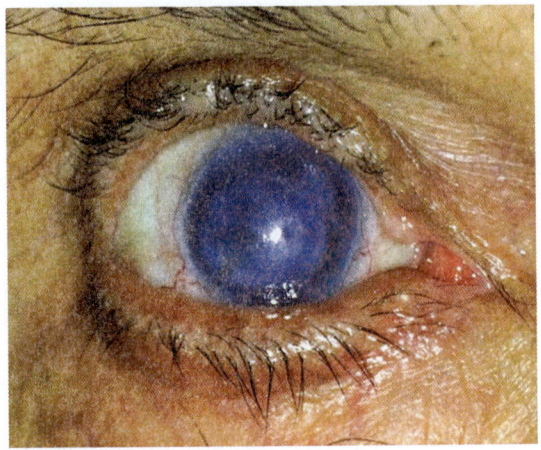

**Fig. 4.14:** Aphakic bullous keratopathy

5. Neovascularization of cornea, increased IOP, vitreous in the anterior chamber and cystoid macular degeneration (CME) may be found.

### Diagnosis

1. History of intraocular surgery
2. Slit-lamp examination can demonstrate epithelial defects, epithelial bullae, endothelial dystrophy, anterior chamber reaction and intraocular lens (IOL) or vitreous touch to the cornea.
3. Dilated fundus examination may show the presence of CME.
4. Fundus fluorescein angiography (FFA) and optical coherence tomography (OCT) can confirm CME.

### Treatment

1. Early corneal edema can be managed by instillations of topical NaCl (5% solution, 5 times a day), corticosteroids (prednisolone 1%, 3–4 times) and use of BCL.
2. Raised IOP is managed by oral acetazolamide (500 mg twice a day).
3. If repositioning of IOL or IOL exchange and vitrectomy are needed, they should be performed early.
4. Pain associated with bullae can be alleviated with anterior stromal puncture or phototherapeutic keratectomy.
5. A conjunctival or an amniotic membrane graft may be considered for painful eye with very poor vision.
6. Endothelial keratoplasty, Descemet's stripping endothelial keratoplasty (DESK) and PKP are other options.

## 4.19 EPITHELIAL CORNEAL DYSTROPHIES

Corneal dystrophies are inherited, bilateral, symmetrical and slowly progressive disorders. They are classified as:
1. Epithelial
2. Stromal
3. Posterior or endothelial.

4

## Corneal Epithelial Basement Membrane Dystrophy

1. In corneal epithelial basement membrane dystrophy (Cogan's microcystic dystrophy), the defect lies in the basement membrane of the epithelium.
2. Initially symptom-free but after the age of 30 years, the patient feels pain in opening the eyes, diplopia (monocular) and impairment of vision due to development of corneal erosions.
3. The dystrophy presents bilateral, cystic, round dot-like or fine refractile linear fingerprint-like lesions.
4. The pattern of lesions often varies with time.
5. Slit-lamp (retroillumination) examination is diagnostic.

## Meesmann's Juvenile Epithelial Dystrophy

1. It is an autosomal dominant epithelial dystrophy.
2. Irritation, photophobia and visual disturbances are common symptoms.
3. Small bubble-like vesicles in the epithelium are seen.
4. They represent degenerated epithelial cells.
5. Epithelial lesions look like whorls.
6. Corneal sensation is reduced.
7. Retroillumination examination is diagnostic.
8. BCL or superficial keratectomy can relieve the symptoms.

## Reis-Buckler Dystrophy

1. Reis-Buckler corneal dystrophy manifests at the age of 5 years. It is an autosomal dominant dystrophy.
2. Recurrent, pain, photophobia, lacrimation and impairment of vision are common complaints.
3. Superficial gray-white reticular corneal opacities are characteristic.
4. Histopathology shows absence of Bowman membrane with scarring.

5. Superficial lamellar keratectomy or excimer laser keratectomy is an effective treatment.

## 4.20 STROMAL CORNEAL DYSTROPHIES

Four main types of stromal corneal dystrophies are described.

## Granular Corneal Dystrophy

1. Granular (*Groenouw's type I*) is the most common stromal dystrophy. It shows a dominant trait and seen in the first decade of life.
2. It is asymptomatic condition in childhood but induces glare and diminution of vision in later life.
3. Breadcrumb-like white, granular opacities are seen in the axial region.
4. The peripheral cornea remains clear.
5. The opacities coalesce and impair the vision in the fourth decade.
6. The granular material represents hyaline degeneration.
7. Slit-lamp examination is helpful in the diagnosis.
8. CLs may improve the vision.
9. Phototherapeutic keratectomy is performed to restore the vision.
10. Recurrence of the dystrophy may occur.

## Macular Corneal Dystrophy

1. Macular (*Groenouw's type II*) dystrophy involves central and peripheral areas of the cornea. It is an autosomal recessive condition.
2. Decreased vision, irritation and watering are common symptoms.
3. Multiple grayish opacities develop in the axial region and impair the vision in the first decade.
4. Gradually, opacities increase in number and size and involve the corneal periphery.
5. Corneal sensation is impaired.

6. The macular corneal opacities contain glycosaminoglycan (GAG).

7. Keratoplasty improves the vision, however, the dystrophy may recur.

## Lattice Corneal Dystrophy

1. Lattice dystrophy appears during the second decade of life. It shows autosomal dominant pattern of inheritance.

2. It manifests in four clinical types. Type 1 Bilber-Haab-Dimmer is most common.

3. Irritation, watering, photophobia and decreased vision occur due to recurrent corneal erosions.

4. The corneal sensation is impaired.

5. The presence of irregularly branching and interlacing filaments is the hallmark of lattice dystrophy of the cornea.

6. Filaments form a lattice net.

7. Numerous dots and stellate opacities are scattered in the net.

8. Lattice dystrophy type 2 is known as Meretoja syndrome.

9. It is characterized by lattice dystrophy, mask face, ear deformities, cranial nerve palsies, loose skin folds and systemic amyloidosis.

10. Lattice dystrophy types 3 and 4 are uncommon and found in advanced age.

11. Slit-lamp retroillumination examination helps in the diagnosis.

12. Amyloid deposit in the stroma may be found on histopathology.

13. PKP can restore the vision.

## Schnyder Crystalline Dystrophy

1. Schnyder crystalline dystrophy is inherited as an autosomal dominant trait.

2. It is presumed to be caused by an error of lipid metabolism.

3. It occurs in childhood but does not impair vision.

4. The presence of golden yellow linear crystals in the central stroma is the hallmark of the dystrophy. The deposition of crystals occurs due to accumulation of abnormal cholesterol and lipid.

5. Later, full-thickness corneal haze and arcus may be found.

6. The dystrophy may be associated with hypercholesterolemia and genu valgum.

7. Slit-lamp examination and serum cholesterol and triglyceride levels help in diagnosis.

8. If vision is deteriorated, laser keratectomy or PKP can restore the vision.

## 4.21 ENDOTHELIAL CORNEAL DYSTROPHIES   4

### Fuchs Endothelial Corneal Dystrophy

1. Fuchs endothelial dystrophy (FED) has an autosomal dominant trait. It manifests after the age of 50 years and is more common in females.

2. The patient may remain asymptomatic but later suffers from glare, blurring of vision and pain due to decompensated cornea.

3. Bilateral asymmetrical corneal guttata first affects the central cornea, then involves the periphery and presents a "beaten silver" appearance.

4. It causes stromal edema.

5. Bullae develop in the central epithelium and rupture of bullae causes severe pain.

6. Later, subepithelial haze and scarring may be seen.

7. Folds in the Descemet's membrane and pigment dusting on the endothelium are often present.

8. IOP may or may not be raised.

### Diagnosis

1. Specular microscopy shows a drop of endothelial cells below $1000/mm^2$.

2. Confocal microscopy can diagnose corneal guttata also.

3. Corneal guttata is best seen with slit-lamp retroillumination.

4. Use of sodium chloride drops (5%) and ointment (6%) and oral carbonic anhydrase inhibitor may reduce the edema.

5. Lubricating drops and soft CLs relieve pain caused by rupture of bullae.

6. DSEK or in the presence of stromal scarring, PKP restores the vision.

### Congenital Hereditary Endothelial Dystrophy

1. Congenital hereditary endothelial dystrophy (CHED) shows both dominant and recessive traits of inheritance. It is linked to chromosome 20.

2. Autosomal recessive CHED is a nonprogressive disease and presents at birth with nystagmus.

3. Autosomal dominant CHED is slowly progressive and shows no nystagmus.

4. Visual symptoms vary depending on the clouding of cornea.

5. Bilateral diffuse milky or ground glass appearance of the stroma associated with marked thickening of the cornea is a classical feature of the dystrophy.

6. Congenital glaucoma should be ruled out.

7. Despite gross edema of the cornea, the epithelial changes are minimal.

8. Histology reveals absence of endothelium with thickening of the Descemet's membrane.

### Treatment

1. PKP may improve the vision.

2. Keratoprosthesis may be tried in failed cases of keratoplasty.

### Posterior Polymorphous Dystrophy

1. Posterior polymorphous dystrophy (PPD) is rare.

2. The posterior surface of cornea shows gray haze, vesicles and bands.

3. Iris abnormalities or iridocorneal adhesions may be seen.

4. IOP may be raised.

5. The histopathology demonstrates multi-layered endothelial cells that act like fibroblasts.

6. Stromal micropunctures or PKP can improve the condition.

## 4.22 KERATOCONUS

### Etiology

1. Keratoconus is an ectatic corneal dystrophy of unknown etiology.

2. It is a familial disorder and has female predominance.

3. A locus for keratoconus is found on chromosome 21.

### Symptoms

1. Progressive decrease in visual acuity, lacrimation, red eye and photophobia are common.

2. Sudden loss of vision, profuse watering and pain can develop due to acute corneal hydrops.

### Signs

1. Keratoconus presents an early sign of scissor red reflex on retinoscopy.

2. Irregular astigmatism and corneal scarring cause poor vision.

3. A conical bulging and thinning of the cornea is seen at the apex of the cone that is situated slightly below the center of the cornea. A conical reflection of light is seen at nasal limbus when the light is thrown from temporal side (*Rizzutti's sign*).

4. On looking down, an indentation in the lower lid by the cone may be seen, known as *Munson's sign*.

5. Corneal opacities and increased visibility of the corneal nerves are seen at the apex of cone (Fig. 4.15).

6. At the base of the cone, a brown ring of pigmentation may be seen; it is called Fleischer ring.

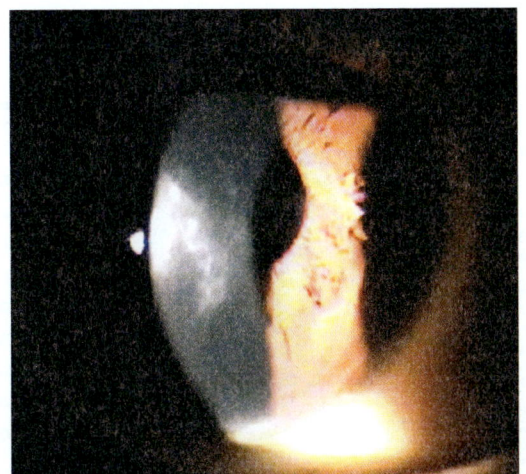

**Fig. 4.15:** Keratoconus with apical scar (*Courtesy:* Dr Prema Padhamanabhan, Sankara Nethralaya, Chennai)

7. Vertical tension lines (*Vogt strae*) are noticed in the posterior corneal stroma.
8. Subclinical keratoconus, *keratoconus forme fruste,* presents difficulty in diagnosis.
9. Keratoconus may be found in association with other eye diseases such as blue sclera, ectopia lentis, vernal conjunctivitis and retinitis pigmentosa.
10. Keratoconus may be one of the features of Down's syndrome, Marfan's syndrome, and von Recklinghausen's disease.

### Differential Diagnosis

Keratoglobus: It is a congenital, bilaterally symmetrical nonprogressive condition. It shows uniform thinning of the cornea maximal in the midperiphery. A central stromal haze (fragmentation of Bowman's membrane) may be present, but apical scar, stress lines and Fleischer's ring are absent. Blue sclera and hyperextensibility of hand and ankle joint may be associated with keratoglobus.

### Diagnosis

1. Slit-lamp examination helps in the diagnosis.
2. The alteration in the curvature of the cornea produces a distortion of the corneal reflex as seen with the Placido's disk.

3. Corneal topography can establish the diagnosis (Fig. 4.16).
4. Subclinical keratoconus (*keratoconus forme fruste*) presents mild inferior steepening and can be detected by performing corneal topography in up gaze.

### Treatment

1. The refractive error should be corrected with glasses or rigid CL.
2. Hydrops should be treated with instillation of hyperosmotic agents and cycloplegics.
3. The use of intracorneal rings (intacs) may be effective in cases of keratoconus.
4. Corneal collagen cross-linkage with riboflavin can arrest progression of keratoconus.
5. PKP improves vision in cases of scarred cornea.

### 4.23 PELLUCID MARGINAL DEGENERATION

### Etiology

1. Etiology of pellucid marginal degeneration is not known. It is a bilateral condition characterized by the thinning of the cornea in the lower and peripheral part in young patients.
2. Connective tissue diseases like rheumatoid arthritis, systemic lupus erythematosus (SLE), Wegener's granulomatosis, polyarteritis nodosa, etc may be associated with the condition.
3. Majority of cases of pellucid marginal degeneration are idiopathic.

### Symptoms

Many patients remain asymptomatic but some may complain of decreased vision, red eye, pain and photophobia.

### Signs

1. Significant thinning occurs in the inferior cornea between 4 o'clock and 8 o'clock positions.
2. A mild buldging of cornea develops just above the thinning resulting in high astigmatism.

4

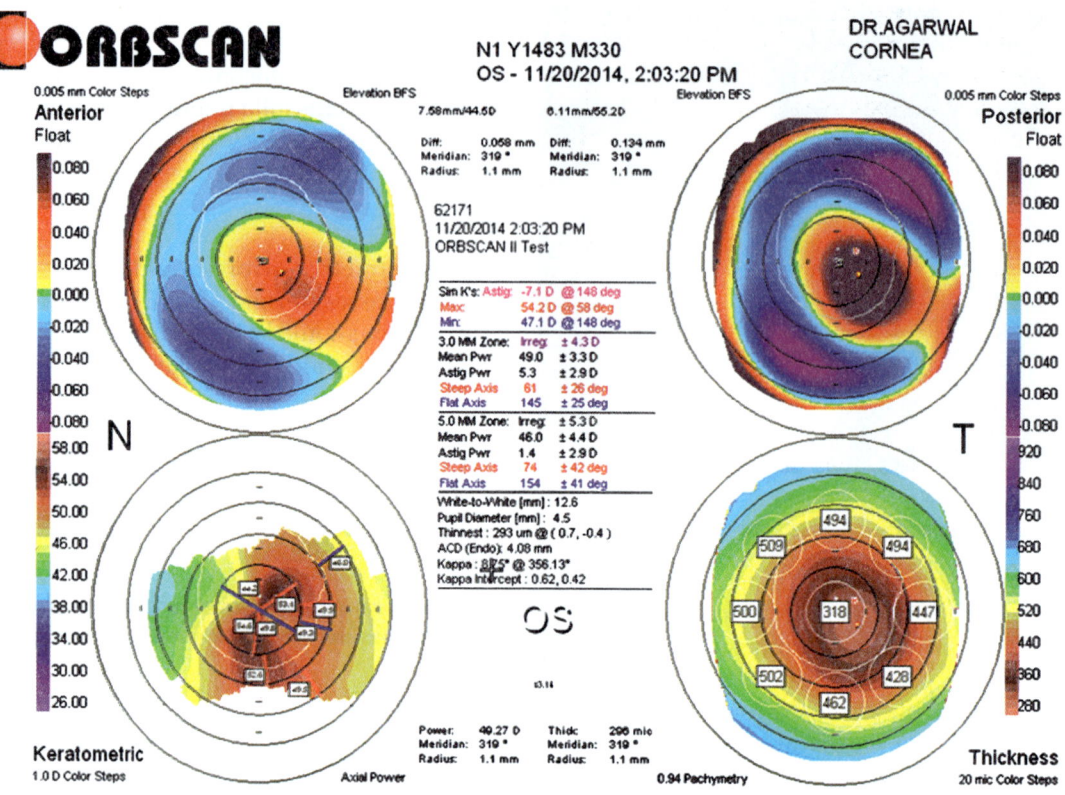

**Fig. 4.16:** Keratoconus: Corneal topography (*Courtesy*: Dr Soosan, Dr Agrawal Eye Hospital, Chennai)

3. Cornea is free of vascularization but the stroma shows scarring.
4. An acute hydrops may develop in some patients.

### Differential Diagnosis

1. VKC
2. Sclerokeratitis
3. Exposure keratopathy
4. Terrien marginal degeneration: A slowly progressive thinning often found in the upper peripheral part of cornea. It may be associated with fine vascularization and yellow lipid infiltration. The degeneration can spread circumferentially and cause irregular astigmatism.
5. Dellen: It is an ellipsoidal corneal thinning seen at the limbus associated with elevation of adjacent conjunctiva and cornea. The causes of dellen include dry eye disease, pterygium, tumor, filtering bleb and postsquint surgery. Use of artificial tears and occasionally patching (if fluorescein staining is positive) are beneficial.
6. Peripheral ulcerative keratitis: It manifests as infectious infiltrates or ulcer and needs culture and serological tests.
7. Mooren ulcer.

### Diagnosis

1. Slit-lamp examination
2. Corneal topography.

### Treatment

1. Correction for astigmatism by glasses or CLs.
2. Lamellar tectonic graft is indicated in some patients.

## 4.24 ADVERSE EFFECTS OF CONTACT LENS

Most of the CL-related problems originate due to infection, toxic reaction, tight lens fitting, overuse of lenses and hypersensitivity reaction.

### Symptoms

The patient may complain of foreign body sensation, itching, watering/discharge, photophobia, pain, decreased vision, CL intolerance, etc.

### Signs

Generally, signs may vary *as per* the cause.

1. Infection
   - Inadequate cleaning, use of old cleaning solution, CL deposits and use of very old contact lenses are risk factors for the infection.
   - Patients with CL may develop bacterial, fungal or *Acanthamoeba* infection.
   - The infection usually starts as corneal infiltrate or superficial ulcer (Fig. 4.17) and later may progress to infectious corneal ulcer.

2. Toxic reaction
   - The preservative solution containing thimerosal or chlorhexidine induces toxicity or hypersensitivity if contact lenses are not thoroughly rinsed before use.
   - Irritation and watering may develop soon after the insertion of the lens.
   - SPK, pseudo-superior limbic kerato-conjunctivitis and corneal infiltrates associated with follicular conjunctivitis and conjunctival injection may be seen.

3. Tight lens syndrome
   - The tight lens syndrome is due to compression of the limbus by the CL that causes early symptoms.
   - Use of dried lens (after dehydration) and overuse of soft lens (lenses are not removed before sleep) can induce SPK, acute corneal hydrops (Fig. 4.18) and anterior chamber reaction.

4. Corneal warpage
   - The long-term use of hard CLs blurs the vision with spectacles but the vision remains good with CL.
   - The blurred vision is due to induction of irregular astigmatism.
   - The discontinuation of CL use resolves the problem.

5. Giant papillary conjunctivitis

6. Displacement of contact lens
   Displacement of lens is not uncommon; it may be displaced in the superior fornix. More frequently, it may fall out of the eye.

7. Other adverse effects
   Other adverse effects of wearing CLs include hyperemia of conjunctiva,

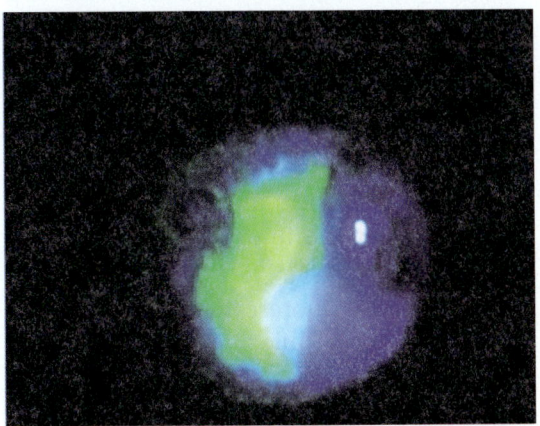

Fig. 4.17: Corneal abrasion caused by contact lens

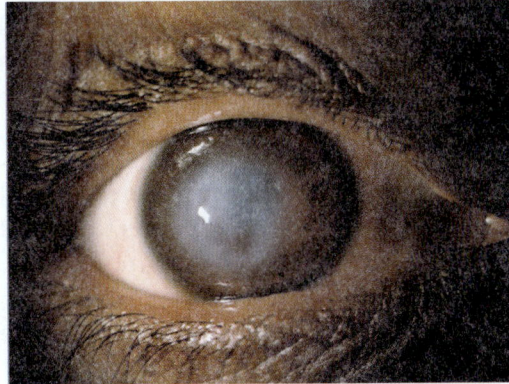

Fig. 4.18: Acute hydrops (*Courtesy:* Dr. Prema Padhamanabhan, Sankara Nethralaya, Chennai)

intolerance, allergic reaction with profuse watering, dry eye, corneal abrasion, superficial corneal vascularization, epithelial irregularity and corneal scarring.

## Diagnosis

1. History: A detailed history must be obtained about the type of lenses, wear time, method of cleaning of lenses and when the present lenses were taken.
2. Evaluate the fitting of the lens and examine the eye on slit-lamp after lens removal and staining with fluorescein.
3. Examine the CL surface for deposits and defects.
4. Smear and culture should be taken from the eye, CL, solutions and lens case in patients with infection.

## Treatment

1. If patient with CL complains of redness and pain, the lens must be removed and eye and CL should thoroughly be examined.
2. Use of CL with deposits should be discontinued and the lens is subjected to proper cleaning or enzyme treatment.
3. Old and damaged CLs need replacement.
4. Discontinue wear of the ill-fitting lenses causing tight lens symptoms. Refit an oxygen permeable lens on resolution of symptoms or prefer daily disposable lens.
5. Frequent use of preservative-free artificial tears has a beneficial effect in patients with dry eye disease.
6. CL associated SPK, corneal infiltrates, SLK, corneal vascularization and hypersensitivity reaction usually respond to topical antibiotic-steroid drops (3 times/day) and mild cycloplegic (once a day).
7. In corneal warpage, discontinue wear of CL for 3–6 weeks and then a gas-permeable lens is fitted.
8. Patients with corneal ulcer and anterior chamber reaction must be treated aggres-sively on the lines of infective keratitis after suspending the wear of CL.

## 4.25 EPISCLERITIS

Episcleritis is an inflammation of episclera present between sclera and Tenon's capsule.

### Etiology

1. *Idiopathic:* No cause of the disease is discernible in large number of patients.
2. *Infective:* Bacterial, fungal and viral (herpes) infection may cause episcleritis.
3. *Hypersensitivity*
4. *Systemic disorders:* Rarely it may be associated with connective tissue disease

### Symptoms

- Redness of eye
- Ocular discomfort
- Pain may or may not be present

### Types

1. Diffuse
2. Nodular

### Signs

- Diffuse episcleritis: It presents as diffuse redness in one or both eyes.
- The episcleral blood vessels running radially are engorged.
- Nodular episcleritis: It is characterized by the presence of a dull pink nodule often situated a few mm away from the limbus (Fig. 4.19).
- The nodule is firm and tender. It can be moved over the underlying sclera after topical anesthesia.
- Occasionally, fluorescein staining may be seen over the nodule.
- Rarely, cornea may be affected and vision gets compromised.
- Recurrences of episcleritis are common.

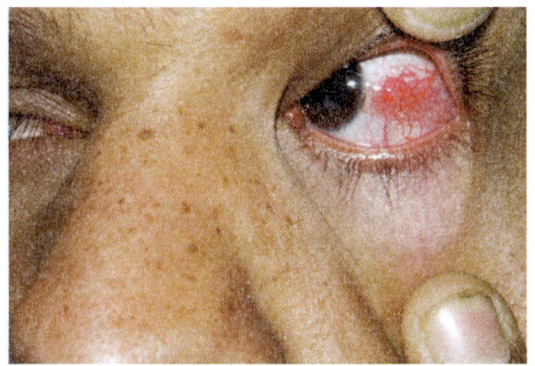

**Fig. 4.19:** Nodular episcleritis

## Differential Diagnosis

1. Conjunctivitis
2. FB granuloma in the bulbar conjunctiva
3. Scleritis

## Diagnosis

1. Diagnosis of episcleritis is usually clinical
2. Slit-lamp examination excludes FB and corneal involvement.
3. Topical phenylephrine (2.5%) blanches the episcleral vessels.

## Treatment

1. Episcleritis may resolve spontaneously.
2. Mild topical corticosteroids like loteprednol (0.5%) or fluorometholone (0.1%) 3–4 times a day provide quick relief.
3. Administration of oral NSAIDs is also effective.
4. Co-existing disease should be treated.

## 4.26 SCLERITIS

Inflammation of sclera proper is known as *scleritis*. Scleritis is far less common than episcleritis. It usually affects adults and elderly persons. The disease is more common in females than males.

## Etiology

1. *Idiopathic:* Etiology of scleritis remains unknown.

2. *Systemic autoimmune collagen and rheumatic diseases:* These diseases contribute to 50% cases of scleritis.
3. *Infections:* Endogenous spread of bacterial, fungal, viral infections (herpes) or parasites may cause scleritis.
4. *Metabolic and endocrine disorders:* Less frequently, scleritis may be found in patients with gout or thyroid disorder.
5. *Postsurgical:* Surgery-induced scleritis is a rare and dreaded complication of pterygium (Fig. 4.20) and retinal reattachment surgeries.

## Classification

Broadly scleritis is classified into two groups—anterior and posterior. The anterior scleritis is subdivided into following four subgroups:

1. Non-necrotizing anterior diffuse scleritis
2. Non-necrotizing anterior nodular scleritis
3. Necrotizing anterior scleritis with inflammation
4. Necrotizing anterior scleritis with minimum or no inflammation

## Symptoms

- Ocular pain is an important symptom. At times, it is so severe that patient wakes up from sleep in the night. Pain often radiates to the forehead.
- Eye is red.

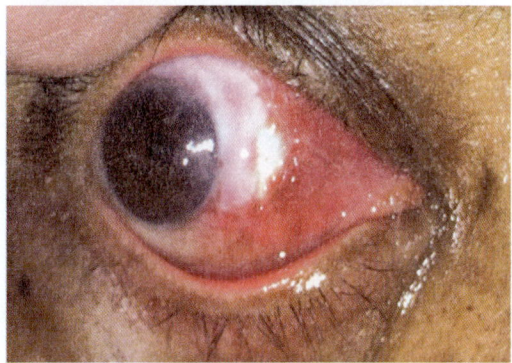

**Fig. 4.20:** Scleral melting following pterygium surgery

- Photophobia and lacrimation are not uncommon.
- Vision may be affected

## Signs

Signs of scleritis usually differ in different types of scleritis

### 1. Non-necrotizing Anterior Diffuse Scleritis

It is characterized by a diffuse injection of deeper episcleral blood vessels either localized in a sector (Fig. 4.21) or in the entire anterior sclera. The eye is tender and looks dull pink or bluish. Both sclera and episclera appear edematous. Corneal involvement is rare.

### 2. Non-necrotizing Anterior Nodular Scleritis

The characteristic feature of non-necrotizing nodular scleritis is the presence of one or two nodules near the limbus (Fig. 4.22). The nodule is raised, 2–4 mm in diameter, red to purple in color, immobile and tender. The nodule is usually surrounded by dilated blood vessels. Occasionally, multiple nodules may be found associated with corneal infiltration and marginal ulcers.

### 3. Necrotizing Anterior Scleritis with Inflammation

It is a severe and destructive type of anterior scleritis caused by vasculitis. The condition is frequently seen in patients with rheumatoid arthritis. White localized area develops due

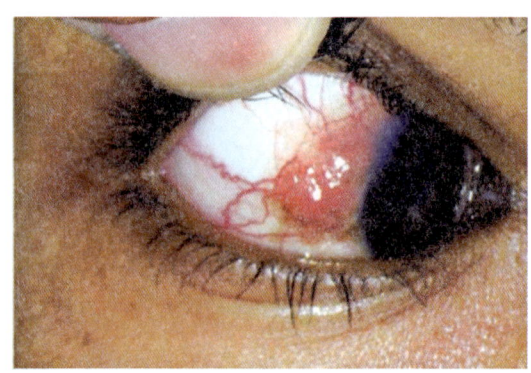

Fig. 4.22: Nodular scleritis

to infarction and the sclera becomes thin, translucent and ectatic. Necrotizing anterior scleritis can cause a number of complications such as sclerosing keratitis, uveitis, secondary glaucoma, cataract and staphyloma.

### 4. Necrotizing Anterior Scleritis with No Inflammation

Necrotizing anterior scleritis with no inflammation is also known as *scleromalacia perforans*. It is a painless condition and does not present signs of inflammation. It is found in patients suffering from long-standing chronic rheumatoid arthritis. Melting and thinning of sclera is common through which the uveal tissue is visible. The globe may rupture following a trivial trauma.

### 5. Posterior Scleritis

The posterior scleritis is relatively a rare condition presenting with pain, proptosis, restricted ocular motility, diplopia and decrease visual acuity. It may occur as an isolated entity or as an extension of the anterior scleritis. It can present as a diagnostic riddle because it manifests as macular edema, exudative retinal detachment, retinal folds, choroidal detachment, papilledema or secondary angle-closure glaucoma.

### Diagnosis

1. Medical examination to diagnose associated systemic disease

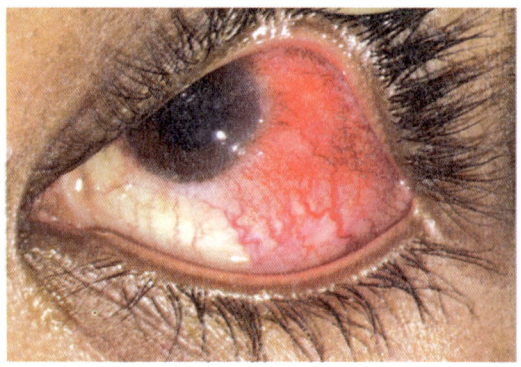

Fig. 4.21: Diffuse scleritis

2. Blood examination: Complete blood count, ESR, C-reactive protein (CRP), blood sugar estimation, thyroid profile, and serum uric acid level.
3. Investigations for collagen and rheumatic diseases: Rheumatoid factor and anti-CCP for rheumatoid arthritis, antinuclear antibodies (ANA), anti-dsDNA and anti-Sm for SLE, and anti-neutrophil cytoplasmic antibodies (ANCA) and cANCA for Wegener's granulomatosis.
4. Rule out tuberculosis and sarcoidosis by lab tests and imaging.

## Treatment

1. Non-necrotizing anterior scleritis is treated with topical corticosteroids
2. Supplementation with oral NSAIDs (indomethacin 75 mg twice a day) gives better results.
3. Non-responding cases need oral cortico-steroids (1 mg/kg/day). It should be gradually tapered to avoid increase in IOP.
4. All cases of necrotizing scleritis should be treated aggressively. Generally, IV methyl-prednisolone (0.5–1g IV infusion with normal saline over 30–60 minutes daily for 3–5 days) is preferred.
5. Necrotizing scleritis associated with rheumatic or connective tissue diseases must be treated with immunosuppressive drugs. These include methotrexate (initially, 7.5 mg/week and increased to 25 mg/week), azathioprine (1.5–2.0 mg/kg/day), cyclophosphamide (oral 1–5 mg/kg/day or 500 mg/mL IV once in 4 weeks).
6. Role of biologics: Infliximab, rituximab and other biologic response modifiers may be tried in necrotizing scleritis where immunosuppressive drugs fail.

4

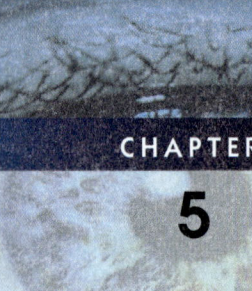

# Diseases of Uvea

## 5.1 ANTERIOR UVEITIS

Depending on the onset, anterior uveitis is usually divided into two categories: (1) acute and (2) chronic.

### Acute Anterior Uveitis

#### Etiology

1. The etiology of uveitis remains idiopathic in about 50% of cases.
2. Approximately, 25–30% of patients with anterior uveitis are positive for HLA (human leukocyte antigen) B27.
3. Common diseases associated with anterior uveitis include ankylosing spondylitis, juvenile idiopathic arthritis (JIA), reactive arthritis, psoriatic arthritis, Crohn disease (inflammatory bowel disease), etc.
4. Patients with ankylosing spondylitis (95% positive for HLA-B27) show bilateral uveitis (80%).
5. Anterior uveitis may be caused by mumps, measles, influenza, adenovirus and *Chlamydia*.
6. It is also found in Lyme disease, leptospirosis, Behçet disease, anterior segment ischemia and Fuchs heterochromia.
7. It can also manifest as postoperative uveitis or lens-induced uveitis.
8. Anterior uveitis may be found associated with retinoblastoma, malignant melanoma, lymphoma, old retinal detachment (RD), rifabutin or cidofovir therapy and topical prostaglandin analogue use.

#### Symptoms

1. Anterior uveitis has an acute onset with photophobia, pain, red eye and decreased vision.
2. Ocular pain is severe at night and usually radiate to forehead and scalp.

#### Signs

1. The circumcorneal injection or ciliary flush is marked.
2. Multiple lymphocytic keratic precipitates (KPs), aqueous flare and aqueous cells are usually seen and in some cases hypopyon develops (Fig. 5.1).

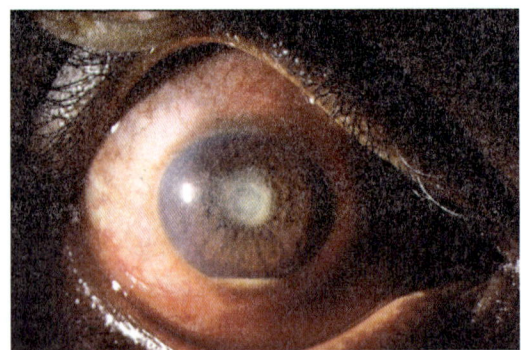

**Fig. 5.1:** Acute anterior uveitis with hypopyon and exudates on the lens (*Courtesy:* Dr J Biswas, Sankara Nethralaya, Chennai)

3. Hyphema may be found in herpes zoster and gonococcal anterior uveitis.

4. The iris appears muddy due to fibrin deposition on its surface.

5. Pupil is constricted and reacts sluggishly.

6. The eye is tender and intraocular pressure (IOP) may be increased or decreased (hyposecretion).

7. Dispersion of pigments on the anterior surface of the lens occurs. Constricted pupil leaves a ring of pigments often seen following dilatation of the pupil (Fig. 5.2).

8. The adhesion of the pupillary margin to the anterior surface of the lens forms posterior synechiae.

9. Later, a ring or annular synechia (*seclusio pupillae*), *iris bombé* and *occlusio pupillae* may get formed. Inflammatory cells are often found in the anterior vitreous.

### Differential Diagnosis

1. Acute conjunctivitis
2. Acute angle-closure glaucoma

### Chronic Anterior Uveitis

#### Etiology

1. Persistence of anterior uveal inflammation more than 3 months is called *chronic anterior uveitis*.

2. The acute uveitis with improper or inadequate treatment may become chronic.

3. Usually, granulomatous infections like tuberculosis, sarcoidosis and syphilis often cause chronic uveitis.

4. Other causes include Vogt-Kayanagi-Harada (VKH) syndrome, sympathetic ophthalmia, herpes simplex virus, varicella zoster virus and connective tissue diseases.

#### Symptoms

The disease may be symptomless or decreased vision may be the only symptom.

#### Signs

1. The patient of chronic uveitis may have ciliary flush or mild ciliary injection and tenderness on pressure.

2. A deep anterior chamber and cells in the vitreous may be found.

3. Presence of stray old KPs or a posterior synechia may be the only sign.

4. Loss of pattern of iris, iris nodules and heavy synechiae are seen (Fig. 5.3).

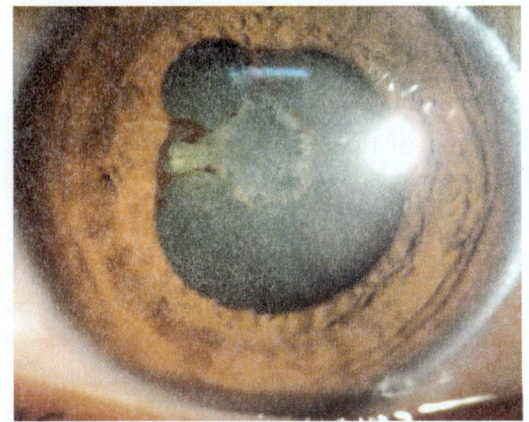

**Fig. 5.2:** Posterior synechiae, pigments on the anterior surface of lens capsule and festooned pupil after dilatation (*Courtesy:* Dr SCL Chandravansi, SS Medical College, Rewa)

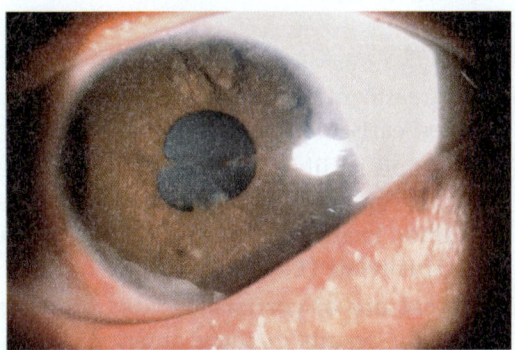

**Fig. 5.3:** Chronic anterior uveitis with nodules on the iris and synechiae (*Courtesy:* Dr J Biswas, Sankara Nethralaya, Chennai)

5. The disease runs a chronic course. Exacerbations and remissions are common.
6. Repeated attacks deteriorate the vision.
7. Complications of chronic uveitis include iris atrophy, neovascular glaucoma, cataract, panuveitis, RD, cyclitic membrane, band keratopathy and rarely phthisis bulbi.

### Diagnosis of Uveitis

1. A definitive diagnosis may be reached only in less than 50% of patients with uveitis
2. A history of eye and systemic disorders and use of medicine must be documented.
3. Slit-lamp examination must be performed.
4. Funduscopy helps in detecting posterior segment lesions.
5. In bilateral granulomatous uveitis, venereal disease research laboratory (VDRL) test, fluorescent treponemal antibody-absorption (FTA-ABS) test, purified protein derivative (PPD) test, angiotensin-converting enzyme (ACE) test, ESR, HLA-B27 and Lyme disease titer, should be evaluated.
6. X-ray or computed tomography (CT) chest, lumbosacral joint or small joints help in the diagnosis of tuberculosis, sarcoidosis, ankylosing spondylitis and JIA.
7. Anterior chamber or vitreous tap is necessary in infective anterior uveitis or endophthalmitis for smear and culture and sensitivity tests.

### Treatment

1. The treatment of anterior uveitis must be started early to prevent complications.
2. The pupil is dilated with cycloplegic like atropine sulfate 1% drops. If the patient is sensitive to atropine, homatropine (2%) or cyclopentolate (1%) should be used.
3. Topical use of corticosteroids produce dramatic results in acute anterior uveitis. Initially, prednisolone drop (1%, 6–8 times/day) is used and then gradually tapered. Corticosteroids can also be administered by subconjunctival, peribular or sub-Tenon routes.

4. Aqueous suppressants are used to lower IOP. Neovascular glaucoma needs special attention.
5. Topical diclofenac sodium (0.1%) or/and ketorolac tromethamine (0.5%) may be used 3 times a day. They do not cause rise of IOP.
6. *Diclofenac* or ibuprofen is useful in relieving the pain. A number of other NSAIDs are also available.
7. Oral prednisolone 60–80 mg per day is administered for 1–2 weeks and then gradually tapered.
8. Specific antibiotic therapy is recommended when the cause of the disease is known. Topical antibiotics may be used to prevent secondary infection.
9. Immunosuppressive therapy should be tried in the steroid-nonresponders.

## 5.2 INTERMEDIATE UVEITIS

### Etiology

1. Etiology of intermediate uveitis (pars planitis) is idiopathic in majority of cases (more than 70%).
2. Other causes include sarcoidosis, multiple sclerosis, syphilis, Lyme disease, inflammatory bowel disease, toxocariasis, Wipple syndrome and lymphoma.

### Symptoms

Presence of floaters is the main symptom. Decreased vision and photophobia may also occur.

### Signs

1. The anterior segment of the eye may not be affected.
2. Cells are seen in the anterior vitreous.
3. Fundus examination reveals white exudates over the inferior retina and over the pars plana. The exudates coalesce to give a typical snow-banking in the inferior vitreous.

4. Peripheral vasculitis, sheathing of vessels, vascular occlusion and vascularization in the retina are usually found.
5. Occasionally, mild inflammatory reaction may be seen in the anterior chamber.
6. Bilateral vitreous hemorrhages may occur.
7. Remissions and exacerbations may be seen.
8. Later, CME, epiretinal membrane, exudative retinal detachment, complicated cataract, secondary glaucoma and band keratopathy may develop.

### Diagnosis

1. The clinical evidence is suggestive.
2. Laboratory tests for sarcoidosis, toxocariasis, syphilis, toxoplasmosis and Lyme disease should be performed.
3. Dilated funduscopy shows the presence of snow-banking at pars plana.
4. Fundus fluorescein angiography (FFA) may confirm vascular occlusion and neovascularization of retina.
5. Optical coherence tomography (OCT) helps in diagnosing cystoid macular edema (CME), retinal vasculitis and epiretinal membrane.
6. MRI of brain for diagnosing MS.

### Treatment

The four-step strategy is recommended for the management of intermediate uveitis:
- *Step 1:* The first line of treatment is corticosteroids. The drug is given by sub-Tenon (every third week), oral prednisolone (1–1.5 g daily, then gradually tapered and given a maintenance dose of 5–10 mg daily) and intravitrial routes.
- *Step 2:* Cryoablation or laser photocoagulation of the pars plana is the second line of therapy if corticosteroids therapy fails.
- *Step 3:* Pars plana vitrectomy, separation of posterior hyaloid and photocoagulation to pars plana are indicated if steps 1 and 2 fail.
- *Step 4:* Systemic immunosuppressive agents should be administered when all the above measures fail.

## 5.3 FUCHS HETEROCHROMIC IRIDOCYCLITIS

### Etiology

The etiology of Fuchs heterochromic iridocyclitis (FHI) is unknown.

### Symptoms

1. FHI is almost a symptom-free condition.
2. Some patients may complain of ocular discomfort or mild blurring of vision.

### Signs

1. A triad of signs consisting of a unilateral heterochromia with iris atrophy (Fig. 5.4), small, round, white KPs scattered all over the endothelium and cells in the anterior chamber and the anterior vitreous, is characteristic.
2. There is absence of posterior synechiae.
3. Neovascularization of the angle is usually seen.
4. Common complications include cataract and glaucoma.

### Treatment

1. Cycloplegics are not required.
2. Topical corticosteroid provides relief alone.
3. Cataract surgery with intraocular lens (IOL) implantation has good prognosis.

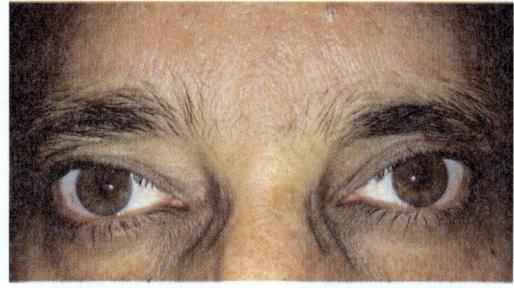

Fig. 5.4: Fuchs heterochromic iridocyclitis

4. Glaucoma does not respond to topical antiglaucoma therapy. Laser trabeculoplasty (LTP) or filtration surgery is effective.

## 5.4 GLAUCOMATOCYCLITIC CRISIS

### Etiology

1. The etiology of glaucomatocyclitic crisis (Posner-Schlossman syndrome) is unknown.
2. Recently, herpes simplex antigen in the aqueous humor has been found and the condition showed favorable response to acyclovir therapy.

### Symptoms

Ocular discomfort, colored halos and photophobia may be the early symptoms.

### Signs

1. Eye is white or shows slight injection.
2. Mild corneal edema is present.
3. Small, white round KPs scattered all over the corneal endothelium.
4. Mild anterior chamber reaction: Flare and a few cells in aqueous humor are seen.
5. Repeated attacks of sudden rise of IOP (40–60 mm Hg) cannot be explained on the basis of mild anterior segment inflammation.
6. Angle of the anterior chamber is open with absence of peripheral anterior synechiae.
7. Hypochromia of iris is present.

### Differential Diagnosis

1. Fuchs heterochromic iridocyclitis (*Refer 5.3*)
2. Uveitic glaucoma: Irregular constricted pupil with synechiae.
3. Pigmentary glaucoma: Marked pigment dispersion and iris transillumination defects (*Refer 6.8*).

### Diagnosis

1. Slit-lamp examination reveals mild anterior uveitis and absence of synechiae.

2. Nearly white eye with episodes of sudden acute rise of IOP.
3. Gonioscopy shows open-angle and absence of peripheral anterior synechiae (PAS).

### Treatment

1. Topical timolol (0.5%, twice a day) or brimonidine (0.15–2%, twice or thrice a day) is effective in lowering the IOP.
2. Oral acetazolamide (500 mg or 1 g) is recommended to control the acute rise of IOP.
3. Topical prednisolone (1%, 3–4 times a day) for 8–10 days controls inflammation. It should be tapered rapidly, otherwise may cause IOP elevation.
4. Topical NSAIDs are used three times a day.
5. Systemic NSAIDs (indomethacin 75–150 mg per day) can also decrease inflammation.
6. If inflammation persists, a mild cycloplegic is used.

## 5.5 POSTERIOR UVEITIS

### Etiology

1. The posterior uveitis is an inflammation of the choroid (choroiditis); the overlying vitreous is often involved.
2. The posterior uveitis (choroiditis) may be infectious or noninfectious in origin.
3. Infection is caused by bacteria, spirochetes, fungus, parasite and viruses.
4. The noninfectious causes include immunologic, allergic, masquerading conditions and idiopathic.

### Symptoms

Decreased vision, multiple floaters, flashes of light, distorted objects (metamorphopsia) and visual loss are common.

### Signs

1. The disease may not be limited to posterior uvea but can involve the entire uveal tract, causing panuveitis in some patients.
2. Signs of posterior uveitis differ depending on the etiology.

## Tuberculous Uveitis

### Etiology

1. *Mycobacterium tuberculosis* often causes a delayed hypersensitivity reaction or rarely a direct infection of the uvea.
2. It should be suspected if patient is old and has a chronic lung infection.
3. Tuberculosis can involve both anterior and posterior uvea.

The involvement of anterior uvea in tuberculosis may occur in the form of acute anterior uveitis or chronic granulomatous anterior uveitis with mutton-fat KPs, iris nodules, thick posterior synechiae and granuloma of angle of the anterior chamber.

Chronic anterior uveitis may cause complicated cataract and secondary glaucoma.

Posterior uveitis, depending on the location, manifests in different forms:

1. Central choroiditis involves macula and causes marked visual loss.
2. Disseminated or multifocal choroiditis is characterized by the presence of small multiple lesions scattered all over the choroid.
3. *Choroidal tuberculoma:* A conglomerate choroidal tuberculoma mimicking a neoplasm may be seen (Fig. 5.5). It is accompanied by vitreous haze and inflammatory signs in the choroid.
4. Multiple miliary tubercles may be seen in advanced stage of meningitis. They are small, pale-white spots found near the disk. They represent hematogenous spread of the organism. Tuberculosis can also present as intermediate uveitis.

### Complications

The posterior uveitis may lead to retinal periplebitis, vascular occlusion, papillitis and subretinal neovascularization.

### Diagnosis

1. X-ray or CT chest

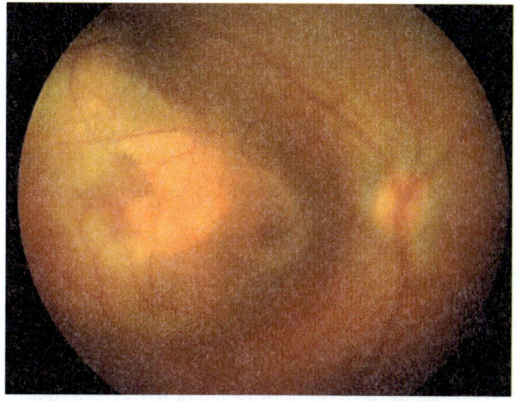

**Fig. 5.5:** Tuberculoma of choroid (*Courtesy:* Dr Dolley Joseph, Tuberculosis, HV Nema et al, editor, Eye in Systemic Disorders, New Delhi, Wiley India, 2015)

2. Tuberculin skin test with purified protein derivative (PPD)
3. PCR helps in the confirmation of the diagnosis.

### Treatment

1. Besides the topical treatment of anterior uveitis, the antitubercular therapy such as rifampicin and isoniazid must be instituted.
2. Patients on ethambutol require frequent check ups for prevention of toxic amblyopia.
3. If needed, corticosteroids can be administered under the cover of the antitubercular treatment.
4. Recurrent choroiditis needs sub-Tenon injections of depot corticosteroid.
5. The systemic administration of antibiotics and corticosteroids often hasten the resolution of the lesion. Once the macula is damaged, the visual prognosis becomes poor.

## Leprotic Uveitis

### Etiology

1. Leprosy is caused by *Mycobacterium leprae*.
2. Uveitis is more common in the lepromatous leprosy than in tuberculoid.
3. Uveitis in leprosy is considered as a manifestation of antigen–antibody deposition.
4. Acute uveitis is usually unilateral.

### Symptoms

Besides systemic disabilities, leprosy can produce a number of ocular symptoms. They include watering, discomfort, dryness, redness, itching, white spot in the eye, pain in the eye and impaired vision or loss of vision.

### Signs

1. Eyebrows and eyelashes are scanty or absent.
2. Limbal leproma, thickening and beading of corneal nerves, corneal anesthesia, SPK, corneal vascularization, interstitial keratitis, corneal ulcer and corneal leukoma are corneal lesions of the disease.
3. The anterior uveitis may be of 2 types: Granulomatous or nongranulomatous. The granulomatous anterior uveitis is marked by the presence of yellow pearl-like iris nodules with minimal inflammatory reaction.
4. The nongranulomatous leprotic iritis causes exudative reaction.
5. Blepharochalasis, trichiasis, entropion, ectropion and inability to close the eye are often seen.
6. Systemic features of leprosy include sensory and motor impairment resulting in contracture deformities of hands and feet.

### Treatment

1. Topical atropine and corticosteroid can contain the anterior uveitis.
2. Systemic sulphones are administered for 1–2 years.
3. Systemic corticosteroids with dapsone (100 mg daily) may control the acute inflammatory reaction.
4. The WHO has recommended clofazimine and rifampicin for the treatment of leprosy. Clofazimine is given 50 mg daily or 100 mg alternate days while rifampicin is administered as a single dose of 600 mg monthly.

## Syphilitic Uveitis

### Etiology

Syphilis is caused by *Treponema pallidum*. Both anterior and posterior uvea can be involved in syphilis.

### Symptoms

Ocular symptoms are photophobia, ocular pain, redness and decreased vision.

### Types

Congenital and acquired.

### Signs

1. *Congenital syphilis*
   - Congenital syphilis is usually bilateral and in majority of cases starts as diffuse iritits with interstitial keratitis.
   - Salt-and-pepper fundus, attenuation of retinal vessels, retinal pigment epithelial degeneration and optic atrophy are the posterior segment manifestations of congenital syphilis.
   - Congenital stigmata of syphilis may be present.
2. *Acquired syphilis*
   - Acquired syphilis is often unilateral. A nongranulomatous iritis is seen in the secondary stage of the disease. It may or may not be accompanied with interstitial keratitis.
   - Argyll-Robertson pupil may be found.
   - A gumma may be found on the iris or ciliary body.
   - Gummatous iritis is characterized by the presence of pink-yellow vascularized nodule at the pupillary border.
   - A focal or multifocal choroiditis (Fig. 5.6) may be seen in the secondary syphilis with juxtapapillary exudates.
   - Retinal vasculitis, exudative retinal detachment, and widespread pigment proliferation are also found in secondary syphilis.

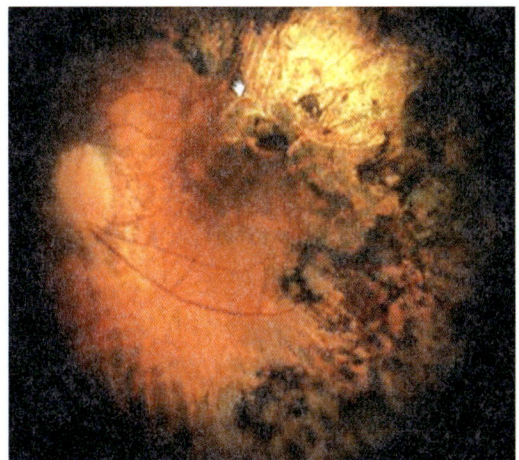

**Fig. 5.6:** Syphilitic retinochoroiditis (*Courtesy:* Dr S Sudarsan, Sankara Nethralaya, Chennai)

### Differential Diagnosis

Retinitis pigmentosa (RP).

### Diagnosis

1. FTA-ABS and microhemagglutination-treponema pallidium (MHA-TP) tests can confirm the diagnosis.
2. In congenital syphilis of newborn, FTA-ABS test of the mother is required.
3. Rapid plasma reagin test is useful in assessing the response to therapy.

### Treatment

1. Besides local therapy with atropine and corticosteroids, systemic administration of benzathine penicillin (50,000–2.4 million U/kg, IM, once) or procaine penicillin (10,000 U/kg, IM daily) for 10 days is recommended.
2. Higher doses of aqueous penicillin (3–4 million U, IV for 10–14 days) are required to treat neurosyphilis.
3. Penicillin-allergic patients below 8 years should be treated with erythromycin and above 8 years with doxycycline.

## Lyme Disease

### Etiology

Lyme disease is caused by *Borrelia burgdorferi.*

### Symptoms

1. Symptoms include blurring of vision, diplopia, ocular pain and photophobia.
2. Headache, malaise, fatigue, fever, chills, facial weakness and joint and muscular pain are general symptoms.

### Signs

1. Ocular signs
   - Involvement of eye occurs in all the three stages of Lyme disease.
   - Keratitis uveitis, vitritis, optic neuritis, cranial nerve palsies, exposure keratitis and endophthalmitis are ocular manifestations of the disease.
2. Systemic signs: The course of disease is divided in three stages:
   - *Stage of early infection* presents a distinctive bull's eye rash at the site of tick bite.
   - Flu-like clinical features are present in the *dissemination stage.*
   - Intermittent joint pain, arthritis, Bell's palsy and cardiac involvement may occur in the *stage of persistent infection.*

### Diagnosis

1. History of tick-bite
2. A high immunofluorescent antibody titer against *Borrelia burgdorferi.*
3. Both ELISA and Western blot tests help in the diagnosis.

### Treatment

1. Doxycycline (100 mg once or twice per day for 10–21 days) or amoxicillin (500 mg three times in a day) is effective.
2. Ceftriazone 2 g IV or penicillin G, 20 million units IV should be administered in patients with neuro-ophthalmic involvement.
3. Topical atropine, antibiotic and corticosteroids are used for managing keratitis and anterior uveitis.

5

## 5.6 HERPETIC UVEITIS

### Etiology

Varicella-zoster virus causes anterior uveitis in about 50% of patients. It can also cause panuveitis.

### Symptoms

Headache, fever, malaise, rashes, watering, red eye, pain and decreased vision may occur.

### Signs

1. A mild anterior uveitis occurs with KPs, flare and a few cells in the anterior chamber.
2. The invasion of live virus in the uveal tissue may result in a severe anterior chamber reaction manifesting as hypopyon or hyphema.
3. The posterior segment involvement manifests as vasculitis, vitritis, chorioretinal exudates, retinal hemorrhages, serous retinal detachment (RD) and peripheral outer retinal necrosis (seen in patients with AIDS).
4. Secondary glaucoma, iris atrophy damage to sphincter pupillae and optic atrophy may occur as sequelae.

### Diagnosis

1. The diagnosis is mostly clinical by history and examination.
2. PCR test of aqueous and vitreous can confirm the diagnosis.
3. The virus can be cultured on human cells.

### Treatment

1. Topical corticosteroids and cycloplegic drops are applied to control uveitis but topical acyclovir is not used.
2. Oral acyclovir (800 mg, 5 times/day for 7 days) is often prescribed.
3. Other anti-viral drugs like oral famciclovir (500 mg, 3 times/day for 7 days) valaciclovir 1 g, 3 times/day for 7 days) are given in low doses and found to be effective especially in postherpetic neuralgia.

## 5.7 CYTOMEGALIC INCLUSION DISEASE

### Etiology

Cytomegalovirus causes cytomegalic inclusion disease. The disease occurs in two forms—congenital and acquired.

### Congenital Cytomegalic Inclusion Disease

#### Symptoms

CID affects the neonates with yellowing of skin and microcephaly.

#### Signs

1. The ocular lesions are multifocal peripheral patches of bush-fire retinochoroiditis, uveitis, optic nerve hypoplasia and microphthalmos.
2. Systemic features are fever, anemia, and hepatosplenomegaly.

### Acquired Cytomegalic Inclusion Disease

#### Symptoms

The patient may complain of floaters, blurring of vision and symptoms of AIDS (in AIDS affected patients).

#### Signs

1. Acquired CID is the most common ocular opportunistic infection in patients with AIDS.
2. All those patients with absolute CD4 cell count of T-lymphocyte of less than 200 cells/mm$^3$ are at a high risk for the infection.
3. An indolent form may show granular opacities with stray hemorrhages in the periphery of retina.
4. Signs of fulminant form of CID include multiple cotton-wool spots, yellow-white exudates giving a pizza pie appearance (Fig. 5.7), patches of retinal necrosis, extensive retinal hemorrhages along the major retinal vascular arcades, vasculitis, vitreous exudates and rhegmatogenous retinal detachment.

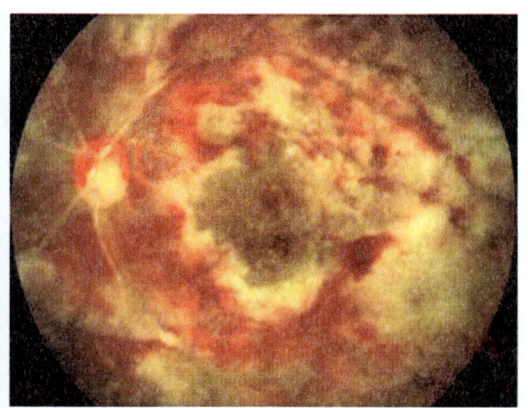

Fig. 5.7: Cytomegalovirus choroiditis showing pizza pie appearance (*Courtesy:* Dr S Shridhran, Sankara Nethralaya, Chennai)

5. The incidence of acquired CID has significantly decreased with the advent of highly active antiretroviral therapy (HAART).

### Diagnosis

1. Typical clinical picture.
2. Demonstration of viral inclusion bodies in urine, saliva and subretinal fluid.
3. Electron microscopy of the retinal tissue for virus particles
4. PCR of aqueous and vitreous fluids confirms the diagnosis.

### Treatment

1. Ganciclovir is a first line drug. It is used in the doses of 5 mg/kg IV, twice daily for 3 times per week and maintained 5 mg/kg IV, once daily, 5 days in a week for long-term.
2. If ganciclovir causes toxicity (neutropenia, thrombocytopenia and renal toxicity), it should be used intravitreally 400 µg/0.1 mL. Ganciclovir 4.5 mg sustained release implant in the anterior vitreous is well tolerated.
3. Foscarnet may be administered 60 mg/kg IV, 8 hourly per week followed by 90 mg/kg daily 5 days/week. It may cause electrolyte imbalance and renal tocixity.

4. Valganciclovir, a prodrug of ganciclovir, can be given orally in the dose of 900 mg twice a day for 3 weeks, then 900 mg once a day. It is as effective as IV ganciclovir. However, it causes renal toxicity.
5. Cidofovir may be administered in the doses of 5 mg/kg, IV weekly for 3 weeks followed by 3–5 mg/kg biweekly. It may be given 20 mg intravitreally every 5th week. The drug can induce hypotony and iritis.
6. HAART should be started early in patients with AIDS.
7. Rhegmatogenous RD (subclinical) with intact macula should be treated with laser delimitation. If macula is involved, pars plana vitrectomy with silicone oil injection is indicated.

## 5.8 TOXOPLASMOSIS

### Etiology

1. Toxoplasmosis is caused by a protozoan, *Toxoplasma gondii*.
2. The protozoan causes a granulomatous necrotic retinochoroiditis.
3. Toxoplasmosis may occur in 2 forms—congenital or acquired.

### Congenital Toxoplasmosis

#### Symptoms

Symptoms include blurring and floating black spots.

#### Signs

1. The congenital toxoplasmosis is more severe.
2. Bilateral punched out macular scar, intracranial calcification and nystagmus form the classical triad of congenital toxoplasmosis.
3. The initial lesion is an exudative focal retinitis (Fig. 5.8).
4. The necrotic inflammation causes destruction of whole thickness of choroid and retina.

5

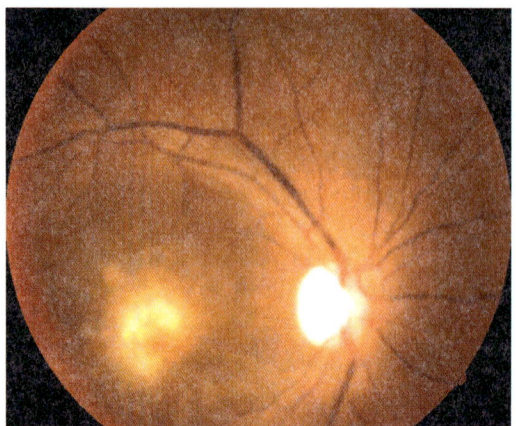

**Fig. 5.8:** Toxoplasmosis, active lesion

5. Reactivation of the healed lesion is attributed to the rupture of retinal cyst which releases parasites.
6. The fresh lesion is whitish-yellow and appears adjacent to the old scar.
7. Vitritis is usually seen along with the retinal lesion.

## Punctate Outer Retinal Toxoplasmosis

1. Punctate outer retinal toxoplasmosis is characterized by the presence of small lesions at the level of RPE near old pigmented scars.
2. These lesions are associated with minimal vitritis.

## Acquired Toxoplasmosis

1. Acquired ocular toxoplasmosis is usually mild.
2. Patients with recently acquired toxoplasmosis do not show scars.
3. Occasionally, a mild anterior uveitis may occur.
4. CNS is not affected.

## Diagnosis

1. Characteristic fundus picture
2. Sabin-Feldman dye test was used in the past to detect Toxoplasma IgG antibodies.
3. In differential agglutination test (AC/HS test): (1) AC antigen found in acute infection and (2) HS antigen seen in later stages of infection. It was used to differentiate between acute and chronic infections.
4. ELISA for toxoplasma IgG and IgM, 6 weeks after infection. It is more sensitive than the dye test and AC/HS tests, therefore, used commonly.
5. Polymerase chain reaction (PCR) amplification is a reliable test for the diagnosis of congenital and acquired toxoplasmosis.
6. CT or magnetic resonance imaging (MRI) to detect CNS lesions.

## Treatment

1. Small lesions of toxoplasmosis resolve spontaneously and may not need treatment.
2. Toxoplasmic anterior uveitis requires use of topical cycloplegic and corticosteroids.
3. Pyrimethamine (daraprim) is a first-line therapy and is administered 25 mg twice a day (after an initial dose of 150 mg) for weeks. Concurrent folinic acid (20 mg daily) should be given to reduce bone marrow toxicity.
4. Trimethoprim-sulfamethoxazole (800 mg twice a day) can be used.
5. Clindamycin (300 mg, 4 times a day, 3–4 weeks) may be used alone or in combination with pyrimethamine. It causes gastrointestinal tract (GIT) disturbances, especially pseudomembranous colitis. In the event of toxicity, the drug can be given either by IV route or intravitreally (0.1 mg/0.1 mL).
6. Atovaquone (750 mg four times a day orally) can be used in place of clindamycin.
7. In severe disease oral prednisolone (60–100 mg, 1 or 2 days after antiprotozoal therapy) should be started to save the macula and optic nerve.
8. Spiramycin (1 g thrice daily) is a safe drug for pregnant or breastfeeding women.
9. Azithromycin or clarithromycin with pyrimethamine is also effective.
10. Neovascularization of retina may need photocoagulation.
11. Pars plana vitrectomy is indicated in the presence of vitreous membranes and RD.

## 5.9 TOXOCARIASIS

### Etiology

1. Toxocariasis is caused by *Toxocara canis* and *Toxocara catis*. The infestation comes from dogs or cats.
2. It is usually unilateral and manifests in following forms:
   - Chronic destructive endophthalmitis
   - Posterior pole granuloma
   - Peripheral granuloma.

### Symptoms

It may be asymptomatic or presents with redness, leukocoria, photophobia, strabismus, decreased vision or loss of vision.

### Signs

1. *Chronic destructive* endophthalmitis presents clouding of vitreous and panuveitis. Later, cyclitic membrane formation and exudative detachment of retina may develop.
2. *Posterior pole granuloma* is unilateral, elevated and 1–2 disk diameter in size. It shows minimal reaction in the retina except tension lines and fibrous tissue strands extending from granuloma to pars plana.
3. *Peripheral granulomas* are hemispherical in shape with connective tissue bands running between them and optic disk (Fig. 5.9)

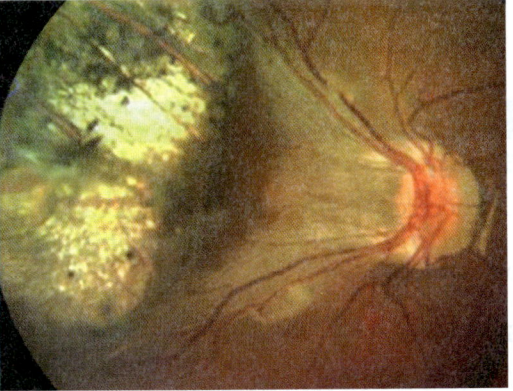

**Fig. 5.9:** Toxocariasis granulomas

through vitreous cavity. The bands may cause hetrotopia of macula (macular dragging).

### Differential Diagnosis

1. Retinoblastoma
2. Retinopathy of prematurity.

### Diagnosis

1. Classical fundus picture
2. Cytology of aqueous tap shows eosinophilia
3. ELISA test.
4. Absence of calcification on CT scan of head and B-scan ultrasonography.

### Treatment

1. Periocular depot methylprednisolone (40–60 mg) is given weekly to prevent loss of vision during active phase of the disease.
2. Systemic corticosteroids with mebendazole (500 mg qid orally) may be tried.
3. Thiabendazole is not effective in ocular disease.
4. Pars plana vitrectomy reduces vitreous traction and prevents RD.
5. Extrafoveal lesions can be destroyed by photocoagulation.

## 5.10 CYSTICERCOSIS

### Etiology

1. Cysticercosis, the most common ocular platyhelminth infestation in humans, is caused by *Cysticercus cellulose*, the larval form of pork tapeworm, *Taenia solium*.
2. Rarely, it is caused by the larvae of beef tapeworm, *T. saginata*.
3. Humans act as the definitive host and pigs and cattle act as intermediate hosts for these parasites.
4. The parasite possibly enters the eye via the choroidal circulation. From choroid, it can

2. It becomes granulomatous during the due course of time and shows moderate flare and mutton-fat KPs.

3. Tags of lens capsule or cortex or hypermature cataract may be seen on slit-lamp examination.

4. The histopathology demonstrates the presence of necrotic area with lens matter with polymorphonuclear cells. Later the picture resembles that of sympathetic ophthalmitis except the necrotic lesion.

**Treatment**

1. Topical and systemic corticosteroids may not improve the condition.

2. Dramatic improvement is usually noticed after removal of all the lens material.

## 5.13 ENDOPHTHALMITIS

1. Inflammation of anterior uvea, vitreous, retina and choroid is called endophthalmitis.

2. The endophthalmitis may be infectious or noninfectious (sterile). The infection may occur either exogenously or endogenously.

3. The exogenous infection may develop after ocular trauma and intraocular operations like cataract surgery, glaucoma surgery (bleb infection), etc.

### Postoperative Bacterial Endophthalmitis

*Etiology*

1. Endophthalmitis is more often bacterial.

2. *Staphylococcus epidermidis, Staphylococcus aureus* and *Streptococcus spp.* are common bacteria that cause acute infection.

3. *Pseudomonas, Proteus* and *Haemophilus influenzae* are less common. *Propionibacterium acne* produces a chronic low grade infection.

4. The bacterial endophthalmitis usually develops within 1–14 days of surgery while infectious blebitis may develop months or years after the trabeculectomy.

5. Endogenous endophthalmitis may occur during septicemia.

*Symptoms*

Blurred vision, lacrimation, ocular pain, redness and loss of vision are common complaints.

*Signs*

1. Bacterial endophthalmitis usually has an acute onset and a stormy course. It presents an unduly increased postoperative reaction.

2. Lid edema, conjunctival and ciliary injections, corneal edema, severe hazy cornea anterior chamber reaction with hypopyon and fibrinous exudates (Fig. 5.11) are usually found.

3. Vitritis, vitreal debris and vitreous abscess may reduce the red fundus reflex and present a dull yellow white reflex.

4. Tenderness of the eye and hypotonia may be noticed.

*Diagnosis*

1. Thorough ocular examination should be conducted to find predisposing factors such as wound leak, vitreous in the section, leaking bleb, etc.

2. If fundus red reflex is lost, B-scan USG is needed to find the status of vitreous and retina.

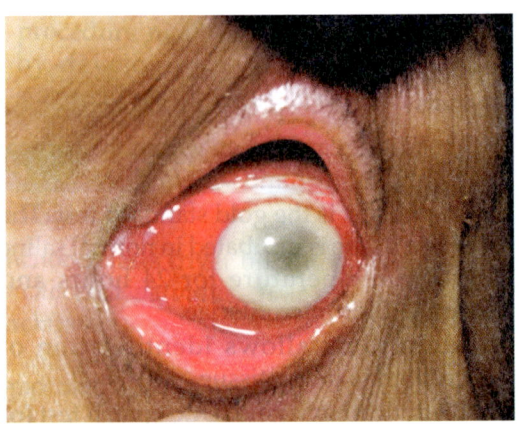

**Fig. 5.11:** Bacterial endophthalmitis

3. It is necessary to get aqueous and vitreous taps for identification of organisms by smear (Fig. 5.12) and culture.

## Treatment

1. Preoperative asepsis, treatment of blepharitis and intraoperative injection of antibiotic are prophylactic measures.
2. Topical moxifloxacin drops (0.5%) or fortified tobramycin and corticosteroids drops (prednisolone 1%) hourly and atropine (1%) three times per day must be instilled.
3. If the etiology is not known, intravitreal 2.25 mg ceftazidime or 400 µg amikacin plus 1 mg vancomycin should be given later, the treatment is modified in the light of culture report.
4. Vancomycin IV or cephalexin IM is used for the treatment of Gram-positive cocci infection.
5. Injection of ceftazidime (2.25 mg) intra-vitreous is given in Gram-negative bacterial infection.
6. Administration of oral corticosteroids 24 hours after the antibiotic therapy may save the eye. They may control eye damage and improve the visual outcome.
7. Endophthalmitis vitrectomy study has advocated the use of vancomycin and amikacin intravitreally, as well as topical. Additionally, vancomycin/ceftazidime should be given subconjunctivally.
8. Patients with severe endophthalmitis need pars plana vitrectomy.

## Fungal Endophthalmitis

### Etiology

1. The fungi which cause endophthalmitis are *Aspergillus, Fusarium, Penicillium, Mucor* and *Candida*.
2. Exogenous endophthalmitis is caused by filamentous fungi.
3. *Candida albicans* usually causes endogenous infection.
4. Fungal endophthalmitis often occurs within 3 months of intraocular surgery.

## Aspergillus Endophthalmitis

1. Aspergillus endophthalmitis is seen in drug addicts and AIDS patients.
2. The clinical picture shows vitritis with fluffy round opacities and diffuse yellowish lesions in the retina with hemorrhages.
3. Occasionally, infection extends anteriorly. The rise of IOP causes perforation of eye at limbus (Fig. 5.13).

## Candida Endophthalmitis

1. Candidiasis is seen in immunosuppressed patients and in those with indwelling catheters.
2. Many yellow-white, fluffy, elevated lesions appear in deep retina and they increase in size with time and involve the vitreous.
3. Vitreous becomes hazy and shows cotton ball opacities or vitreous abscess.
4. Retinal hemorrhages and retinal detach-ment are not uncommon.

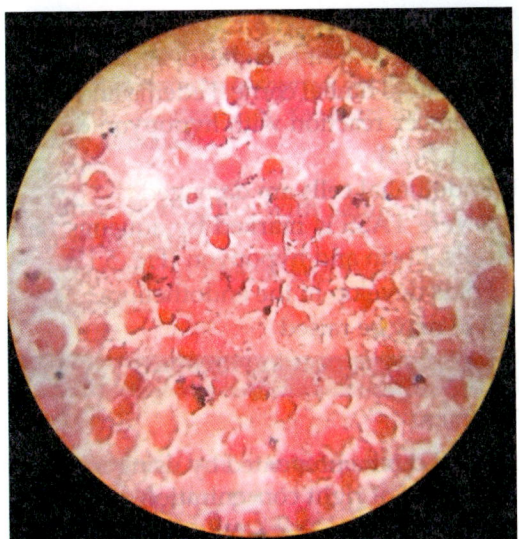

**Fig. 5.12:** Vitreous tap: Smear stained with Gram stain shows cocci

## Symptoms

Mucopurulent discharge, red eye, blurring of vision, diarrhea and joint pain may occur.

## Signs

1. Nonspecific conjunctivitis, urethritis and polyarthritis from the triad of Reiter's syndrome.
2. The conjunctivitis is mucopurulent.
3. In about 30% of cases recurring anterior uveitis may be found.
4. Arthritis (95%) of hands and feet and non-gonococcal urethritis (75%) are common.
5. Keratoderma blennorrhagica of palms and soles and balanitis circinata are important components of clinical diagnosis.

## Diagnosis

1. Besides classical triad of urethritis, poly-arthritis and conjunctivitis, presence of keratoderma blennorrhagicum and circinate balanitis help in diagnosis.
2. Patients are positive for HLA-B27
3. X-ray or CT of joints for arthritis.

## Treatment

1. Reiter's syndrome is a self-limiting disease.
2. Topical cycloplegics and topical, periocular or systemic corticosteroids are effective.
3. Tetracycline 250 mg, four times a day or doxycycline 100 mg, twice a day for 3–6 weeks yield good results.
4. Oral NSAIDs are helpful in ameliorating the joint swellings.

## 5.18 BEHÇET'S DISEASE

### Etiology

1. Behçet's disease is an obliterating vasculitis.
2. It is more common in young adults of Japan and Turkey and is considered as an idiopathic chronic disease.
3. The incidence of HLA-B5 phenotype and its subtype HLA-BW51 is significantly higher in patients with Behçet's disease.

## Symptoms

1. Patients may complain of multiple floaters, photophobia, ocular pain and sudden decrease in vision.
2. Pain in mouth and swellings on skin are other complaints.

## Signs

The characteristic sign is acute bilateral anterior uveitis with hypopyon.

1. In spite of the severe anterior uveitis, fibrin never appears in the anterior chamber, hence hypopyon remains mobile.
2. The posterior uveal lesions include vitritis, periphlebitis retinae (Fig. 5.18A and B), central retinal vein occlusion, posterior vitreous detachment (92%), thromboangiitis obliterans, frosted branch angiitis, retinitis, exudative retinal detachment papillitis, papilledema, ischemic optic neuropathy and choroidal infarcts.
3. Retinal atrophy and attenuation of retinal vessels are seen in late stages along with massive retinal exudation and detachment.
4. The common earliest lesions are aphthous ulcers of mouth, gums or lips. They are recurrent, multiple and painful. Genital ulcers may develop on penis and scrotum in males and vulva and vagina in females.
5. The skin manifestations are erythema nodosum acne vulgaris, rashes and dermatographia.
6. Arthritis can develop in 30–50% of patients.
7. Seizures, idiopathic intracranial hyper-tension, deafness, cranial nerve palsies, hemipareses, cerebellar ataxia, pyramidal and extrapyramidal signs, peripheral neuropathies, confusion and hallucinations are CNS manifestations of the disease.

## Differential Diagnosis

1. Spondyloarthritis—associated with recurrent anterior uveitis
2. Reiter's disease
3. Sarcoidosis

6. Imaging (chest X-ray, CT chest, MRI brain)
7. Complete blood count, erythrocyte sedimentation rate and C-reactive protein.

## Treatment

1. Uveitis may not respond to routine therapy.
2. Early use of systemic corticosteroid (prednisolone 1–2 g per day) combined with azathioprine is likely to prevent blindness.
3. Biologicals should be used as a first line therapy for Behçet's uveitis.
4. Keep interferon, cyclosporine, tacrolimus and infliximab for resistant cases.

## 5.19 VOGT-KOYANAGI-HARADA SYNDROME

### Etiology

1. The etiology of VKH syndrome is not known. It affects persons of Asian ancestry and native Americans between 30 years and 50 years of age.
2. The uveal melanin plays some role in the etiology of the disease.
3. HLA-DR4, HLA-MT3 and HLA-BW54 testing is positive in patients with VKH syndrome.

### Symptoms

1. Bilateral decreased vision, photophobia, distortion of images, red eyes and pain may be the presenting symptoms.
2. Symptoms of meningism like headache, rigid neck, nausea, vomiting and fever may be associated with tinnitus, hearing loss and dysacusis.

### Signs

1. A bilateral granulomatous panuveitis is the hallmark of VKH syndrome.
2. Signs of posterior uveitis include bilateral diffuse vitritis, multiple-elevated patches of choroiditis, exudative detachment of retina inferiorly, papillitis and neovascularization of retina and optic disk.

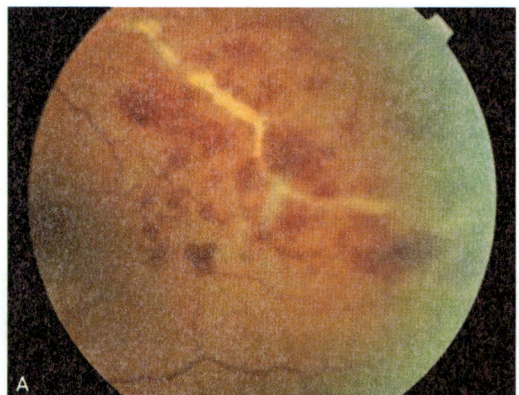
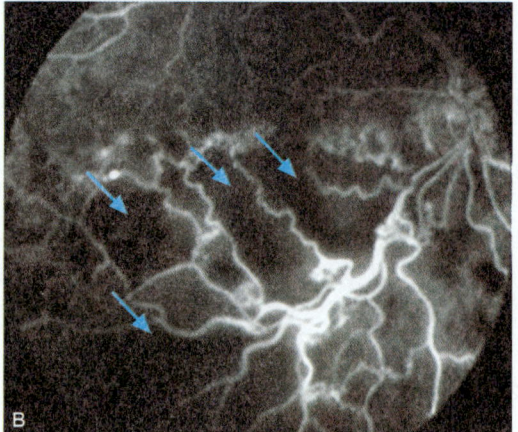

**Fig. 5.18A&B:** Behçet's disease (*Courtesy:* Dr Upender Wali)

4. Systemic lupus erythematosus
5. Intermediate uveitis.

## Diagnosis

1. Presence of recurrent painful oral aphthous ulcers, inflammatory eye disease, genital ulceration and skin lesions helps in diagnosis.
2. Pathergy or Behcetin test (formation of a local postule on skin puncture by a needle).
3. Presence of HLA-B5 and HLA-BW51.
4. Granular-staining antineutrophilic cytoplasmic antibody to rule out Wegener's granulomatosis (WG).
5. Fluorescein angiography (FA) and indocyanine green angiography (ICGA) for retinal lesions.

3. The anterior uveitis is characterized by the presence of mutton fat KPs, cells in the anterior chamber, iris nodules, shallow anterior chamber, peripheral anterior synechiae and secondary glaucoma.

4. The chronic phase begins with resolution of exudative retinal detachment.

5. Depigmentation of RPE results in the "sunset-glow" fundus appearance. Multiple round depigmented lesions may be found.

6. Perilimbal vitiligo may be present.

7. Ocular complications of VKH include secondary glaucoma, cataract, extraocular muscle palsy and phthisis bulbi.

8. The extraocular signs include vitiligo, alopecia and poliosis (about 30%), hearing loss, ataxia and cranial neuropathy.

## Differential Diagnosis

1. Sympathetic ophthalmia: Patients give history of ocular trauma

2. Sarcoidosis: Presents multisystem involvement

3. Multifocal placoid pigment epitheliopathy: Here there is no involvement of the anterior segment.

## Diagnosis

1. The diagnosis is primarily clinical.

2. FFA shows multiple leaks at retinal pigment epithelium level and subretinal vascularization

3. HLA typing

4. Lumbar puncture may show pleocytosis in VKH

5. MRI to rule out CNS disorders.

## Treatment

1. Topical cycloplegic agents and corticosteroids must be administered early.

2. Posterior subtenon depot steroids are used periocularly.

3. Systemic prednisolone 60–80 mg daily and gradually tapered.

4. Immunosuppressive therapy (azathiozone, methotrexate, cyclosporine) is essential for the treatment of VKH syndrome.

5. Subretinal vascular network is destroyed by photocoagulation.

## 5.20 ACUTE POSTERIOR MULTIFOCAL PLACOID PIGMENT EPITHELIOPATHY

### Etiology

1. The etiology of acute posterior multifocal placoid pigment epitheliopathy (APMPPE) is unknown.

2. It may be caused by inflammatory obstruction of blood supply to choriocapillaris.

3. APMPPE is seen in young HLA-B27 positive healthy adults.

4. Patients with APMPPE may have concurrent thyroiditis, cerebral vasculitis and erythema nodosum suggesting an autoimmune reaction.

### Symptoms

Patients remain symptom-free or complain of floaters and decreased vision.

### Signs

1. Funduscopy presents multiple cream color lesions about one disk diameter under the retina. They may become confluent.

2. Both pigmented and depigmented areas are found in the retina.

3. Vitreous cells, periphlebitis, optic neuritis and optic disk edema may occur.

### Diagnosis

1. Typical posterior segment lesions with sparing of the anterior segment.

2. In the active stage of the disease, FFA shows blocked fluorescence in the early stage and with hyperfluorescence of margins of the lesion in the late stages.

3. HLA-B27 positivity.

## Treatment

Systemic corticosteroids are reported to be effective in cases with macular involvement. Most patients recover vision.

## 5.21 BIRDSHOT RETINOCHOROIDOPATHY

### Etiology

1. The etiology of birdshot retinochoroidopathy is not known.
2. The disease is more common in females than males and seen in forties.
3. The disease shows HLA association and perhaps autoimmunity plays some role in etiology.

### Symptoms

Blurring of vision, color deficiency and night blindness.

### Signs

1. Fundus examination reveals presence of multiple, cream-colored or depigmented lesions distributed all over the retina and their distribution pattern is like a scatter from a shotgun (Fig. 5.19).
2. Other fundus changes include periphlebitis, attenuation of retinal arteries, papilledema, optic atrophy, cystoid macular edema, subretinal choroidal neovascularization and surface wrinkling retinopathy.
3. Vitritis is common but involvement of the anterior segment may be minimal.
4. Birdshot retinochoroidopathy is a chronic disease. It shows exacerbations and remissions.

### Diagnosis

1. Characteristic fundus appearance
2. FFA reveals peripapillary leakage, papilledema and cystoid macular edema. The lesions show early hypofluorescence and late staining. ICGA gives more information than FFA.

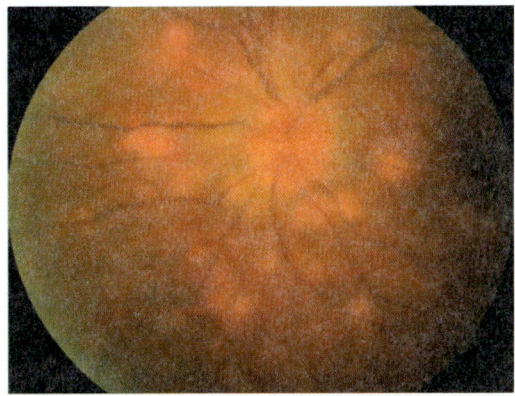

**Fig. 5.19:** Birdshot choroidopathy

3. HLA-A29 positivity (80–96%)
4. Retinal autoantigen reactivity.

### Treatment

1. The disease responds poorly to NSAIDs therapy.
2. Periocular, intravitreal and systemic steroids can control inflammation and cystoid macular edema.
3. Immunosuppressive agents (cyclosporine, mycophenolate mofetil, azathioprine, etc) are effective in resolution of retinal lesions and improving the visual prognosis.

## 5.22 SERPIGINOUS CHOROIDOPATHY

### Etiology

1. Serpiginous choroidopathy or geographical helicoid peripapillary choroidopathy (GHPC) is a disease of obscure etiology.
2. It affects HLA-B7 positive persons between the ages of 40 years and 60 years.

### Symptoms

Blurred vision is the most common symptom.

### Signs

1. The disease is characterized by multiple cream colored lesions in the retinal periphery (Fig. 5.20A).

2. They all heal by scaring.

3. Active yellow-gray and edematous lesions may be present.

4. New lesions appear in contiguous to the previous scars in a tongue-shaped or snake-like pattern.

5. Vitreous may be minimally involved.

6. Retinal vascular sheathing, detachment of retinal pigment epithelium, macular choroiditis and neovascularization of disk may be found.

## Diagnosis

1. Clinical picture of the disease
2. HLA-B7 positivity
3. FFA shows blockage of the dye by active lesions (Fig. 5.20B), while inactive lesions transmit the dye without staining.

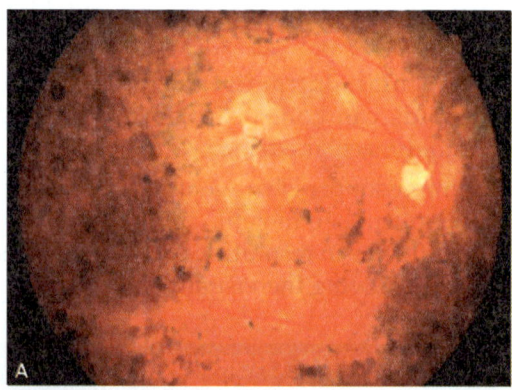

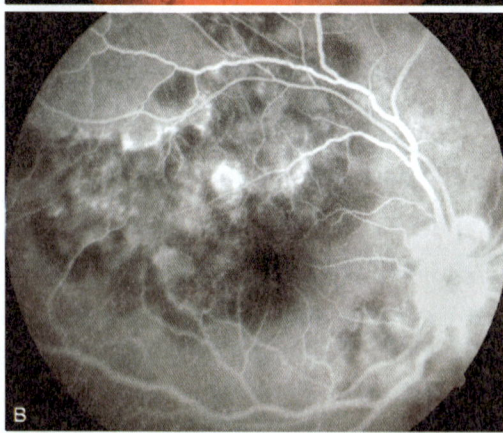

**Fig. 5.20A&B:** Serpiginous choroidopathy (*Courtesy:* Dr A Bhargav, Retina Hospital, Indore)

## Treatment

1. The disease may not respond to cortico-steroids and immunosuppressants.

2. Sub-Tenon steroid and systemic cyclo-sporine are recommended if there is threat to macula.

## 5.23 CHOROIDAL DETACHMENT

### Etiology

1. Choroidal detachment may be seen following ocular trauma, cataract, glaucoma or retinal detachment surgeries and photocoagulation.

2. It may occur in uveal effusion syndrome, carotid-cavernous fistula, VKH syndrome and malformed eye.

3. Rarely, choroidal detachment develops spontaneously.

### Symptoms

Patient may be asymptomatic or there can be decreased vision, pain and redness.

### Types

Choroidal detachment may be serous or hemorrhagic.

### Signs

1. Bullous elevation of the retina and choroid.

2. It appears orange-brown and smooth.

3. Extensive globular detachment makes ora serrata visible without scleral depression (Fig. 5.21).

4. Anterior chamber is always shallow with mild cells and flare.

5. Serous detachment is characterized by low IOP and a positive transillumination test.

6. Hemorrhagic detachment is marked by increased IOP and a negative transillumination test.

### Differential Diagnosis

1. RD
2. Malignant melanoma of choroid.

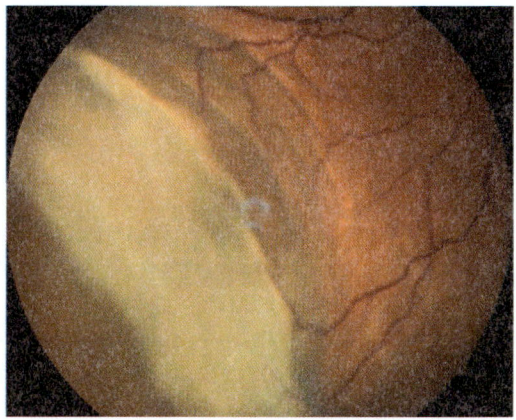

**Fig. 5.21:** Choroidal detachment

## Diagnosis

1. History of trauma or operation.
2. Characteristic clinical picture on dilated fundus examination.
3. Seidel test to check wound leak.
4. Gonioscopy to rule out cyclodialysis cleft.
5. Transillumination test to know about type of detachment.
6. B-scan ultrasonography to exclude malignant melanoma and RD.
7. OCT is helpful.

## Treatment

1. Repair the wound leak with cyanoacrylate glue or suturing.
2. Cyclodialysis cleft should be repaired.
3. Cycloplegic and corticosteroid therapy for anterior uveitis.
4. Systemic corticosteroids seem beneficial in serous detachment.
5. Surgical drainage of suprachoroidal fluid/hemorrhage should be performed with or without vitrectomy.
6. RD requires surgical repair.

## 5.24 MALIGNANT MELANOMA OF CHOROID

### Etiology

1. Malignant melanoma (MM) of choroid, an intraocular tumor, occurs between 50 years and 70 years of age.

2. It is usually unilateral and affects both sexes equally.
3. MM affects white races more commonly and has a predilection for the temporal half of the choroid.
4. Melanosis oculi and nevus of Ota are considered as risk factors.

### Symptoms

1. The symptoms depend on the location and size of MM. The patient remains symptom-free for a long time if it is situated in the periphery of retina, whereas centrally (near macula) situated tumor presents early visual symptoms.
2. A large tumor causes floaters and flashes of light due to RD and pain in the eye.

### Types

Clinically, MM is of two types:

1. The *circumscribed melanoma* is usually single and pigmented.
2. The *diffuse melanoma*.

### Modified Callender's Classification

1. Spindle cell nevus
2. Spindle cell melanoma
3. Epithelioid melanoma
4. Mixed-cell (mixture of spindle and epithelioid cells).

### Stages of Malignant Melanoma

1. *Quiescent stage:* A flat or lens-shaped, brown or yellow mass grows from choroid and pushes the retina. Presence of drusen over MM indicates an inactive tumor, whereas orange patches (lipofuscin) represent an active growth. The growth assume mushroom shape with the rupture of Bruch's membrane. It is associated with detachment of retina (Fig. 5.22A). A diffuse infiltrating melanoma presents a slaty-gray pigmentation unassociated with RD.

2. *Glaucomatous stage:* It is characterized by ocular pain, rise of IOP and inflammatory reaction in the anterior chamber. The IOP is increased due to compression of vortex veins, forward push of iris by the tumor growth and blocking of trabeculum by tumor cells.

3. *Stage of extraocular extension:* The MM spreads to the orbit sclera and the retina.

4. *Stage of metastasis:* MM spreads to liver through blood stream.

### Differential Diagnosis

1. Choroidal nevus
2. Hemangioma of the choroid
3. Rhegmatogenous RD

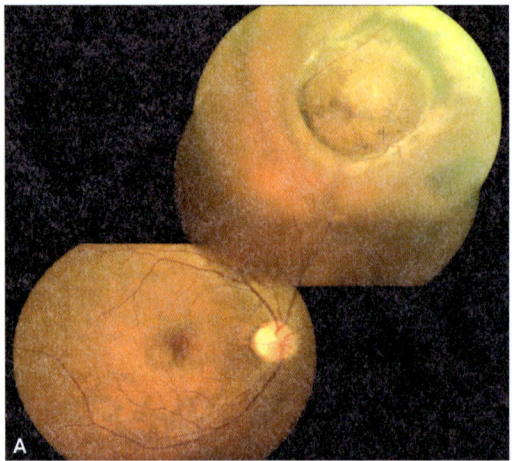

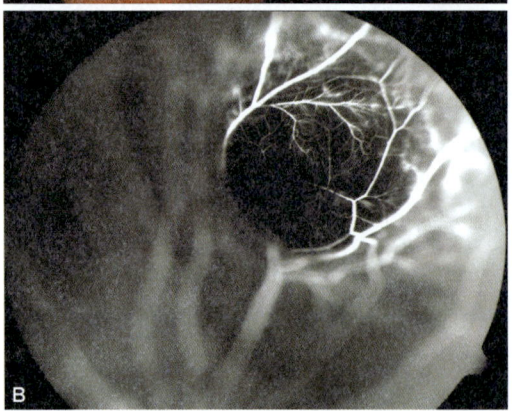

**Fig. 5.22A&B:** Malignant melanoma (*Courtesy:* Dr Khetan, Sankara Nethralaya, Chennai)

4. Detachment of choroid
5. Choroidal cyst
6. Old choroidal hemorrhage.

### Diagnosis

1. Dilated funduscopy
2. Slit-lamp biomicroscopy with fundus contact lens
3. Transillumination test
4. FFA to identify leakage, neovascularization and characteristic double circulation (Fig. 5.22B).
5. Indocyanine green angiography may reveal double circulation within melanoma
6. Fundus autofluorescence to differentiate from choroidal nevus
7. Enhanced depth imaging OCT
8. B-scan ultrasonography is helpful especially when media are hazy. It is the most important diagnostic modality and shows a choroidal mass with orbital shadowing.
9. Estimate the levels of alkaline phosphate, lactate dehydrogenase, asparate and alanine aminotransferases for systemic metastasis.
10. CT or MRI of orbit and liver for metastases.

### Treatment

1. A close follow-up supported with stereoscopic colored fundus photographs.
2. Photocoagulation is advised if MM is not located near fovea and it is small (<10 mm) and flat.
3. A full-thickness resection can be performed in selected cases.
4. A combination of radioactive plaque therapy (cobalt-60 or ruthenium-106) with thermotherapy is effective.
5. Enucleation or exenteration is indicated for extraocular metastatic tumors.
6. Patients with systemic metastasis are treated with chemotherapy.

# Glaucoma

## 6.1 PRIMARY OPEN-ANGLE GLAUCOMA

### Etiology

1. The etiology of primary open-angle glaucoma (POAG) is not known.
2. A rise in intraocular pressure (IOP) occurs as a result of increased resistance to aqueous outflow in spite of open angle of the anterior chamber.
3. Increased IOP (above 21 mmHg), old age, family history of glaucoma (10% of the first degree relatives), myopia, diabetes and hypertension are risk factors for the POAG.
4. The incidence of disease is higher in black Africans.

### Symptoms

1. Initially, a symptom-free condition but later patients may present with mild headache and ocular discomfort.
2. Difficulty in reading or doing close work and frequent changes of glasses (early onset presbyopia) are common.
3. Patients may complain of difficulties in night driving and color identification and decrease in vision.
4. Loss of vision and visual field defects grossly handicap the affected person.

### Signs

1. IOP is usually elevated more than 21 mmHg.
2. IOP shows diurnal variations and large fluctuations in IOP are common.
3. The depth of the anterior chamber is normal.
4. Initially, the pupil is briskly reacting to light but later becomes sluggish.
5. The angle of the anterior chamber is open (Fig. 6.1).
6. Optic disk appears pale and cupped.
7. The vertical cup/disk ratio is high because neuroretinal rim notching occurs early at the upper and lower poles of the disk (Fig. 6.2).

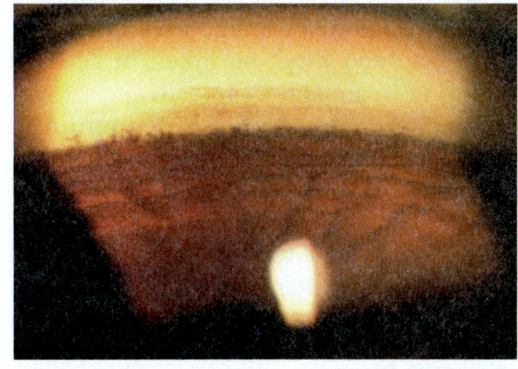

**Fig. 6.1:** Open angle (*Courtesy:* Prof. R Ramakrishnan, Aravind Eye Hospital, Tirunelveli, TN)

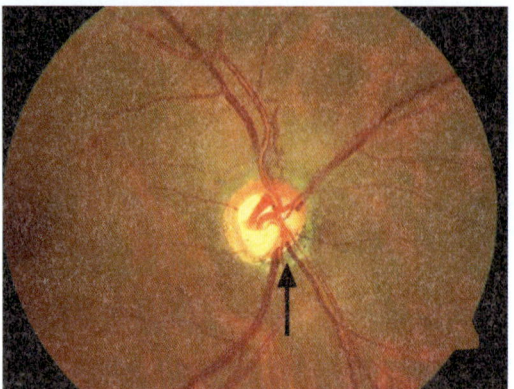

**Fig. 6.2:** Prominent inferior notch in the optic disk (*Courtesy:* Prof. R Ramakrishnan, Aravind Eye Hospital, Tirunelveli, TN)

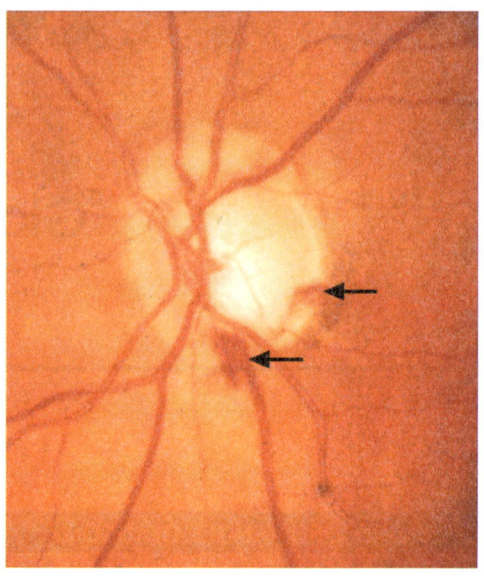

**Fig. 6.3:** Inferior notch and two splinter hemorrhages (black arrows) are present at the lower optic disk margin (*Courtesy:* Prof. R Ramakrishnan, Aravind Eye Hospital, Tirunelveli, TN)

8. Normally, the neuroretinal rim is pink in color and is widest in the inferior disk region. The width of the rim decreases in descending order in the superior, the nasal and the temporal disk region (ISNT rule).
9. A thinning of neuroretinal rim is seen in long-standing cases.
10. An asymmetry of more than 0.2 cup/disk ratio between normal and eye with POAG is often found.
11. The loss of nasal nerve fibers causes displacement of blood vessels nasally.
12. Deepening of the cup leads to double angulation of the blood vessels (*bayoneting sign*).
13. Splinter hemorrhage may be seen near the disk in patients with POAG (Fig. 6.3). The presence of hemorrhage indicates active disease and must be taken in account during treatment.
14. Peripapillary atrophy is common in POAG.
15. The retinal nerve fiber loss appears as slit-grooves or wedge-defects.
16. Paracentral scotoma, arcuate scotoma (Fig. 6.4), nasal step or glaucoma hemifield defect may be found as visual field defects.

### Differential Diagnosis

1. Ocular hypertension

2. Chronic angle-closure glaucoma [presence of shallow anterior chamber and peripheral anterior synechiae (PAS) differentiates it from POAG]
3. Primary optic atrophy (optic atrophy causes greater visual loss and pallor of the disk)
4. Secondary open-angle glaucoma
5. Chiasmal tumors
6. Optic nerve drusen.

### Diagnosis

1. Visual acuity, color vision and amplitude of accommodation are recorded.
2. Baseline IOP is measured. Asymmetry in the IOP between the two eyes of 5 mmHg or more is suggestive of the disease.
3. Diurnal variation of more than 10 mmHg suggests the presence of glaucoma.
4. Central corneal thickness (CCT) is measured by pachymetry. CCT affects measurement of IOP; an increased CCT gives higher and a decreased CCT a lower IOP measurements.

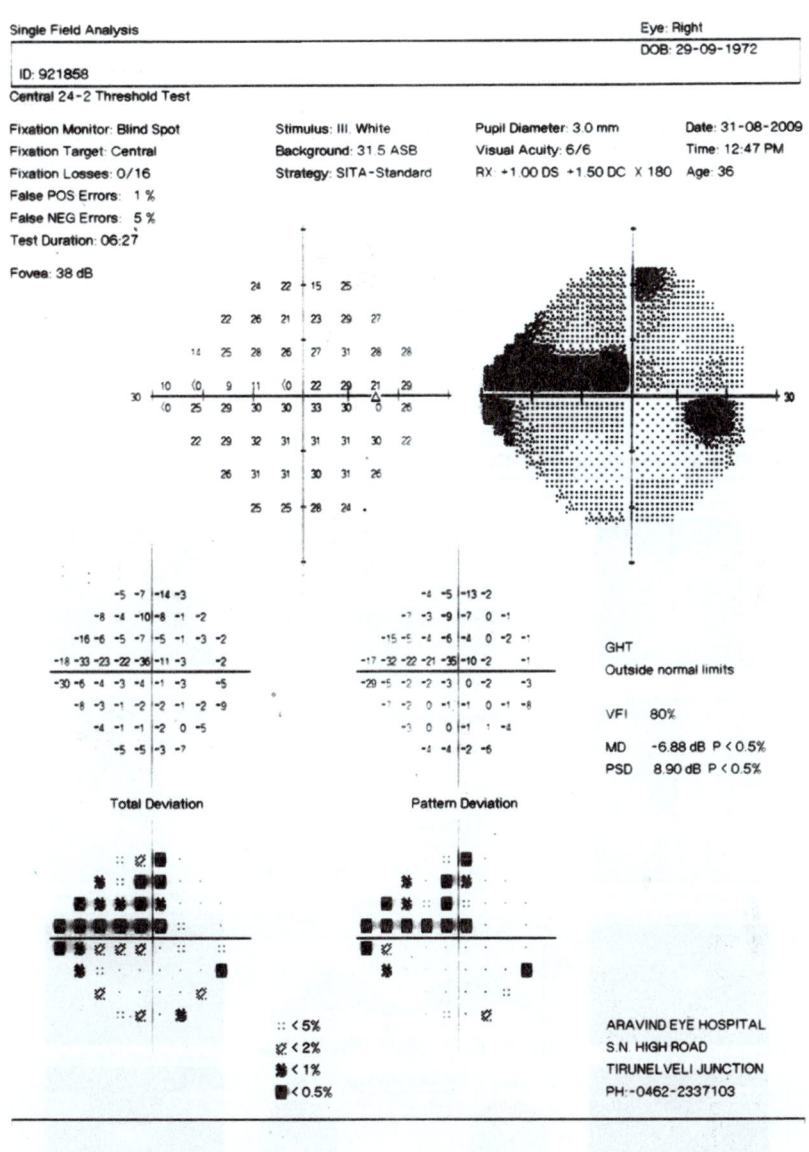

**Fig. 6.4:** Single field analysis of the right eye of a patient showing superior arcuate scotoma (*Courtesy:* Prof. R Ramakrishnan, Aravind Eye Hospital, Tirunelveli, TN)

5. Slit-lamp examination can exclude secondary open-angle glaucoma.

6. Gonioscopic examination is essential to differentiate between primary and secondary glaucoma as well as between POAG and primary angle-closure glaucoma (PACG).

7. Evaluation of optic disk is important to assess enlargement of cup, damage to neuroretinal rim and to look for congenital and acquired disk anomalies.

8. Imaging of the optic disk by Heidelberg retina tomogram (HRT) II measures the

area and volume of the optic disk, cup, and rim.

9. The retinal nerve fiber layer is measured quantitatively with the help of GDx nerve fiber analyzer or optical coherence tomography (Fig. 6.5).

10. Both central and peripheral visual fields should be determined under standardized conditions.

11. To exclude neurological disorders causing optic neuropathy computed tomography (CT) or magnetic resonance imaging (MRI) of brain is needed.

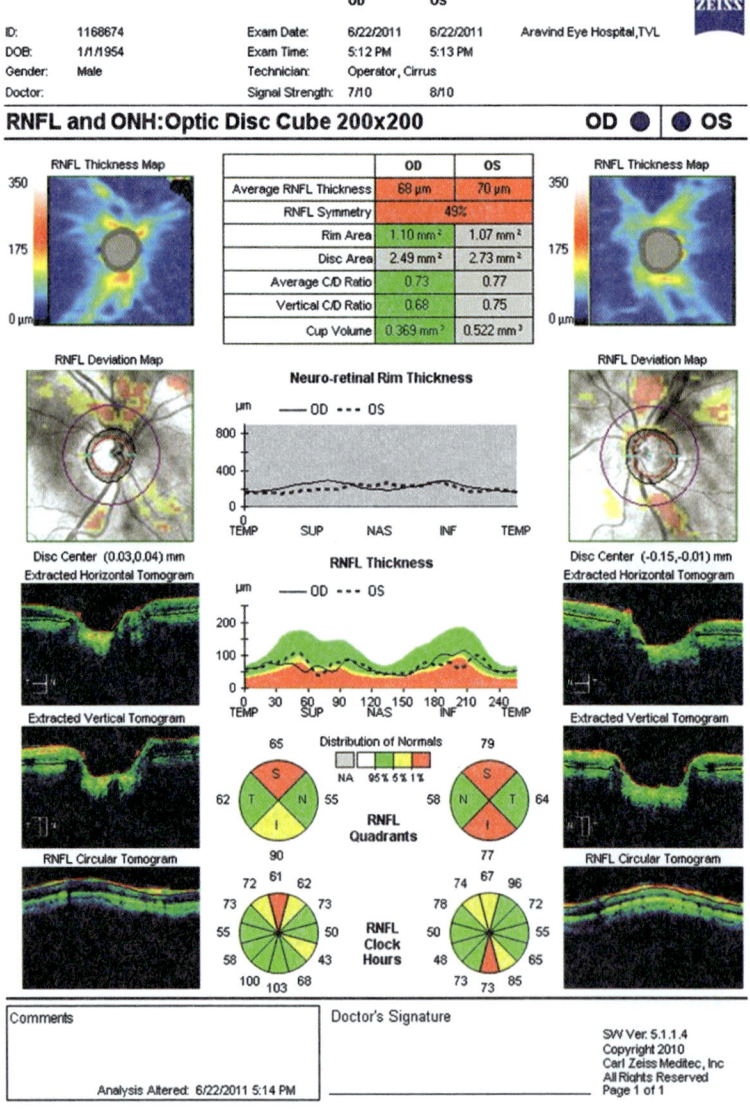

**Fig. 6.5:** Cirrus OCT of a POAG patient showing bipolar neuroretinal rim thinning and superior and inferior retinal nerve fiber layer thinning in both eyes (*Courtesy:* Prof. R Ramakrishnan, Aravind Eye Hospital, Tirunelveli, TN)

12. Provocative test: Water-drinking provocative test does not provide a definitive diagnosis.

## Treatment

1. Medical therapy
   - The main aim of treatment of open-angle glaucoma is to decrease IOP at a target level which does not cause damage to the retinal nerve fibers.
   - Use one of the prostaglandin agonists [latanoprost (0.004%), bimatoprost (0.03%), travoprost (0.004%)] once at bedtime as first line of treatment.
   - Beta-blocker, timolol maleate (0.25–0.5%, twice a day) is most widely used worldwide. It is contraindicated in respiratory disorders, congestive cardiac failure (CCF) and depression.
   - Selective alpha 2-receptor agonist— brimonidine tartrate (0.15–0.2%, 2–3 times in a day) decreases the IOP significantly. It should be avoided in children below 5 years of age.
   - Topical carbonic anhydrase inhibitors (CAIs), dorzolamide (2%, 3 times a day) or brinzolamide (1%, 3 times a day) reduce IOP moderately (14–17%).
   - Systemic CAIs (acetazolamide 250 mg, 4 times a day, 500 mg, once or twice a day, methazolamide 25–50 mg, 2–3 times a day) are used in patients with high pressure.
   - Miotic, pilocarpine (0.5–2%, 2–3 times a day) is less frequently used.
2. Surgical therapy
   - Argon laser trabeculoplasty (ALT) decreases IOP in about 75% of patients.
   - Selective laser trabeculoplasty uses lower energy. It is a safe and effective procedure.
   - Trabeculectomy is indicated if maximal medical therapy fails to achieve target IOP. It may or may not be combined with the use of antifibrotic agents like 5-flurourocil or mitomycin C (MMC).

## Follow-up

1. A close periodic (3–6 months interval) reevaluation of all cases of POAG is mandatory to check the progression of the disease.
2. On each follow-up, vision, tonometry, gonioscopy, visual fields, and dilated fundus examination should be performed to monitor response to treatment.

## 6.2 NORMAL PRESSURE GLAUCOMA

### Etiology

1. The etiology of normal pressure glaucoma (NPG) is unknown.
2. It is considered a multifactorial disease and associated with vascular insufficiencies (ischemic vascular diseases, vasospasm and Raynaud's disease), thyroid disease, sleep apnea, autoimmune diseases and coagulopathies that contribute to low perfusion pressure.
3. Patients with NPG have thinner lamina cribrosa and low CSF pressure.
4. The disease is common in females.

### Symptoms

Patients remain symptom-free for a long time, frequent changes of glasses, early onset of presbyopia, decreased vision, difficulty in fixation, and loss of vision can gradually develop.

### Signs

1. In spite of a low or normal IOP, patients with NPG may present signs of POAG.
2. The optic disk shows pallor and notch at the inferior pole (Fig. 6.6).
3. There is thinning of neuroretinal rim inferiorly.
4. Splinter hemorrhage(s) (40%) may be found on the disk (Fig. 6.6) and an acquired pit can appear on the disk.
5. Beta peripapillary atrophy with narrow vessels may be seen.

6

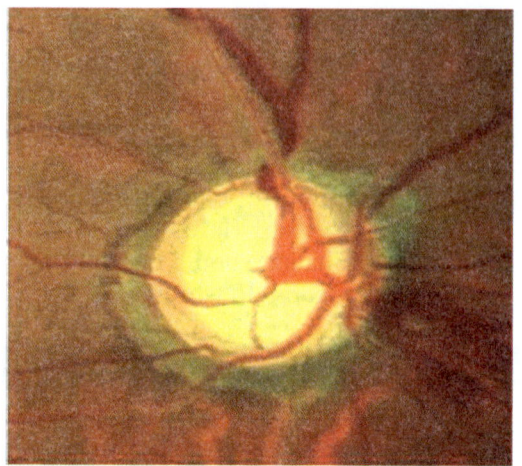

**Fig. 6.6:** Fundus photograph of a patient with normal tension glaucoma showing advanced cupping with pallor of the rim and disk hemorrhage (*Courtesy:* Prof. R Ramakrishnan, Aravind Eye Hospital, Tirunelveli, TN)

6. The visual field defects in NPG are relatively more deeper and near the fixation point than POAG. A dense paracentral or arcuate scotoma is typical (Fig. 6.7).
7. In normal pressure glaucoma, a low IOP occur as a result of low scleral rigidity or lower CCT.
8. Two eyes may have asymmetrical IOP.
9. The eye with higher pressure shows greater damage.

### Differential Diagnosis

1. Primary open-angle glaucoma
2. Coloboma of the optic nerve head
3. Tumor of optic chiasma
4. Anterior ischemic optic neuropathy

### Diagnosis

The workup of patients with NPG is on the lines of POAG:
1. History of migraine, vasospasm, hypotension, hypertension, autoimmune disorders and loss of autoregulation is helpful.
2. Antinuclear antibody and extractable nuclear antigens can help in the diagnosis of autoimmune collagen vascular disorders.

3. Record diurnal variations of IOP to check fluctuations.
4. Gonioscopy for excluding other types of glaucoma—angle recession and angle-closure
5. CT and MRI of brain to rule out optic nerve compression and central nervous system (CNS) disorders
6. Carotid Doppler ultrasonography to rule out carotid insufficiency
7. Imaging studies such as OCT, HRT, and GDx are not only helpful in the diagnosis but also in the treatment and progression of the normal-pressure glaucoma.

### Treatment

1. NPG is treated on the lines of POAG.
2. The target pressure is usually kept relatively low (10–12 mmHg).
3. The use of calcium channel blockers (nifedipine, nimodipine, brovincamine, etc) may be beneficial in stabilizing the visual fields.

## 6.3 OCULAR HYPERTENSION

### Etiology

1. Ocular hypertension has an elevated IOP (more than 2–3 standard deviations from the mean) in the absence of optic neuropathy and field defects.
2. It is seen in 6–10% of population above the age of 40 years.
3. Glaucoma may develop in 5% cases of ocular hypertension on follow up.
4. Higher baseline IOP, reduced CCT, diabetes, POAG in the fellow eye, thyroid dysfunction, asymmetry of optic cup and family history of glaucoma are important risk factors for the development of glaucoma.

### Symptoms

Patients with ocular hypertension remain symptom-free.

6

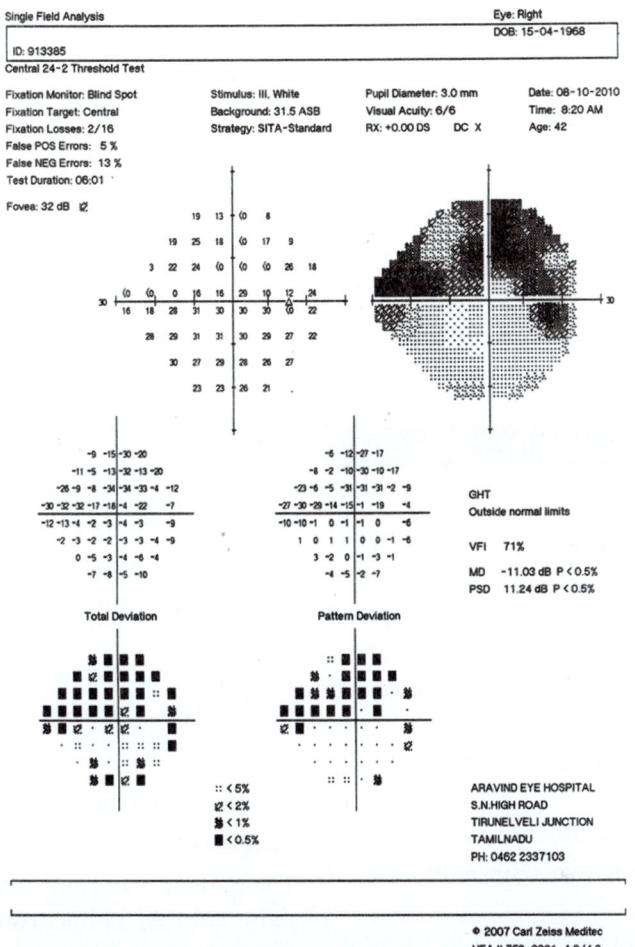

**Fig. 6.7:** Single field analysis of the right eye of a patient with normal tension glaucoma showing superior arcuate scotoma (*Courtesy:* Prof. R Ramakrishnan, Aravind Eye Hospital, Tirunelveli, TN)

## Signs

1. IOP is increased (more than 21 mmHg) in both eyes on more than two occasions and shows wide variations (between 20 and 40 mmHg).
2. Angle of the anterior chamber is open.
3. The optic disk and retinal nerve fiber layer appear normal.
4. Visual fields do not show any defect.

## Diagnosis

1. IOP is always elevated (more than 21 mmHg) on repeated measurements.

2. In spite of increase in IOP (more than 30 mmHg), optic disk and visual fields appear normal.
3. Diurnal variation of IOP shows a fluctuation of more than 8 mmHg.

## Treatment

1. Patients with mild increase in IOP (20–25 mm Hg) do not need any treatment unless the fellow eye has POAG.
2. A careful follow-up is necessary at 3–6 monthly interval to assess further rise in baseline IOP, glaucomatous damage to

optic disk and retinal nerve fiber layer, and visual field defects.

3. Young or middle-aged patients with an IOP of more than 30 mmHg need medical treatment to reduce IOP by 20–25% from the baseline pressure.

4. Ocular Hypertension Treatment Study reported that despite treatment, 4.5% of patients with ocular hypertension develop glaucoma as compared to 9.5% of patients without treatment.

## 6.4 PRIMARY ANGLE-CLOSURE GLAUCOMA

### Etiology

1. Primary angle-closure glaucoma (PACG) is common among Asians.

2. The prevalence of PACG increases in old age.

3. PACG is more common in females than in males (ratio 4:1).

4. The first degree glaucoma relatives are at a greater risk.

5. The predisposing factors for PACG are:
   - Small, hyperopic eye with a short axial length
   - Shallow anterior chamber (1.8–2.1 mm)
   - The iris is inserted anteriorly on the ciliary body.
   - The lens is thick.
   - A close contact of the sphincter pupillae with the anterior surface of the lens blocks the circulation of aqueous from the posterior to the anterior chamber resulting in a relative pupillary block. The peripheral iris bows forward (iris bombe') and causes appositional angle-closure and obstruction to the aqueous outflow.

### Classification

The angle-closure glaucoma may show four stages which may or may not be sequential:
1. Angle-closure suspect

2. Intermittent angle-closure
3. Acute angle-closure
4. Chronic angle-closure

### Angle-closure Suspect

1. Generally, the term angle-closure suspect is applied to a predisposed eye with shallow anterior chamber, normal IOP and occludable angle.

2. Prophylactic peripheral laser iridotomy is the treatment of choice.

### Intermittent Angle-closure

1. The patient may present with transient blurring of vision and colored halos around light.

2. Clinical features include sudden increase in IOP, shallow anterior chamber and occludable angle.

3. In between attacks, the eye appears normal.

4. It is also managed with peripheral laser iridotomy.

### Acute Angle-closure

#### Symptoms

The patient may complain of sudden onset of pain, colored halos around lights (rainbow vision), watering, red eye, photophobia, profound diminution of vision, frontal headache, nausea and vomiting.

#### Signs

1. Edema of lids and conjunctiva, ciliary flush, steamy and insensitive cornea are often present.

2. There is dusting of corneal endothelium with iris pigments.

3. The anterior chamber is extremely shallow with aqueous flare and the angle is closed (Fig. 6.8).

4. Pupil is dilated, vertically oval. It is non-reactive to light and accommodation. The iris appears edematous and atrophic.

5. The IOP is very high (60 mmHg).

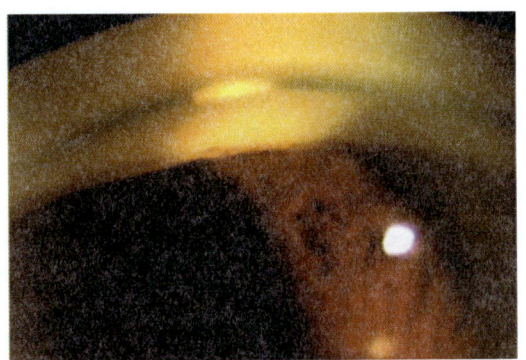

**Fig. 6.8:** Gonioscopic view showing closed angle with only the Schwalbe's line visible (*Courtesy:* Prof. R Ramakrishnan, Aravind Eye Hospital, Tirunelveli, TN)

6. Repeated attacks form peripheral anterior synechiae.
7. The fellow eye shows a narrow or occludable angle.
8. Opacities in the anterior lens cortex, glaukomflecken may be found.
9. Funduscopy may show hyperemic and swollen optic disk, with hemorrhages pulsations of the retinal artery and occasionally, retinal vascular occlusion.

### Differential Diagnosis

1. Acute conjunctivitis
2. Acute anterior uveitis
3. Secondary glaucoma.

### Diagnosis

1. A positive history of risk factors and typical onset of the disease is often available.
2. Clinical evidence of corneal edema, very high IOP, angle-closure and dilated, vertically oval, nonreacting pupil.
3. The compression gonioscopy can differentiate between a reversible and irreversible angle-closure.
4. Ultrasound biomicroscopy and anterior segment OCT can help in the diagnosis and understanding the pathomechanism of the disease.

### Treatment

1. The medical treatment is aimed to reduce the IOP to prevent visual loss and make the eye suitable for laser iridotomy.
2. Intensive topical timolol maleate (0.5%, every 15 minutes) is used till IOP is reduced. If timolol is contraindicated brimonidine (0.15%), prostaglandin analog or darzolamide (2%) may be used.
3. Administration of oral or IV acetazolamide (500 mg twice a day) or mannitol 1–2 g/kg body weight, IV can reduce the IOP early.
4. Prednisolone (1%, 4 times a day) to prevent ocular damage.
5. Pilocarpine (1–2%, 3–4 times a day) should be started after reduction of iris ischemia and lowering of IOP because sphincter pupillae does not respond to the drug if IOP is very high.
6. Later, laser iridotomy must be considered in the absence of peripheral anterior synechia or an iridoplasty can be performed.
7. In the presence of goniosynechiae, trabeculectomy is indicated.

### Fellow Eye

A peripheral laser iridotomy must be performed in the fellow eye with occludable angle.

### Follow-up

All patients with glaucoma need a periodical checkup of IOP, angle of the anterior chamber, stereo-disk photographs and visual fields to monitor the treatment.

## 6.5 CHRONIC PRIMARY ANGLE-CLOSURE GLAUCOMA

### Etiology

1. Chronic PACG can develop following recurrent attacks of subacute PACG.
2. Repeated attacks can cause a permanent closure of a large segment of the angle by PAS and produce damage to trabecular meshwork.

6

3. An angle-closure caused by a slow circumferential PAS formation is known as *creeping angle-closure*.

## Symptoms

Patients are asymptomatic or complain of headache and decrease in vision.

## Signs

1. The anterior chamber is shallow and the chamber angle is usually closed.
2. The indentation gonioscopy shows permanent PAS.
3. The IOP is moderately increased.
4. Glaucomatous optic neuropathy is often seen.
5. Characteristic visual field defects of POAG may be found.

## Differential Diagnosis

Chronic open-angle glaucoma

## Diagnosis

1. Clinical picture resembling chronic open-angle glaucoma with moderate rise of IOP
2. A closed-angle on gonioscopy
3. Indentation gonioscopy shows presence of permanent PAS.

## Treatment

1. In the presence of extensive PAS, laser iridotomy is not effective.
2. Majority of patients with chronic PACG are managed by trabeculectomy.

## 6.6 UVEITIC GLAUCOMA

### Etiology

1. The IOP may be raised in anterior uveitis due to obstruction of trabeculum by inflammatory cells and debris, trabeculitis, plasmoid aqueous and trabecular endothelial cells dysfunction.
2. The secondary glaucoma in chronic anterior uveitis may result from extensive peripheral anterior synechiae or pupillary block (seclusio pupillae and occlusiopupillae).

## Symptoms

Red eye, photophobia, mild pain, and decreased vision may occur.

## Signs

1. Characteristic signs of acute anterior uveitis such as ciliary flush, keratic precipitates (KPs), flare and cells in the aqueous are usually present.
2. The miotic irregular pupil, posterior synechiae, iris bombé and an increased IOP are important features.
3. The angle of the anterior chamber is open with occasional peripheral anterior synechiae (Fig. 6.9) and trabecular pigmentation.
4. In chronic cases, extensive PAS, ring synechia, occlusio pupillae, high pressure glaucoma and typical glaucomatous optic atrophy may develop.

## Differential Diagnosis

1. Steroid glaucoma (*Refer* 6.7)
2. Fuchs heterochromic iridocyclitis (*Refer* 5.3)
3. Glaucomatocyclitic crisis (*Refer* 5.4)

## Diagnosis

1. History may point at the nature of uveitis and secondary glaucoma
2. Clinical evidence of anterior uveitis and baseline IOP.

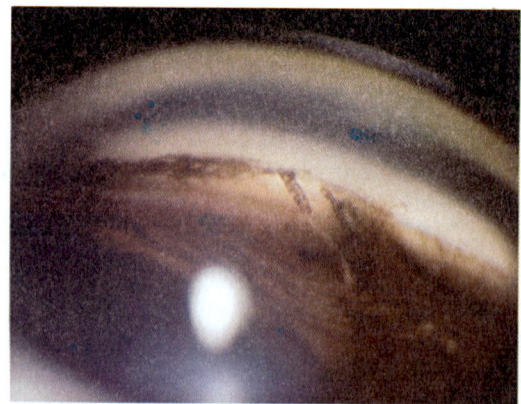

**Fig. 6.9:** Peripheral anterior synechiae

## Treatment

1. Use cycloplegic (twice a day) in spite of raised IOP
2. Topical prednisolone (1%, 4 times a day) is often used in the treatment of acute anterior uveitis. It should be gradually tapered.
3. In steroid responder glaucoma, steroid must be tapered during a short period and additional pressure lowering therapy should be instituted.
4. Topical timolol (0.5%, twice a day) or brimonidine (0.15–0.2%, thrice a day) or dorzolamide (2%, thrice a day) is used to reduce the IOP.
5. The use of pilocarpine and prostaglandin analogs is contraindicated in active uveitis.
6. If pressure is high, oral acetazolamide (500 mg twice a day) or mannitol 20% (1–2 g/kg, IV, over 45 minutes) should be administered.
7. If patient (with extensive PAS) is not responding to maximal medical therapy, trabeculectomy with adjunct antifibrotic agent (MMC) is indicated.

## 6.7 STEROID-INDUCED GLAUCOMA

### Etiology

1. Steroid administered topically, periocularly, orally or intravitreally causes an elevation of IOP in 5% of the general population.
2. The myocilin gene of POAG has some role in responsiveness to steroids.
3. Dexamethasone causes higher rise of IOP as compared to soft steroids.
4. The mechanism of rise of IOP after the use of corticosteroids is due to reduced facility of outflow of the pigmented trabeculum.
5. Accumulation of polymerized glycosaminoglycans (GAG) in the trabeculum, suppression of phagocytic activity, and inhibition of synthesis of prostaglandins are implicated in reduced aqueous outflow and rise in IOP.
6. Patients with POAG, high myopia, diabetes, and individuals with family history of glaucoma are at a higher risk of developing glaucoma.

### Symptoms

1. Patients are symptom-free initially
2. Some of them may present with marked pain, colored halos, blurred vision, lacrimation and redness.

### Signs

1. Eye remains white in spite of increased IOP.
2. The angle of the anterior chamber is open.
3. Long-standing cases show characteristic changes of POAG in the optic nerve head.
4. Similarly, typical visual field defects of POAG are found.
5. Patients with sudden and acute rise of IOP show ciliary flush and corneal edema.
6. Signs of associated inflammatory ocular disease, for which steroids are prescribed, are also present.

### Differential Diagnosis

1. POAG
2. Open-angle inflammatory glaucoma.

### Diagnosis

1. History of use of steroids and positive family history
2. Slit-lamp examination to exclude inflammatory glaucoma
3. Fundus examination for classical optic disk changes
4. Visual field defects.

### Treatment

1. Defer use of potent water soluble corticosteroids (dexamethasone or betamethasone) for minor eye ailments.
2. Less potent steroids like medrysone, loteprednol or fluromethalone should be preferred.
3. Topical NSAIDs [ketorolac (0.4–0.5%) or diclofenac (0.1%)] can be used in place of corticosteroids.

6

4. Topical beta-blockers and/or systemic acetazolamide effectively lower IOP.

5. If medical therapy cannot control IOP following depot steroid injection, the steroid may be excised.

6. Similarly, intravitreal triamcinolone can be removed by pars plana vitrectomy.

7. Trabeculectomy should be performed if hypotensive drugs fail to control high IOP.

## 6.8 PIGMENT DISPERSION GLAUCOMA

### Etiology

1. Pigment dispersion glaucoma (PDG) is a secondary open-angle glaucoma that affects mostly young myopic males (65%) in third to fifth decades.

2. It is inherited in autosomal recessive manner and gene responsible for PDG is mapped on the long arm of chromosome 7 (7q35–36).

3. The pathomechanism of pigment dispersion is not clear. It is presumed that pigment granules are shed from the posterior surface of the iris due to rubbing with zonules.

4. The trabecular meshwork is blocked by the released pigments.

### Symptoms

Patients with PDS are initially asymptomatic but later complain of headache, colored halos around lights especially after exercise or dilation of pupil and blurring of vision.

### Signs

1. Presence of vertically-oriented pigment granules (Krukenberg spindle) on the corneal endothelium.

2. Pigment cells may be seen in the aqueous humor.

3. The plane of the iris may appear concave.

4. Midperipheral iris transillumination defects in a radial spoke-like pattern corresponding to the irido-zonular contact.

5. IOP is elevated and shows large fluctuations.

6. Gonioscopy shows open-angle with homogeneous heavy pigmentation of the trabecular meshwork (Fig. 6.10) and pigment dusting along the Schwalbe's line. It may also reveal a more posterior insertion of the iris and concave appearance of iris.

7. Pigment deposition may be seen on the posterior equatorial lens surface (Scheie line), at the junction of zonules with the posterior capsule (Scheie strip) and on the hyaloid face.

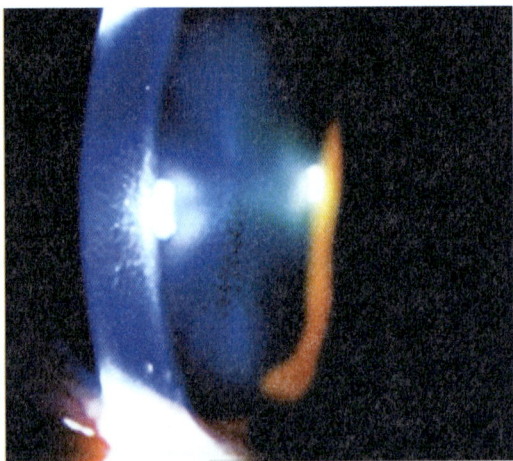

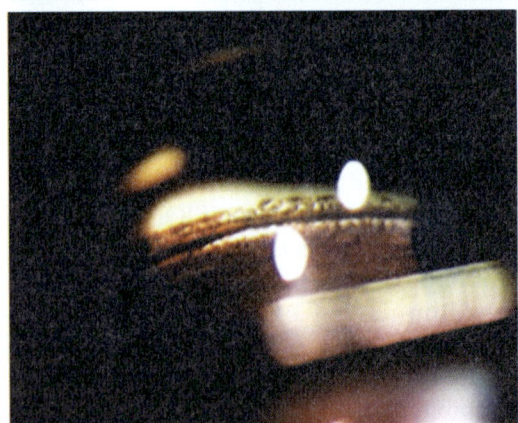

Fig. 6.10: Pigment dispersion glaucoma: Pigmentary dispersion in the AC and heavy pigmentation in the trabeculum (*Courtesy:* Dr Rajul Parikh, Shreeji eye care, Mumbai)

8. Glaucomatous optic neuropathy can develop if IOP is not controlled.

9. Lattice degeneration (20%) and retinal tears (11.7%) are more frequent in patients with PDS.

### Differential Diagnosis

1. Anterior uveitis
2. Pseudoexfoliation syndrome

### Diagnosis

1. Slit-lamp examination for Krukenberg spindle
2. Transillumination test
3. Tonometry
4. Gonioscopy for pigmentation in the angle
5. Dilated fundus examination
6. Ultrasound biomicroscopy (USM) for concave configuration of iris.

### Treatment

1. Pilocarpine is effective in reducing the IOP, and minimizing irido-zonuar contact. It should be used with caution in eyes with lattice degeneration.
2. Beta-blockers and CAIs can control the pressure.
3. Laser iridotomy can lower IOP, reverse pupillary block and the posterior bowing of iris.
4. Selective laser trabeculectomy is a preferred technique to control IOP in PDS.
5. Filtration surgery may be needed in those patients where other treatment modalities fail to reduce IOP.

## 6.9 PSEUDOEXFOLIATION GLAUCOMA

### Etiology

1. Pseudoexfoliation is an age-related disorder of extracellular matrix of basement membrane of unknown etiology. The pseudoexfoliative material is basically a fibrillar elastotic material produced in pre-equatorial lens epithelial cells, nonpigmented ciliary epithelium and trabecular endothelium due to oxidative stress.

2. Prevalence of pseudoexfoliation increases with age and it is more common in males.

3. The incidence of pseudoexfoliation is high in Scandinavian and some European countries.

4. Pseudoexfoliation (PEX) syndrome is inherited in an autosomal dominant manner.

5. Sequence variation in the lysyl oxidase-1 protein (LOXL1) gene is implicated in its etiology because it catalyzes the formation of elastin fibers.

6. Glaucoma in pseudoexfoliation occurs due to obstruction of drainage channels by the material.

7. Open-angle glaucoma may be found in about 50% cases of pseudoexfoliation syndrome.

### Symptoms

Initially, the condition is symptom-free but subsequently symptoms of increased IOP may develop.

### Signs

1. *Lens:* The dandruff-like material deposited on the anterior capsule of lens is the most consistent feature (Fig. 6.11). The material forms three distinct zones: (1) a homogeneous zone near the pupillary margin, (2) a granular peripheral zone and (3) a clear zone separating the two due to rubbing of iris. Nuclear opacities, phakodonesis and spontaneous subluxation or dislocation of lens are common.

2. *Iris:* Pseudoexfoliative material is prominently seen on pupillary border. The pupil becomes rigid to dilatation due to dilator muscle atrophy. Pigment loss from iris leads to iris transillumination defects.

3. *Angle of anterior chamber:* A dense pigment deposition on the trabecular meshwork is found more marked inferiorly than

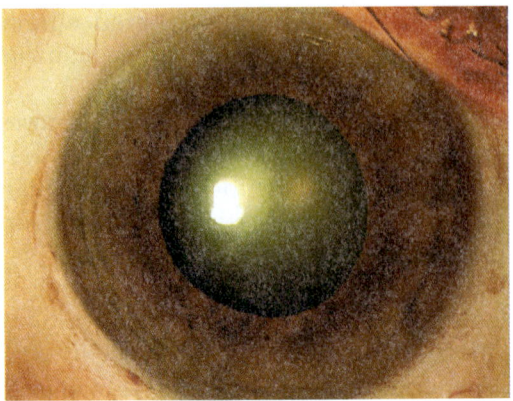

**Fig. 6.11:** Pseudoexfoliative material on the iris and lens (*Courtesy:* Dr Sushmita Kaushik, Associate Professor, PGI, Chandigarh)

superiorly. The pigments are arranged in a linear fashion anterior to Schwalbe's line (*Sampaolesi's line*). The magnitude of IOP elevation is correlated to the amount of pigmentation and exfoliated material.

4. Cornea: The corneal endothelium cell count is lower than normal and white flakes of the material may be found on it.
5. Zonules and ciliary body: Cycloscopy may reveal deposition of pseudoexfoliative material on zonules and ciliary body earlier than lens deposits making zonules more friable.
6. Vitreous and retina: The material may be detected in vitreous and on the retinal surface.
7. Optic nerve: Optic disk in patients with pseudoexfoliative glaucoma is small and shows bilateral asymmetrical optic neuropathy.

### Differential Diagnosis

1. True exfoliation or capsular delamination: It occurs due to trauma or exposure to intense heat seen in cases of glass blowers cataract. The condition is not associated with secondary glaucoma.
2. Uveitic glaucoma
3. Pigment dispersion glaucoma
4. POAG.

### Diagnosis

1. The clinical evidence of deposition of pseudoexfoliative material on iris, anterior capsule of the lens and trabecular meshwork.
2. An elevated IOP
3. Transillumination defects in iris
4. Exclude pigmentary, uveitic glaucomas and true exfoliation
5. Increased concentration of transforming growth factor (TGF-1) in aqueous.

### Treatment

1. Treatment of glaucoma associated with pseudoexfoliation is difficult.
2. Pilocarpine is the first line of treatment because it increases the aqueous outflow and clears the pseudoexfoliative material and pigments from the angle. It controls pigment liberation by miosis. A combination of pilocarpine with timolol has an additive effect.
3. Laser trabeculoplasty or selective laser trabeculoplasty can be effective.
4. Pseudoexfoliative glaucoma with PACG is often dealt with laser iridotomy.
5. The nonresponsive cases can be managed with trabeculectomy.
6. PEX syndrome patients with cataract if subjected to cataract extraction with IOL implantation may develop complications such as subluxation of lens, vitreous loss, and decentering of IOL due to weak zonules.

### 6.10 PLATEAU IRIS SYNDROME

### Etiology

1. Anatomically, the iris plane is flat and peripheral iris is very close to trabecular meshwork.
2. In plateau iris syndrome, the ciliary processes are situated anteriorly. They push the peripheral iris forward and cause crowding of the angle of the anterior chamber.

3. A tendency for pupillary block is not a predominant mechanism.

4. Dilatation of pupil may precipitate angle-closure due to crowding of the peripheral iris and obstruct the angle.

5. The glaucoma is seen in young (between 30 and 50 years) hyperopic females who have undergone even the laser iridotomy.

## Symptoms

More often it is an asymptomatic condition but pain, redness, watering and blurring of vision can manifest with acute rise of IOP.

## Signs

1. Anterior chamber is deep in the center and shallow in the periphery due to convexity of the peripheral iris.

2. Moderate rise of IOP with chronic angle-closure and high IOP during acute attack (after dilatation of pupil) are seen.

3. Gonioscopy shows crowded angle with double hump sign on indentation (the first hump is the normal convexity of iris and the second due to anterior rotation of ciliary body).

## Differential Diagnosis

Acute angle-closure glaucoma.

## Diagnosis

1. Deep anterior chamber in the center with flat iris in young people with increased IOP.

2. Bilateral anteriorly placed ciliary processes and convex peripheral iris on gonioscopy.

3. UBM of the angle structures.

4. Evaluation of optic disk.

5. Visual fields.

## Treatment

1. All cases of plateau iris should be closely examined for the development of acute attack of closed-angle glaucoma.

2. Periodic examination of IOP, gonioscopy and optic nerve is mandatory.

3. Patients with a tendency for angle-closure glaucoma should undergo argon laser peripheral iridoplasty.

4. Acute angle-closure glaucoma should be managed by medical treatment with pilocarpine.

5. If extensive PAS are formed, trabeculectomy should be preferred.

## 6.11 PHACOGENIC GLAUCOMA

Lens-induced or phacogenic glaucoma can be seen with both open-angle and closed angle of the anterior chamber.

## Types

Lens-induced open-angle glaucoma can be of following types:

1. Phacolytic
2. Lens particle glaucoma
3. Phacomorphic glaucoma
4. Glaucoma associated with dislocation of lens.

### Phacolytic Glaucoma

#### Etiology

Phakolytic glaucoma is caused by leaking lens proteins in the anterior chamber from hypermature cataract. The liberated proteins are phagocytosed by macrophages; they block the trabeculum.

#### Symptoms

Ocular pain, redness, watering, photophobia, blurring of vision and colored halos are common.

#### Signs

1. Phacolytic glaucoma has rapid onset with acute rise of IOP.

2. Corneal epithelial edema with heavy flare and a few cells seen in the aqueous.

3. Circulating iridescent particles, small white tags of lens material, and macrophages may be found in the anterior chamber.

4. White patches (macrophages) on the anterior capsule of the cataractous lens may appear.

5. Gonioscopy may reveal clumps of swollen macrophages in the open-angle of the anterior chamber.

### Differential Diagnosis

1. Lens particle glaucoma
2. Uveitic glaucoma
3. Acute angle-closure glaucoma.

### Diagnosis

1. Characteristic clinical picture
2. Presence of macrophages in the open-angle of the chamber in the inferior part
3. Demonstration of engorged macrophages with engulfed lens material in the aqueous tap.

### Treatment

1. Use a mild cycloplegic [homatropine (2%)]
2. Topical timolol (0.5%, twice/day) or brimonidine (0.15–0.2%, thrice/day) helps to reduce IOP.
3. Topical prednisolone (1%) is frequently used for a short-time
4. Majority of patients need oral acetazolamide (500–1,000 mg/day) and/or mannitol (1–2 g/kg IV)
5. If IOP does not come under control with maximal medical therapy, cataract extraction is performed after paracentesis.

### Lens Particle Glaucoma

### Etiology

1. Lens particle glaucoma is caused by liberation of the lens particles in the anterior chamber following extracapsular cataract surgery or trauma.
2. The liberated lens material blocks aqueous outflow channels and cause elevated IOP.

### Symptoms

Symptoms include ocular pain, red eye, watering, blurred vision and photophobia.

### Signs

1. Conjunctival and ciliary congestions with corneal edema
2. Presence of white fluffy particles of lens cortex in the anterior chamber with cells and flare
3. Increased IOP
4. A break in the anterior capsule is found in patients with a history of trauma.
5. The angle of anterior chamber is open.

### Differential Diagnosis

Phacolytic glaucoma.

### Diagnosis

1. History of trauma or surgery
2. Lens particles in the aqueous humor
3. Increased IOP with open-chamber angle.

### Treatment

1. Timolol (0.5%, 2 times/day) or brimonidine (0.15–0.2%, 3 times/day) can reduce the IOP.
2. Oral acetazolamide (500–1,000 mg/day) is often given to control high IOP.
3. In nonresponding cases, surgical removal of cortical lens matter is indicated.

### Phacomorphic Glaucoma

### Etiology

1. The phakomorphic glaucoma is caused by a combination of relative closure of the angle of anterior chamber as a result of swelling of lens during intumescent stage of cataract and forward displacement of lens-iris diaphragm resulting in pupillary block.
2. The disease is common in old age and affects patients with small hyperopic eyes.

## Symptoms

Symptoms include pain, redness and decreased vision.

## Signs

1. Conjunctival and ciliary injections
2. Corneal edema and significant loss of a number of corneal endothelial cells
3. Shallow anterior chamber due to progressive swelling of lens
4. Sudden rise of IOP
5. Intumescent cataract with progressive increase in A-P diameter of lens.
6. Long-standing attack can lead to synechial closure of the angle.
7. Optic neuropathy develops in untreated cases.
8. Occasionally, an anterior chamber inflammatory reaction may be found.

## Differential Diagnosis

Primary closed-angle glaucoma.

## Diagnosis

1. Clinical evidence of shallow anterior chamber, large size of lens, forward displacement of iris-lens diaphragm, angle closure and increased IOP help in diagnosis.
2. UBM is helpful in showing actual size and position of lens, and configuration of the angle of the anterior chamber.

## Treatment

1. The management of phacomorphic glaucoma includes medical control of IOP with topical timolol 0.5%, twice daily, oral CAIs and hyperosmotic agents.
2. Control of inflammation by topical corticosteroid and hypertonic saline for corneal edema.
3. A laser iridotomy may prevent angle-closure attack.
4. Once IOP is controlled and eye becomes quiet, cataract surgery is performed.
5. The patient of phacomorphic glaucoma with extensive PAS needs cataract extraction with trabeculectomy.

6. Nonresponding cases need glaucoma valve implantation to decrease IOP.

## Glaucoma Associated with Subluxated or Dislocated Lens

### Etiology

1. The etiology of subluxation or dislocation of lens is congenital or acquired.
2. Congenital subluxation of lens is usually found in ectopia lentis, Marfan syndrome, Weill-Marchesani syndrome and homocystinuria.
3. Acquired causes include trauma, high axial myopia, pseudoexfoliative glaucoma, etc.
4. The dislocated lens, especially in Weill-Marchesani syndrome, causes pupillary block.

### Symptoms

Monocular diplopia, loss of vision, red eye, and ocular pain may develop.

### Signs

1. A subluxated lens presents irregular depth of anterior chamber, segmental iridodonesis, phakodonesis and monocular diplopia (Fig. 6.12).
2. A dislocated lens in the anterior chamber may block the outflow of aqueous humor at the pupil and cause acute rise in IOP.
3. A dislocation of the lens into the vitreous cavity induces inflammation. The inflammatory cells or degenerated lens material in the anterior chamber can block the trabecular meshwork resulting in the rise of IOP.

### Diagnosis

1. Slit-lamp examination can diagnose anterior dislocation or subluxation of lens
2. Dilated funduscopy
3. B-scan ultrasonography
4. UBM of the anterior segment
5. OCT helps in evaluation of macula and examining the anterior segment structures.

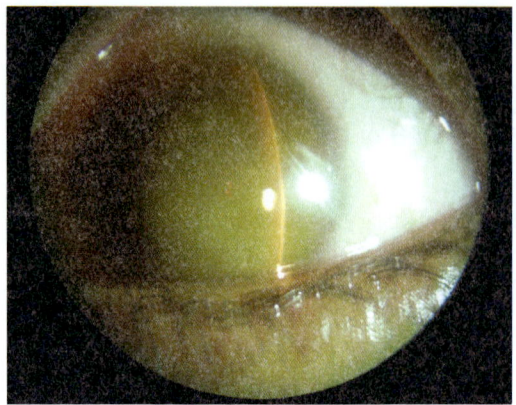

**Fig. 6.12:** Secondary glaucoma due to subluxation of lens

## Treatment

1. Dislocation of the lens into the anterior chamber warrants early removal to prevent endothelial damage.
2. A laser iridotomy relieves the pupillary block.
3. In patients with subluxated lens extraction with intraocular lens (IOL) implantation with capsular tension ring is indicated to restore the vision.

## 6.12 TRAUMATIC ANGLE-RECESSION GLAUCOMA

### Etiology

1. A blunt trauma may cause recession of the angle of the anterior chamber.
2. Unilateral nontraumatic angle recession of unknown etiology may also occur.
3. Hyphema causes early onset glaucoma while late onset glaucoma is the result of development of PAS and trabecular fibrosis.

### Symptoms

Initially, the condition is asymptomatic but later ocular discomfort and decreased vision or loss of vision may present.

### Signs

1. The angle recession glaucoma is usually a chronic disease.

2. It is a unilateral open-angle glaucoma with moderate to severe rise of IOP.
3. Gonioscopy shows a broad angle recess, retroflexion of torn iris, a depression in trabeculum and scleral spur.
4. Later the angle of the anterior chamber may show fibrosis of trabecular meshwork and extensive PAS.
5. Other findings include corneal edema, iris atrophy, sphincter tear, cataract and optic atrophy.

### Diagnosis

1. History of trauma
2. Classical gonioscopy picture
3. UBM can confirm the recession of the angle of anterior chamber.

### Treatment

1. A moderate rise of IOP following recession of the angle can be managed by aqueous suppressants, hypotensive lipids and carbonic anhydrase inhibitors.
2. In severe cases, medical therapy is ineffective and a filtering operation becomes necessary.

## 6.13 HEMOLYTIC AND GHOST CELL GLAUCOMA

### Etiology

1. Hemolytic and ghost cell glaucoma are caused by vitreous hemorrhage. IOP is elevated due to blockage of trabeculum by hemoglobin-filled macrophages and ghost cells.
2. In old vitreous hemorrhage, the red blood cells degenerate to form ghost cells. The ghost cells are hollow in appearance, khaki colored and rigid. They block trabecular meshwork and produce *ghost cell glaucoma*.
3. The ghost cell glaucoma is mostly seen in aphakic eyes.

### Symptoms

Symptoms are ocular pain, decreased vision and colored halos.

## Signs

1. Tan-colored cells in the aqueous humor
2. Increased IOP and the angle of the anterior chamber is open
3. Presence of ghost cells in the chamber angle
4. Old hemorrhage in the vitreous.

## Diagnosis

1. History of trauma or intraocular surgery causing vitreous hemorrhage
2. Gonioscopy shows ghost cell in the angle.

## Treatment

1. Medical therapy with aqueous suppressants is effective.
2. Some patients may need anterior chamber irrigation, or pars plana vitrectomy to clear the vitreous hemorrhage.
3. In nonresponding cases with increased IOP, a filtering surgery is recommended.

## 6.14 POSTOPERATIVE PSEUDOPHAKIC GLAUCOMA

### Etiology

1. A transient rise of IOP is seen following cataract surgery due to retained viscoelastic material, mild hyphema, pigment dispersion, particles of lens matter and mild inflammatory reaction to surgery.
2. Pupillary block can also occur after anterior chamber IOL implantation.

### Symptoms

Ocular discomfort, watering, pain, and blurred vision or loss of vision may occur.

### Signs

1. Shallow irregular anterior chamber
2. Increased IOP
3. Iris bombé
4. Posterior synechiae with IOL
5. Retained cortex
6. Uveitis glaucoma hyphema (UGH) syndrome can develop in patients with IOL implantation in the anterior chamber.

## Diagnosis

1. History of cataract operation
2. Characteristic clinical picture
3. UBM shows pupillary block and position of lens.

## Treatment

1. Postoperative inflammation is managed by topical use of cyclopentolate (1%, 2–3 times a day) or phenylepherine (2.5%, 3–4 times), and prednisolone (1%, 4–6 times a day).
2. Topical timolol (0.5%, twice a day) or brimonidine (0.15–0.2%, 3 times a day) is used to lower the IOP.
3. If IOP is very high and does not respond to timolol and brimonidine, oral acetazolamide (500 mg twice a day) should be added.
4. Pupillary block can be managed by multiple laser iridotomies.
5. A persistent postoperative flat anterior chamber should be reformed without any delay to prevent corneal endothelial damage.
6. In patients with UGH syndrome, IOL exchange may be considered.
7. Vitreous hemorrhage may require pars plana vitrectomy.

## 6.15 MALIGNANT GLAUCOMA

### Etiology

1. Malignant glaucoma follows surgeries for angle-closure glaucoma, cataract, retinal detachment, etc in patients with relatively small anterior segment.
2. It is caused by the anterior rotation of ciliary processes resulting in posterior misdirection of aqueous humor.
3. Accumulation of aqueous in the vitreous cavity results in a forward shift of iris-lens or IOL diaphragm. It is also known as *posterior aqueous diversion syndrome*.

### Symptoms

Moderate to severe ocular pain, redness, watering and photophobia are common.

## Signs

1. The anterior chamber is very shallow or flat. Lens or vitreous bulges forward.
2. Ciliary processes are visible through iridectomy hole.
3. An acute increase in IOP
4. An aqueous zone may be visible in the vitreous.

## Differential Diagnosis

1. Acute angle-closure glaucoma
2. Pupillay block glaucoma
3. Choroidal detachment or hemorrhage
4. Postoperative wound leak.

## Diagnosis

1. History of operation on an eye with small anterior segment
2. Flat anterior chamber with forward bulge of iris-lens (IOL) diaphragm
3. Slit-lamp examination can reveal the status of iridotomy/iridectomy (open or plugged)
4. Seidel test to rule out wound leak
5. B-scan USG to locate aqueous pockets in vitreous and rule out choroidal detachment
6. UBM can confirm the anterior rotation of ciliary processes.

## Treatment

1. Topical atropine (1%, 3 times a day)
2. Topical timolol (0.5%, twice a day) and brimonidine (0.15–0.2%, 3 times a day) are used to reduce IOP.
3. Acetazolamide (oral 250 mg, 4 times a day or IV 500 mg, twice daily) is an effective hypotensive agent.
4. If IOP is still raised after giving acetazolamide, mannitol 20%, 1–2 g/kg IV should be used.
5. A peripheral iridectomy is likely to break the attack of malignant glaucoma with deepening of the anterior chamber.
6. In recalcitrant cases, disrupt the posterior capsule of the lens and anterior hyaloid face

by YAG laser to restore normal flow of aqueous.
7. Vitrectomy helps in cutting the anterior hyaloid face, removing aqueous pockets and endophotocoagulation of the ciliary processes.

## 6.16 NEOVASCULAR GLAUCOMA

## Etiology

1. Neovascular glaucoma (NVG) is caused by a growth of fibrovascular membrane over anterior chamber angle associated with neovascularization of iris.
2. In patients with central retinal vein occlusion, diabetic retinopathy, Eales disease, ocular ischemic syndrome and intraocular tumors, vascular endothelial growth factors are released due to ischemia, causing neovascularization.

## Symptoms

Initially, patients remain asymptomatic. Later complain of pain, redness, photophobia, floaters, decreased vision or even sudden loss of vision.

## Signs

1. In early stage, new vessels appear along the pupillary margin and over the trabecular meshwork of open-angle (Fig. 6.13).
2. After sometime, new vessels appear on the surface of the iris (*rubeosis iridis*)
3. Moderate to acute rise of IOP occurs
4. Ciliary injection and corneal edema appear
5. A few cells and flare are seen in the aqueous humor
6. Recurrent hyphema may occur.
7. Gonioscopically, a fibrovascular membrane covering the trabecular meshwork is seen.
8. The membrane drags the peripheral part of iris and forms synechiae at the level of Schawlbe's line resulting in partial closure of the angle.

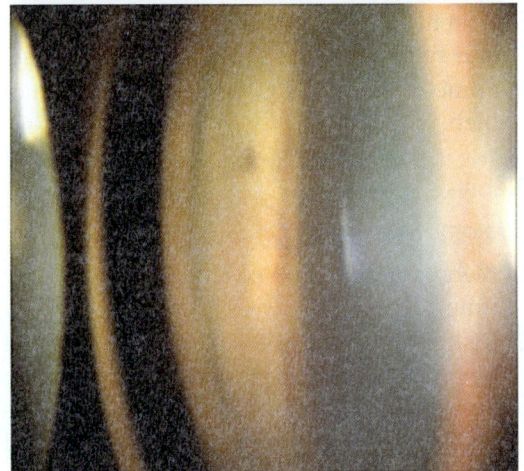

**Fig. 6.13:** Neovascular glaucoma: Neovascularization of iris and the angle of the anterior chamber (*Courtesy:* Dr Rajul Parikh, Shreeji Eye care, Mumbai)

9. Untreated cases develop optic nerve damage and visual field defects.

### Differential Diagnosis

1. Uveitic glaucoma
2. Acute angle-closure glaucoma.

### Diagnosis

1. History of diabetes mellitus (DM) or ocular vascular disorders
2. Presence of neovascularization of iris and fibrovascular membrane in the angle, and increased IOP
3. Dilated fundus examination for PDR, long standing RD, and other retinal vascular or malignant conditions

4. Fundus fluorescein angiography (FFA) confirms the retinal pathology
5. Carotid Doppler to rule out carotid stenosis
6. If media are opaque, B-scan USG can diagnose intraocular hemorrhage and retinal detachment and other ocular conditions responsible for NVG.

### Treatment

1. Topical prednisolone (1%, 4 times/day) and atropine (1%, 3 times/day) reduce inflammation and pain.
2. Topical timolol (0.5%), brimonidine (0.15%, 3 times/day) and oral acetazolamide (500 mg twice a day) may reduce IOP.
3. Retinal ischemia can be treated by panretinal photocoagulation and direct goniophotocoagulation with green laser.
4. Regression of neovascularization of iris and angle should be attempted by ranibizumab or bevacizumab injection.
5. Tube-shunt procedure like (Ahmed, Molteno valve implantation) may control IOP.
6. In blind and painful eye an external or endocyclophotocoagulation or trans-scleral cyclocryopexy may help to reduce IOP and relieve pain. The procedure may be complicated by phthisis bulbi.

## 6.17 POSTOPERATIVE COMPLICATIONS OF BLEB

The important complications of bleb are:
1. Nonfiltering bleb
2. Overfiltering bleb
3. Blebitis.

### Nonfiltering Bleb

#### *Etiology*

Two main causes of nonfiltering bleb after trabeculectomy are:
1. A tight suturing of trabeculectomy flap can cause occlusion of external filtration.
2. Internal filtration from sclerostomy may be blocked by iris, vitreous, blood-fibrin clot or viscoelastic material.

6

## Symptoms

Postoperative ocular discomfort with decrease vision may occur.

## Signs

Anterior chamber is deep and IOP is increased.

## Treatment

1. Apply point pressure on the anterior edge of the bleb
2. Tight flap sutures should be released by laser suturolysis or surgically
3. Blocked sclerostomy by blood or fibrin gets cleared with time. However, intracameral injection of tissue plasminogen (10 µg) may clear it early.
4. Blocked sclerostomy can be cleared by YAG laser.

## Overfiltering Bleb

### Etiology

A large thin bleb, leaking bleb, and rupture of bleb are not infrequent with the use of MMC or 5-fluorouracil during trabeculectomy.

### Symptoms

The patient complains of decreased vision and is not comfortable even 6–8 weeks after surgery.

### Signs

1. A large bleb is associated with deep anterior chamber and stable IOP.
2. Gradually, the anterior chamber becomes shallow with decrease in IOP.
3. The anterior chamber is flat with no bleb.
4. Gonioscopy may reveal cyclodialysis cleft.
5. Dilated fundus examination often shows presence of serous choroidal detachment and hypotony maculopathy and optic neuropathy.

## Treatment

1. Use of topical atropine (1%, 2 times/day), and autologous blood injection in a large bleb may check the overfiltration.
2. If anterior chamber is very shallow, attempt should be made to reform the chamber with intracameral viscoelastic material and use topical atropine.
3. Leaking wound should be repaired.
4. Cyclodialysis cleft is managed by laser application.
5. Urgent drainage in choroidal detachment and reformation of the anterior chamber.
6. Some of the patients may need revision of bleb.

## Blebitis

### Etiology

1. Blebitis or infection of bleb may occur any time.
2. Risk factors for blebitis include presence of blepharitis, conjunctivitis, thin and cystic bleb, bleb leak, use of antimetabolite in the surgery, contact lens wear and location of bleb at the lower limbus.
3. Early infection is commonly caused by *Staphylococcus epidermidis* and *Staphylococcus aureus.*
4. Organisms responsible for late infection include *Streptococcus, Haemophilus, Pseudomonas, Moraxella*, etc.

### Symptoms

1. Mild blebitis causes red eye, discharge, ocular discomfort and photophobia.
2. Blebitis associated with postoperative endophthalmitis produces severe symptoms such as intense pain, and marked swelling of eye, photophobia, decreased vision or loss of vision.

### Signs

1. Mild blebitis presents localized injection of conjunctival vessels around the bleb, and

bleb appears dull with some collection of mucopus which may leak from it (Fig. 6.14).

2. Moderate blebitis is often associated with anterior chamber reaction such as flare and cells in the aqueous and hypopyon.

3. Severe blebitis presents a picture of postoperative endophthalmitis.

### Differential Diagnosis

1. Episcleritis
2. Anterior uveitis (*Refer 5.1*)
3. Endophthalmitis (*Refer 5.13*).

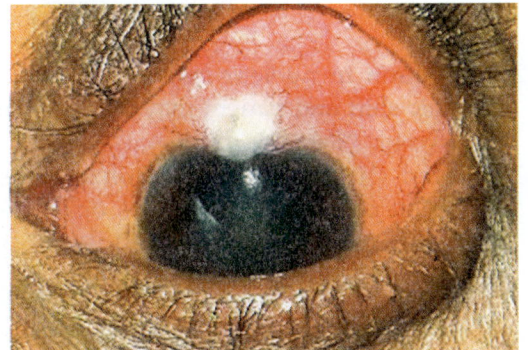

**Fig. 6.14:** Blebitis (*Courtesy:* Dr RP Mourya, Department of ophthalmology, IMS, BHU, Varanasi)

### Diagnosis

1. Slit-lamp examination of bleb, anterior chamber and vitreous
2. Seidel test to find bleb leak
3. Dilated fundus examination
4. Smear and culture from bleb discharge
5. B-scan USG is useful in finding the severity of vitreous involvement if corneal clarity is compromised.

### Treatment

1. Topical fortified cefazolin and amikacin used initially every 5 minutes followed by hourly can control mild to moderate blebitis.

2. Topical atropine (1%, twice a day) and systemic antibiotic based on culture-sensitivity of organism(s) should be added in patients with moderate blebitis. Topical steroids should be started one day after commencing the antibiotic therapy.

3. Severe blebitis is treated on the lines of postoperative endophthalmitis.

6

# Cataract and Optics

## 7.1 ACQUIRED CATARACT

### Etiology

1. The etiology of acquired cataract is not known. The cataract formation may occur due to hydration, denaturation of lens proteins and degeneration or slow sclerosis.
2. Genetic mutations may cause cataracts in families.
3. Intraocular inflammation, degeneration, ischemia, metabolic disorders can cause cataract.
4. Wilson's disease and skin diseases are often associated with cataract.
5. Senility, smoking, diarrhea, ocular trauma, X-rays, gamma rays, neutrons, infrared, ultraviolet rays, microwave, laser radiations, and drug toxicity are known risk factors.

### Symptoms

1. Initially, almost all patients remain symptom-free.
2. Glare, spots, multiple moons, distorted shape of objects and colored halos are symptoms.
3. A variable degree of visual impairment and difficulty in night driving are common.

### Signs

1. Fundus view becomes dull.

2. Refraction in nuclear cataract shows a myopic shift and patient may give up the presbyopic glasses.
3. Dilated slit-lamp examination reveals different configuration of lens opacities depending on types and etiology as described below.

### Senile Cataract

1. Senile cataract is the most common and usually seen in people above 60 years of age.
2. It manifests in three forms:
   - Cortical
   - Posterior subcapsular
   - Nuclear
   - **Senile cortical cataract:** It may present five stages:
     - *Stage of lamellar separation* is marked by the hydration of lens which separates lens fibers.
     - *Incipient stage* presents wedge-shaped opacities in the lens cortex.
     - *Intumescent stage* is characterized by progressive hydration swelling and opacification (Fig. 7.1).
     - *Mature cataract* presents a complete opacification of the lens (Fig. 7.2).
     - *Hypermature cataract* presents a soft and practically liquefied cortex and the hard nucleus may or may not sink to the bottom (Fig. 7.3).

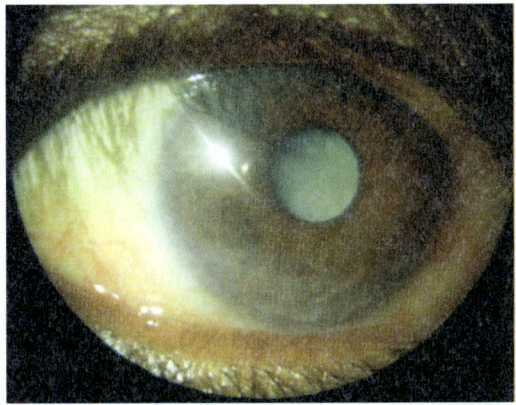

Fig. 7.1: Intumescent cataract

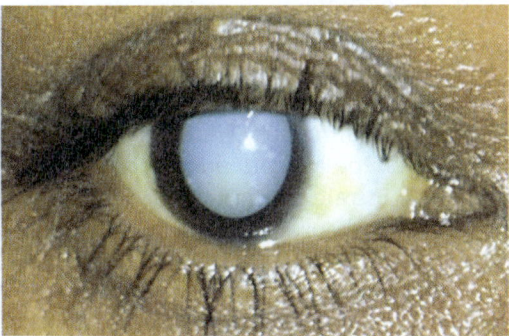

Fig. 7.2: Mature cataract

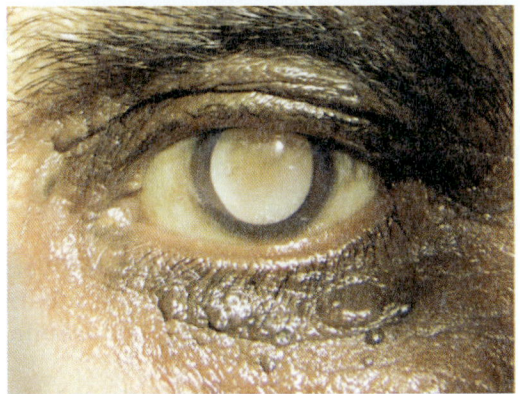

Fig. 7.3: Hypermature cataract

- It causes glare and poor vision.
- Slit-lamp examination reveals a granular or a plaque-like opacity (Fig. 7.4).

■ **Senile nuclear cataract**
  - Senile nuclear cataracts are often bilateral, and develop due to progressive sclerosis (Fig. 7.5).
  - Gradually the nucleus becomes hard and yellow.
  - The central part of the lens becomes completely opaque and later the opacity may also involve the peripheral cortex.
  - The lens may become brown, *cataracta brunescence* (Fig. 7.6) or black *(cataracta nigra)*.

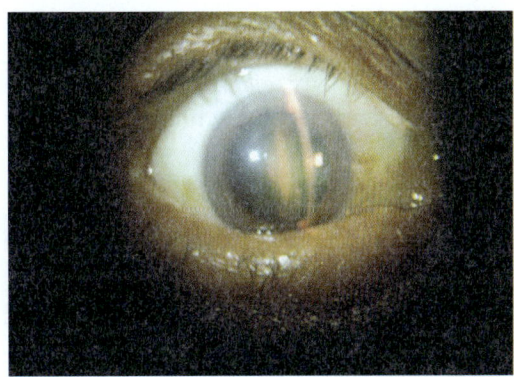

Fig. 7.4: Posterior subcortical cataract

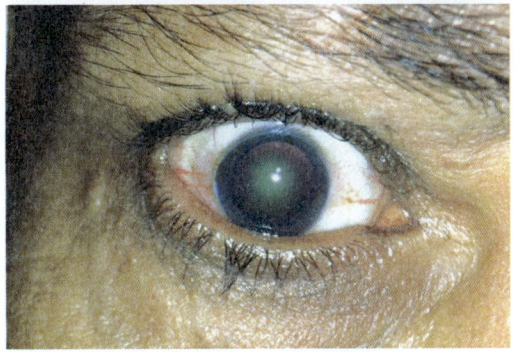

Fig. 7.5: Nuclear cataract

■ **Posterior subcapsular cataract**
  - Posterior subcapsular cataract is seen in the posterior cortex and situated axially.

7

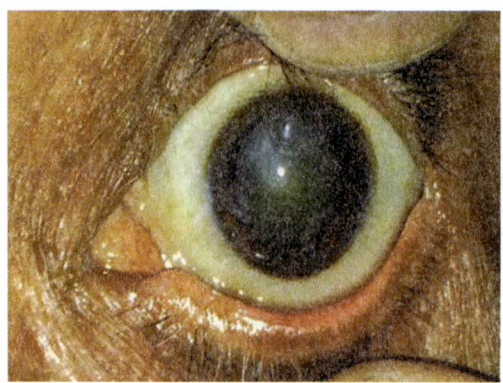

**Fig. 7.6:** Brown cataract

## Complicated Cataract

### Etiology

1. Both inflammatory and degenerative diseases of the eye can cause complicated cataract. Anterior uveitis is the main cause. Degenerative diseases include retinitis pigmentosa, high myopia, etc (Fig. 7.7).
2. Small lens opacity, *glaukomflecken*, may be seen after an attack of acute angle-closure glaucoma.

### Symptoms

Besides decrease in vision, symptoms of causative disease such as pain, watering and red eye in iridocyclitis, or night-blindness in retinitis pigmentosa (RP) are associated.

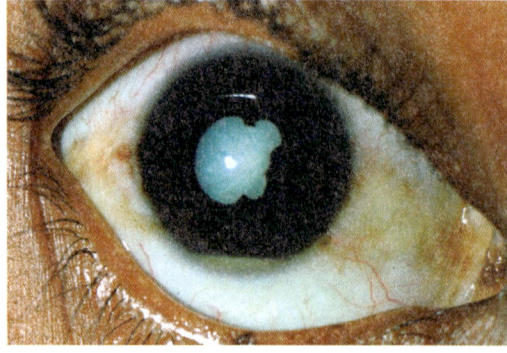

**Fig. 7.7:** Complicated cataract (*Courtesy:* Dr SR Rathinam, AEH, Madurai)

### Signs

1. Complicated cataract is situated near posterior pole resulting in marked impairment of vision.
2. Lens opacity shows irregular margins and polychromatic luster.
3. The complicated cataract may remain confined to the posterior cortex or occasionally, involve the entire lens.
4. A mature complicated cataract has a tendency for hypermaturity.

## Traumatic Cataract

### Etiology

1. Mechanical, electrical and chemical injuries can cause cataract.
2. A blunt injury to the eye can produce Vossius ring, cataract and dislocation of lens.
3. A concussion cataract takes a rosette- or stellate-shape and often located axially.
4. A small intralenticular foreign body may cause a focal cortical cataract.
5. The delayed effect of alkali burn is known to cause cortical cataract.
6. Open globe injury causes swelling of the lens and total cataract in a short-time.

## Radiation-Induced Cataract

1. Radiation can induce punctate opacities in the posterior capsule and cortex and feathery opacities in the anterior subcapsule.
2. The heat of infrared radiation can produce true exfoliation of capsule.

## Metabolic Cataract

1. Cataract can occur in metabolic disorders like diabetes, hypocalcemia and inborn errors of metabolism (galactosemia, Wilson's disease).
2. *Diabetic cataract* occurs in juvenile diabetes due to accumulation of sorbitol and fructose in the lens. It is progressive and characterized by the presence of snow-flake opacities in the anterior and posterior subcapsular regions.

3. *Tetanic cataract* is characterized by small, white, iridescent and discrete opacities in the cortex. These coalesce to form flakes.

4. *Wilson's disease cataract* has a sunflower pattern and appears in the anterior capsular region.

### Dermatogenic Cataract

1. *Atopic dermatitis* may show bilateral anterior subcapsular cataract in about 25% of young patients.

2. *Rothmund's syndrome* presents bilateral zonular cataract more frequently in females.

3. *Werner's syndrome* is characterized by premature senility, endocrine disturbances and bilateral posterior subcapsular cataract.

### Drug-Induced Cataract

1. *Corticosteroid cataract* can develop after prolonged use of topical, subconjunctival or systemic corticosteroids. They may be posterior subcapsular or cortical.

2. *Phenothiazine cataract* represents toxicity to the drug; it causes pigmented opacities in lens epithelium.

3. *Miotic cataract* can develop after prolonged topical pilocarpine therapy in about 20% glaucoma patients.

### Cataract in Myotonic Dystrophy

Red and green fine dust-like opacities develop in the lens cortex. They form stellate cataract known as Christmas tree cataract.

### Diagnosis and Evaluation of Cataract

- Visual loss should correspond to degree of lens opacity. Accompanying glaucoma or optic neuropathy can cause a dispropor-tionate visual loss.
- Color vision should be tested.
- Projection of light and pin-hole test or laser interferometry may help in assessing prognosis.
- Pupillary reactions and IOP must be recorded.

- Assess the grade of cataract after the dilatation of pupil to plan operative strategies.
- Exclude corneal dystrophy, pseudoex-foliation and phakodonesis by slit-lamp examination.
- Dilated fundus examination should be performed to evaluate status of macula, optic nerve and retina.
- B-scan ultrasonography is recommended if cataract is dense and fundus examination is not possible.
- Calculates the intraocular lens power for transplantation with the help of biometry.
- Specular microscopy determines the endothelial cell count. A preoperative low cell count may cause postoperative corneal decompensation.
- Patient's written consent must be obtained after informing risks and benefits of the cataract surgery.

### Treatment

1. Cataract surgery is the only treatment to restore vision.
2. Cataract extraction with IOL implantation is the operation of choice.

## 7.2 SUBLUXATION OR DISLOCATION OF LENS

### Etiology

1. When lens is not in its normal anatomical position, it is called subluxated or dislocated.

2. In subluxation the lens remains in the pupillary area, while the dislocated lens comes either in the anterior chamber or floats in the vitreous.

3. The lens may be found dislocated in ocular conditions like trauma, aniridia, ectopia lentis, ectopia lentis pupillae, buphthalmos and iris coloboma.

4. It may be subluxated in systemic disorders such as Marfan syndrome, Wiell-

Marchesani syndrome, homocystinuria and Ehlers-Danlos syndrome.

## Symptoms

Monocular diplopia, decreased vision and pain in eye may occur.

## Signs

1. The depth of the anterior chamber is irregular
2. Tremulousness of iris (iridodonesis)
3. Phacodonesis
4. Miotic rigid pupil
5. Presence of phakic and aphakic pupillary areas or complete absence of the lens
6. Presence of lens in the anterior chamber or in the vitreous, or rarely in the sub-conjunctival space
7. The displacement may be seen in any direction (Fig. 7.8).
8. It is displaced inferotemporally in ectopia lentis et pupillae and inferonasally in homocystinuria.
9. The lens is small in Weill-Marchesani syndrome (spherophakia) and it is displaced either anteriorly or inferiorly. Anterior displacement may cause pupillary block.
10. Intraocular pressure (IOP) may be raised.

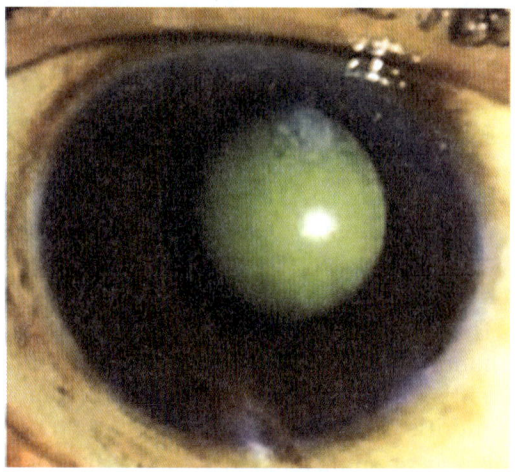

**Fig. 7.8:** Subluxated lens

## Diagnosis

1. Dilated retinoscopy reveals phakic and aphakic areas.
2. Slit-lamp examination can locate the site of dislocated lens.
3. Dilated funduscopy may detect the presence of lens in the posterior segment as well as retinal pathology.
4. B-scan ultrasonograhy and ultrasound bio-microscopy (UBM) are helpful in locating the lens and associated congenital anomalies.
5. Radiology is used to study skeletal abnor-malities found in Marfan and Weill-Marchesani syndromes.
6. Diagnosis of homocystinuria is confirmed by detecting disulfide including homo-cystine in the urine.

## Treatment

1. Patient with subluxated clear lens and dec-reased vision is given a spectacle correction.
2. Dislocated lens in the anterior chamber should be removed on emergency basis.
3. Dislocated lens in the vitreous body needs pars plana vitrectomy for lens removal.
4. Subluxated cataractous lens is operated using a capsular tension ring.

## 7.3 PSEUDOPHAKIA

1. An artificial intraocular lens (IOL) is usually implanted after cataract extraction, the condition is known as *pseudophakia*.
2. The refractive power of the lens is calcu-lated preoperatively to make the eye almost emmetropic (refractive cataract surgery).
    - *Types of IOL*
        - The implanted lens may be monofocal or bifocal or multifocal.
        - Monofocal IOLs correct mostly the distant vision while bifocals correct both distance and near vision.
        - Multifocal IOLs have an additional advantage of seeing at intermediate distance also.

- *Material of IOLs*
  - Lenses are made up of polymethyl methacrylate (PMMA), silicone or acrylic. Hybrid lenses are also available.
  - Poor quality material of the lens often induces intraocular reaction.
- *Design of IOLs*
  - IOLs have undergone many modifications to achieve improvement in implantation and obtaining excellent results.
  - The haptic is changed from J-curve to C-curve for better fixation contact.
  - Variable optic sizes from 5 mm to 7 mm to suit individuals.
  - Dialing holes are eliminated to reduce glare.
  - Biconvex optics and laser ridges to reduce posterior capsule opacification.
  - Soft foldable lens for small incision.
  - Bifocal, multifocal or accommodative lenses.
- *Sites of implantation*
  - *Anterior chamber:* Anterior chamber intraocular lenses (AC IOLs) are fixated on iris by clips or their flexible loops are rested in the chamber recess (Fig. 7.9).
  - *Posterior chamber implantation in the capsular bag* (Fig. 7.10): It is the most common site of implantation to gain excellent visual results with minimal complications.
  - *Sulcus:* IOL may be implanted in ciliary sulcus if in-the-bag implantation is not possible. The haptic may be sutured with the sclera or fixed with the glue.
- *Techniques of cataract removal*
  - Generally, small incision cataract surgery with phacoemulsification is commonly used technique for cataract removal.
  - Phacoemulsification is performed under the following steps:

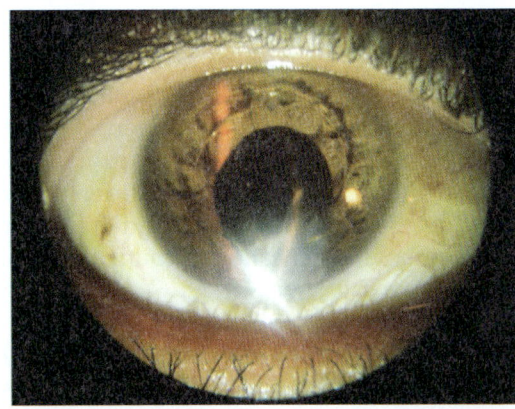
**Fig. 7.9:** Pseudophakia with AC IOL in a traumatic cataract

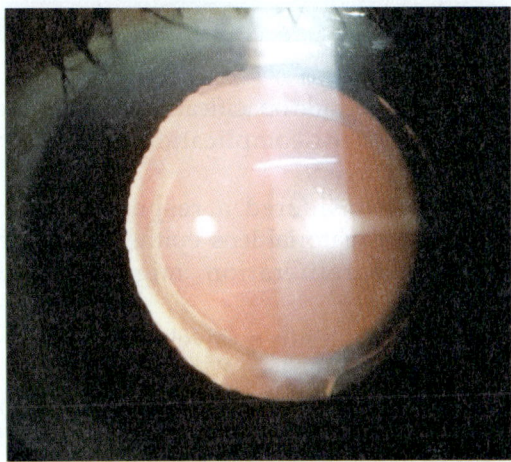
**Fig. 7.10:** PCIOL in the bag (*Courtesy:* Dr SCL Chandravanshi, SS Medical College, Rewa)

7

- ❖ A triplanar self-sealing 2.5–2.8 mm limbal incision
- ❖ Capsulorrhexis
- ❖ Removal of lens after hydrodissection, hydrodelineation and emulsification
- ❖ Irrigation and aspiration for removal of soft cortex
- ❖ Implantation of IOL
- ❖ Closure of wound.
- *Common complications*
  - *ACIOL:* The lenses may cause complications like uveitis, glaucoma and

hyphema (UGH) syndrome and a high incidence of corneal decompensation and cystoid macular edema (CME), therefore, they are not preferred.

- *Posterior chamber intraocular lens (PCIOL):* PCIOLs have tendency for decentering (Fig. 7.11) and posterior capsule opacification in young patients.

### Diagnosis

Slit-lamp examination after dilatation of pupil can confirm the IOL *in situ* or its decentration.

### 7.4 POSTERIOR CAPSULE OPACIFICATION

### Etiology

1. Posterior capsule opacification (PCO) is the most frequent complication of modern cataract surgery.
2. PCO is considered a response of the residual equatorial lens epithelial cells to undergo proliferation, migration and metaplasia.
3. Almost all children develop PCO post-operatively.
4. Several risk factors such as coexisting ocular or systemic diseases, surgical technique and IOL design influence the incidence of PCO.

5. Patients with cataract associated with uveitis, high myopia, diabetes, pseudoexfoliation and RP have greater tendency for opacification.
6. Meticulous cleaning of cortex, polishing posterior capsule and smaller curvilinear capsulorrhexis (CCC) than the diameter of optics can reduce PCO.
7. Implantation of hydrophobic acrylic lenses or sharp edge or continuous 360° square edge IOL may delay or decreased the possibility of PCO by decreasing the migration of epithelial cells.

### Types of PCO

1. Fibrotic type: Proliferation and metaplasia of residual lens epithelial cells cause PCO. Continuous formation of lens fibers can produce a ring of Soemmering (Fig. 7.12). Deposition of collagen results in white fibrotic opacities.
2. Elsching's pearls type: The equatorial subcapsular lens cells proliferate and form balloon-like cells instead of lens fibers.

### Symptoms

1. The main symptom of PCO is progressive decrease in visual acuity.
2. Patients may complain of lines or distortion of object with wrinkles and folds.

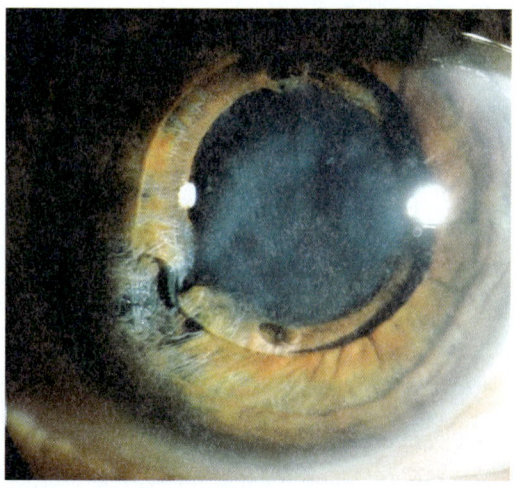

**Fig. 7.11** Decentered IOL

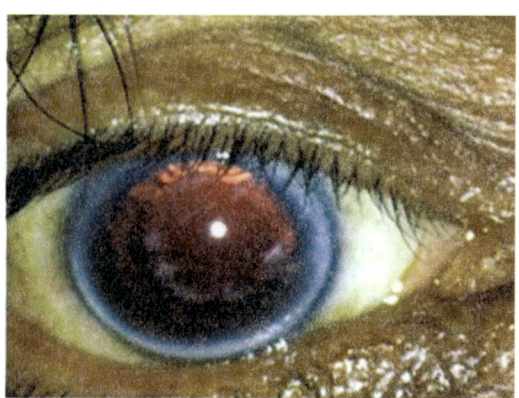

**Fig. 7.12:** Soemmering's rings

## Signs

1. In early postoperative period, a gray band representing left over cortical lamellae may be visible on slit-lamp examination.
2. Later, a dense fibrous plaque or diffuse fibrosis of the posterior capsule may be seen (Fig. 7.13).

## Management

1. Neodymium: Yttrium aluminium garnet (Nd: YAG) laser posterior capsulotomy is performed in adult patients.
2. The laser treatment can produce IOL damage, subluxation of IOL, retinal detachment and increase in IOP in some cases.
3. YAG laser may not create a proper opening in some cases (Fig. 7.14).
4. A pars plana membranectomy may be required in children with thick membrane.

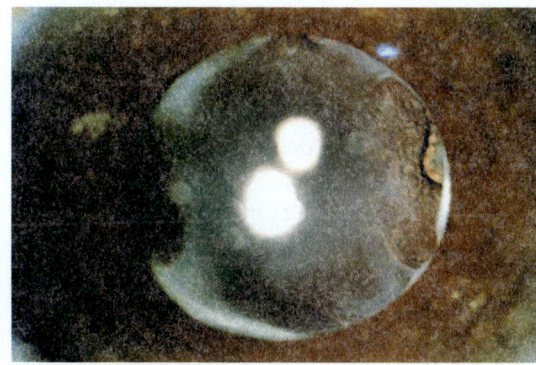

**Fig. 7.13:** Thick PCO (*Courtesy:* Dr Soosan Jacob, Dr Agrawal Eye Hospital, Chennai)

## 7.5 APHAKIA

### Etiology

1. Surgical removal of acquired or congenital cataract is the most frequent cause of aphakia.
2. Dislocation of the lens, couching, and absorption of the lens in children following injury are some of the other causes.
3. The aphakia may be congenital.

### Symptoms

Decrease in vision for near and distance, photophobia and difficulty in reading or close work are common.

### Signs

1. Classical signs of aphakia include deep anterior chamber, iridodonesis and a jet-black pupil (Fig. 7.15).
2. A scar mark at the limbus, an iris coloboma and loss of Purkinje's third and forth images may be seen.
3. Eye becomes highly hyperopic with astigmatism against the rule.
4. There is loss of accommodation.

### Diagnosis

1. Diagnosis is mostly clinical
2. Refraction reveals high hyperopia with astigmatism.

7

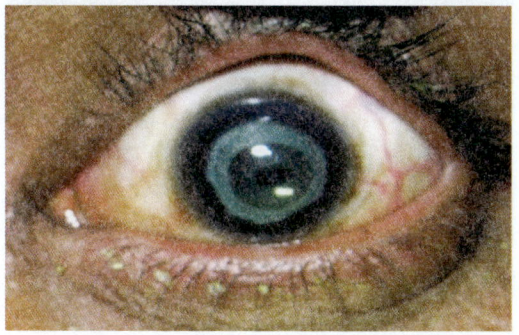

**Fig. 7.14:** Failed YAG capsulotomy for PCO

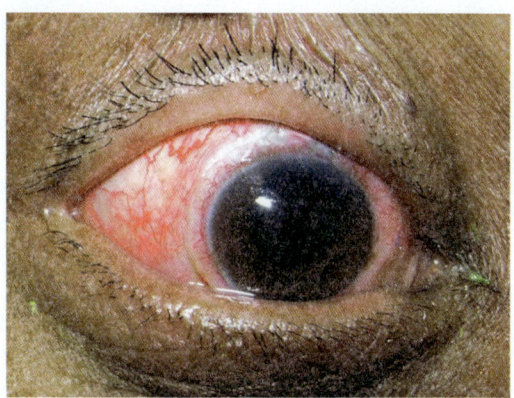

**Fig. 7.15:** Aphakia

## Treatment

1. Aphakic glasses and contact lenses.
   - Aphakic spectacles are usually not accepted in monocular aphakia due to enlargement of image (25–30%) in the aphakic eye.
   - Contact lenses are often acceptable as they improve the vision and cause a magnification of about 7%.
2. Secondary IOL implantation is preferred.
3. Almost all cases with cataract are operated with primary lens implantation to obtain emmetropia (refractive cataract surgery).
4. The loss of accommodation after cataract surgery can be managed by implanting multifocal or accommodating IOL or by prescribing bifocal or progressive glasses.

## 7.6 MYOPIA

### Etiology

1. Myopia can be caused by an increased axial length or abnormal curvature of the cornea or lens.
2. High myopia has a strong hereditary tendency. It is more common in females than males.

### Symptoms

The symptoms include inability to see distant objects, reading the book at a close distance, eyestrain, headache, black spots or floaters and flashes of light.

### Signs

1. The refractive error rapidly increases during the period of active growth.
2. Refraction may be more than −6.0 D and the axial length exceeds 26 mm. [one mm increase in axial length three diopters (3D) of myopia]
3. Vision may not be improved fully with optical correction.
4. The eyes are prominent with mildly dilated pupils.
5. An apparent convergent squint may be present on account of a large negative angle kappa.
6. Vitreous degeneration and opacities are often seen.
7. Funduscopy reveals the presence of a big optic disk with crescent temporally or all around the disk (Fig. 7.16) and nasal supertraction.
8. The insertion of the optic disk may be oblique or tilted with or without vertical elongation.
9. The patches of chorioretinal atrophy, choroidal sclerosis, yellow subretinal streaks (lacquer cracks), hyperpigmented lines and Foster-Fuchs spot at macula are found.
10. Retinal hemorrhages, posterior vitreous detachment, posterior staphyloma and lattice degeneration are found in high myopia.
11. There is a risk for retinal detachment, choroidal neovascular membrane (Fig. 7.17) and complicated cataract.
12. Open-angle glaucoma may be associated with high myopia.
13. Visual field defects may be found.

### Differential Diagnosis

1. Age-related macular degeneration
2. Toxoplasmosis
3. Presumed ocular histoplasmosis syndrome
4. Gyrate atrophy.

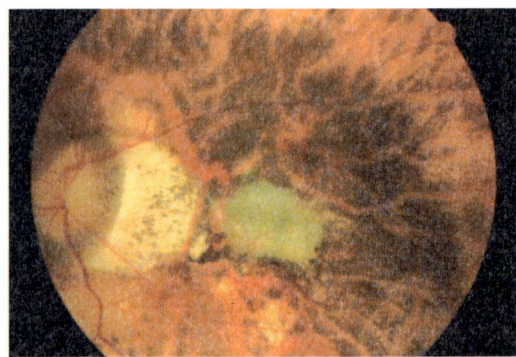

**Fig. 7.16:** Myopia showing macular scarring

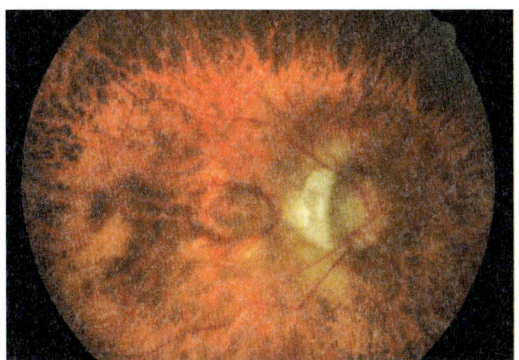

**Fig. 7.17:** Myopia with CNVM

## Diagnosis

1. Refraction reveals a high myopic error.
2. Dilated fundus examination may detect the presence of typical myopic changes like large pale-tilted disk, lattice degeneration, retinal pigmentation, posterior staphyloma, etc.
3. Slit-lamp examination of macula with 60 or 90 D can find Fuchs spot, subretinal fluid, hemorrhage or neovascularization (CNV).
4. If CNV is suspected, indocyanine green angiography (ICGA) will confirm the lesion.
5. Optical coherence tomography (OCT) can identify foveal schisis or detachment over the posterior staphyloma, and also the CNV.
6. The blind spot is enlarged and peripheral visual field is generally constricted.

## Treatment

1. Patients with high myopia are advised to avoid straining and take all precautions against ocular trauma.
2. Areas of lattice degeneration and retinal breaks must be sealed by photocoagulation or cryotherapy.
3. CNV associated with myopia should be managed by laser photocoagulation, photodynamic therapy and/or intravitreal injections of antivascular endothelial growth factor (anti-VEGF).

4. Optical correction can improve the vision in majority of patients.
5. Contact lenses are useful in high myopia as they eliminate the peripheral distortion caused by thick lenses.
6. Low vision aid may help patient with high myopia not benefitted by other modes of therapy.
7. A number of refractive surgical techniques are employed to obtain an emmetropic status in myopic patients. Techniques include:
   - Photorefractive keratectomy (PRK)
   - Intracorneal rings (ICR) or corneal inlays
   - Laser-assisted *in situ* keratomileusis (LASIK)
   - Phakic lens implantation
   - Refractive lens exchange.
8. Genetic counseling may stop hereditary propagation of myopia in certain patients who are legally blind.

## 7.7 ANOMALIES OF ACCOMMODATION

Anomalies of accommodation are presbyopia, spasm of accommodation, insufficiency of accommodation and paralysis of accommodation.

### Presbyopia

#### Etiology

1. Presbyopia is a progressive decrease in accommodation due to decrease in the elasticity of the lens after the age of 40 years.
2. Hypofunction of ciliary muscle is also implicated.
3. Presbyopia usually sets in above the age of 40–45 years with a decline in an individual's amplitude of accommodation.
4. The onset of presbyopia is usually late in myopia and early in hypermetropia.
5. A person should possess amplitude of accommodation nearly double to that of accommodation required for routine comfortable near work.

7

## Symptoms

1. Difficulty in reading small letters and doing close work, blurring of near vision, heaviness of eyes, or tiring of eyes on prolonged near work, occasional headache and intermittent diplopia.
2. Symptoms are exaggerated during fatigue, debilitating conditions and illness.

## Signs

1. The patient's distant vision is normal (20/20) but he/she keeps reading materials at a greater distance than usual.
2. Some patients may have associated ametropia.
3. The patient fails to focus on close work.
4. Presbyopic subject requires more illumination for near visual task.
5. The amplitude of accommodation is reduced.

## Diagnosis

1. *Donder's push-up method*: The near point of accommodation is measured by moving a fixed print size type chart toward the eye until the print blurs. The point of blur is measured in centimeters.
2. *Krimsky Prince near point accommodation rule* consists of a reading card with a ruler calibrated in centimeters and diopters. With this bifurcated rule, readings of accommodation near point and convergence near point can be measured.
3. The binocular amplitude of accommodation is usually greater than monocular by 0.5–1 D.
4. Refraction should be performed.

## Treatment

1. Optical correction: In emmetropic patients, generally weakest convex (+ 0.75 D) lenses are prescribed at the age of 40 years to read smallest letters of near vision chart.
2. Additions are needed for advancing ages, for example, +1.5 to +1.75 D for 45–50 years, +2.0–2.25 D for above 50–55 years and +2.5–2.75 for above 55–60 years.
3. Presbyopic spectacles can either be single vision reading glasses or bifocals, trifocals or progressive lenses.
4. Initially, ametropia is corrected and a presbyopic correction is prescribed over it.
5. Presbyopia can also be managed surgically. Surgical procedures for correcting presbyopia include:
   - Conductive keratoplasty
   - Photorefractive keratectomy
   - LASIK
   - Implantation of multifocal IOLs or accommodative IOLs.

## Spasm of Accommodation

### Etiology

1. Spasm of accommodation is seen in young females engaged in close work.
2. The spasm can be precipitated following instillation of strong miotics [pilocarpine (4%), echothiophate iodide (1.25% to 0.25%)].
3. Fatigue, stress, neurosis, uncorrected refractive error or astigmatism and prolonged reading in poor illumination are risk factors.

### Symptoms

1. Sudden bilateral decrease in vision, fluctuating vision and blurred vision may occur.
2. Eyestrain, diplopia and mild headache are common.

### Signs

1. High degree of myopia.
2. Ciliary muscle has a physiological tone of about 1D; but in spasm of accommodation, it becomes much greater.

3. Myopia is substantially less on cycloplegic refraction than refraction without cycloplegia.

4. Spasm of accommodation is usually associated with excessive convergence and miosis.

5. Accommodational spasm may be triggered while testing ocular movements.

### Differential Diagnosis

Anterior uveitis.

### Diagnosis

Refraction under cycloplegia is diagnostic.

### Treatment

1. Eliminate precipitating risk factors.

2. Near work must be curtailed and cycloplegic agent is prescribed for a short period to relax spasm.

3. Refraction under atropine indicates the actual error which should be carefully corrected.

## Insufficiency of Accommodation

### Etiology

1. Early onset of lenticular sclerosis

2. Weakness of ciliary muscles due to general debility.

3. Open-angle glaucoma.

### Symptoms

Eyestrain, particularly during near work.

### Signs

Range of accommodation is poor.

### Treatment

1. Improve general health of the patient

2. Prescribe the weakest convex lens which facilitates near work and stimulates the accommodation.

## Paralysis of Accommodation

### Etiology

1. Paralysis of accommodation or cycloplegia may be seen in diphtheria, trauma, midbrain disease, diabetes and alcoholism.

2. Most commonly it is seen after the application of a cycloplegic drug such as atropine and homatropine.

### Symptoms

Photophobia, blurred vision and difficulty in reading and near work are common symptoms.

### Signs

1. Pupils are dilated and nonreacting to light and near stimulation.

2. Pupils do not constrict with 1% pilocarpine.

### Treatment

1. Recovery occurs in pharmacological paralysis.

2. Prescribe convex lenses for near work.

3. Use of dark glasses relieves photophobia.

## 7.8 CONVERGENCE INSUFFICIENCY

### Etiology

1. It is idiopathic in children and typically affects students.

2. Head trauma, viral encephalitis, progressive supranuclear palsy, Parkinson disease, uveitis and use of spectacles with base-out prism can cause convergence insufficiency.

3. Debilitating diseases and fatigue are precipitating factors.

### Symptoms

1. Blurred vision and fatigue and eyestrain on reading.

2. Occasional diplopia on near work.

## Signs

1. Exophoria occurs due to poor near-fusional convergence. It is greater for near focus than for distance; the difference may exceed 10 prism diopters.
2. AC/A ratio is low
3. Near point of convergence recedes.

## Differential Diagnosis

1. High refractive error
2. Presbyopia
3. Convergence paralysis.

## Diagnosis

1. Measure the near point of convergence and record the distance at which diplopia occurs.
2. Refraction to rule out error.
3. Exclude insufficiency of accommodation with 4-diopter-in prism.
4. Measure the exophoria for near and distance with the help of Maddox wing and rod respectively.
5. Poor fusional ability for near can be measured with prism bar.

## Treatment

1. Correct refractive error; full correction of myopia and under correction of hyperopia is recommended.
2. Pencil push-ups exercises are useful.
3. Exercise with base-out prism is effective.
4. If above measures are not effective, base-in prisms should be provided.

7

# Retina and Vitreous

## 8.1 HYPERTENSIVE RETINOPATHY

### Etiology

1. Hypertension is the most common cardio-vascular disorder observed in general population. Its incidence varies from 10 to 15%.
2. Advance age, male sex, smoking, alcohol intake, diabetes mellitus (DM), high serum cholesterol and obesity are known risk factors.
3. Majority of patients suffer from essential or primary or idiopathic hypertension (92–94%). Heredity plays an important role in hypertension and is often associated with increased vascular resistance.
4. About 5–6% of patients have secondary hypertension and have a known cause. The major causes of secondary forms of hypertension include renal parenchymal disease, eclampsia, coarctation of aorta and endocrine disorders.

### Symptoms

1. Headache in the early morning, dizziness, palpitation, weakness, epistaxis, hematuria and blurring of vision are common.
2. Later, angina and dyspnea can develop.
3. Secondary hypertension often presents symptoms of underlying disease.

### Signs

1. Fundus examination reveals increased arterial reflex, copper wire or silver wire appearance of the retinal arteries due to retinal arteriolar narrowing.
2. Arteriovenous crossing changes are often seen. They indicate the chronicity of hypertension.
3. Later cotton-wool spots, flame-shaped hemorrhages and macroaneurysms are found (Fig. 8.1).
4. Small branch arteriolar or vein occlusion with or without neovascularization of

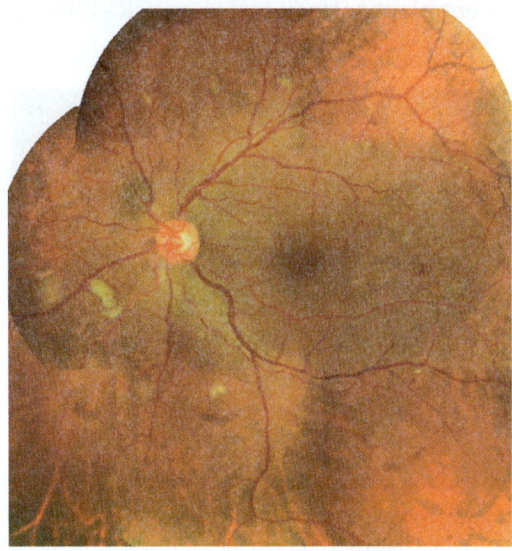

**Fig. 8.1:** Grade 3 hypertensive retinopathy

141

retina, focal chorioretinal atrophy from choroidal infarcts (Elschnig spots) and optic nerve head edema may occur.

## Classification

Scheie's classification of hypertensive retinopathy includes also the changes of arteriosclerosis:
1. Grade 0: No changes
2. Grade 1: Visible arteriolar narrowing
3. Grade 2: Obvious arteriolar narrowing with localized irregularities and arteriovenous crossing changes such as concealment of vein under artery, banking of vein distal to arteriovenous crossing (*Bonnet's sign*), tapering of vein on either side of the crossing (*Gunn's sign*) and right-angled deflection of vein (*Salus' sign*).
4. Grade 3: Cotton-wool spots, exudates and flame-shaped hemorrhages are present in addition to grade 2 changes.
5. Grade 4: It is known as malignant hypertensive retinopathy characterized by edema of the optic disk, macular star and changes of grade 3 (Fig. 8.2).

## Differential Diagnosis

1. Diabetic retinopathy (DR) (*Refer* 8.2)
2. Central retinal vein occlusion (CRVO) (*Refer* 8.3)
3. Branch retinal vein occlusion (BRVO) (*Refer* 8.4)
4. Collagen vascular diseases (CVD).

## Diagnosis

1. History of hypertension
2. Increased blood pressure (BP); systolic above 140 mmHg and diastolic more than 90 mmHg.
3. Dilated fundus examination presents characteristic changes of hypertension in the retina.
4. In the presence of papilledema, order computed tomography (CT) or magnetic resonance imaging (MRI) to exclude central nervous system (CNS) disorders.

## Treatment

1. Control hypertension in consultation with a physician
2. If the diastolic pressure is high (110–120 mmHg) and the patient has chest pain or breathing difficulty, treatment is warranted on an emergency basis.
3. Neovascularization of the retina is managed by laser photocoagulation and/or intravitreal injections of antivascular endothelial growth factor (anti-VEGF) agents.

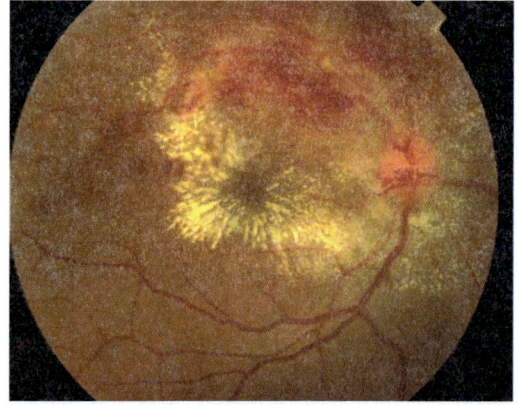

**Fig. 8.2:** Hypertensive retinopathy: Grade 4 showing disk edema, hemorrhages and exudates (*Courtesy:* Dr Meena Chakrabarti, Trivandrum)

## 8.2 DIABETIC RETINOPATHY

### Etiology

1. Diabetic retinopathy (DR) is one of the leading causes of blindness worldwide.
2. Diabetes is of two types:
   - Type I diabetes is juvenile onset and considered autoimmune (destruction of insulin secreting cells of pancreas). It has a high risk for proliferative diabetic retinopathy (PDR).
   - Type II diabetes is more common and has an adult onset. There occurs normal production of insulin but receptor cells are insulin-resistant.

8

3. Early onset and long duration of disease, pregnancy, hypertension and poor glycemic control can significantly increase the risk of development of retinopathy (Diabetes Control and Complications Trial).
4. DR is a microangiopathy leading to both microvascular occlusion and leakage.

### Classification

DR is conventionally classified into two broad categories:
1. Nonproliferative (background)
2. Proliferative
   ▪ Diabetic maculopathy can occur with both nonproliferative or proliferative DR

### Symptoms

Decreased vision, distortion of shape of objects, color vision defect, floaters and loss of vision.

### Signs

1. *Nonproliferative DR*
   ▪ Nonproliferative diabetic retinopathy (NPDR) may range from mild to very severe in severity.
   ▪ Presence of microaneurysms is the earliest sign of NPDR. They appear in clusters as minute multiple dots at the end of vascular twigs especially at the posterior pole (Fig. 8.3).
   ▪ Additional signs include venous dilatation, yellow-white waxy-looking hard exudates, intraretinal hemorrhages and macular edema.
   ▪ The exudates may form irregular big plaques and cause visual impairment.
   ▪ Arteriolar attenuation, flame-shaped hemorrhages and cotton-wool spots are seen in diabetic patients with associated hypertension.
   ▪ Pre-PDR or severe NPDR is graded by 4:2:1 rule:
      • Microaneurysms/hemorrhages are seen in all the quadrants of the fundus.

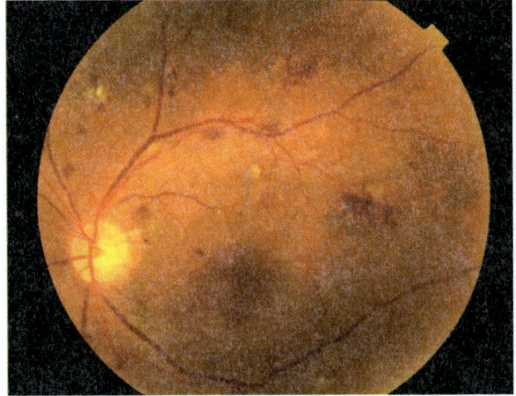

**Fig. 8.3:** Nonproliferative diabetic retinopathy showing microaneurysms and hard exudates

      • Venous beading in two quadrants
      • Intraretinal microvascular abnormalities in one quadrant.
   ▪ Presence of at least two abnormalities indicate the presence of very severe NPDR that has a risk of 10–50% progression to PDR in 1 year.
2. *Proliferative DR*
   Proliferative diabetic retinopathy is seen in approximately 5% of diabetic population.
   ▪ Retinal changes in PDR are preretinal as well as vitreal.
   ▪ Neovascularization is the characteristic feature of PDR (Figs 8.4 and 8.5). It may be either of the optic disk (NVD) or elsewhere (NVE) in the retina. Vitreous may

**8**

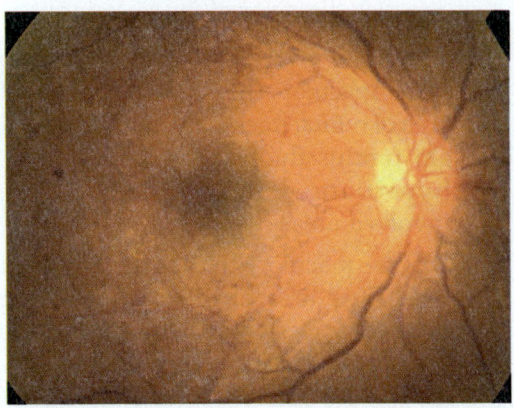

**Fig. 8.4:** Proliferative diabetic retinopathy (*Courtesy:* Dr Dhananjay Shukla, Aravind Eye Hospital, Madurai)

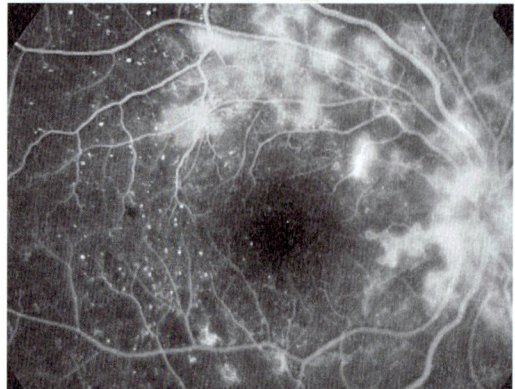

**Fig. 8.5:** FFA proliferative diabetic retinopathy

show vitreous hemorrhage, liquefaction, detachment and collapse.

- The fibrovascular tissue in the vitreous may contract and lead to tractional retinal detachment (TDR).

3. *Diabetic maculopathy*
   - Clinically significant diabetic macular edema (CSME) may be present in any of the stage of DR and is the most common cause for decreased vision.
     - CSME occurs due to leakage from dilated capillaries around macula. It is marked by the appearance of exudates and edema within 500 microns of the foveal center or edema greater than one disk diameter is present in any part of one disk diameter of the foveal center.
   - Diabetic maculopathy can be:
     - Focal maculopathy shows a localized area of retinal thickening in the macula. On fundus fluorescein angiography, hyperfluorescence is seen in the involved area.
     - Diffuse maculopathy is characterized by diffuse area of retinal thickening invariably involving the center of the fovea. On fluorescein angiography (FA), there occurs a diffuse leakage of the dye in the late phase of angiogram that sometime forms a flower-petal

appearance typical of cystoid macular edema (CME).

- Ischemic maculopathy presents with profound diminution of vision in an otherwise normal looking macula. In some cases, macular edema may occur concurrently. On FA, capillary non-perfusion is seen in the macular area with enlargement of FAZ.

**Differential Diagnosis**

1. CRVO
2. BRVO
3. Hypertensive retinopathy
4. Ocular ischemic syndrome
5. Sickle cell retinopathy
6. Radiation retinopathy
7. Retinopathy of systemic lupus erythematosus.

**Diagnosis**

1. Blood examination: Fasting and postprandial blood sugar, glycosylated hemoglobin and lipid profile.
2. Slit-lamp examination for CSME, NVD, NVE or anterior segment neovascularization in the iris and angle of anterior chamber.
3. Dilated fundus examination for features of DR.
4. Biomicroscopy with the help of fundus contact lens to look for diabetic vitreous changes.
5. Optical coherence tomography (OCT) for the presence and extent of macular edema and vitreoretinal interface changes.
6. FA is a useful test for knowing areas of nonperfusion, foveal ischemia, subclinical neovascularization and assessing need for focal photocoagulation for macular edema.
7. B-scan ultrasonography is needed to diagnose tractional macular detachment in eyes with dense vitreous hemorrhage.

## Treatment

1. Tight glycemic control and treatment of associated hypertension or other associated conditions like hyperlipidemia may prevent the progression of DR.
2. All leaking microaneurysms, 500 microns away from the center of fovea need focal laser photocoagulation.
3. Macular edema patients are treated with intravitreal injection of anti-VEGF drugs or triamcinolone acetonide (4 mg/0.1 mL).
4. Diabetic maculopathy with diffuse capillary leak may be managed by grid laser photo-coagulation.
5. Panretinal photocoagulation (PRP) is advised in patients with NVD and NVE.
6. Dense vitreous hemorrhages, premacular hemorrhage, nonclearing vitreous hemor-rhage, epiretinal membrane, vitreoretinal fibrovascular proliferation and traction retinal detachment benefit from early vitrectomy.

## Follow-up

1. All cases of treated or untreated DR must be subjected to periodic follow-up examination.
2. Patients who have undergone either focal laser photocoagulation or PRP should be screened every 3 months to monitor the effect of treatment. Many of them may require an additional photocoagulation or an alternative treatment.
3. Patients with mild to moderate DR need dilated fundus examination at an interval of 6–9 months to document the progress of DR.

## 8.3 CENTRAL RETINAL VEIN OCCLUSION

### Etiology

1. CRVO is seen in elderly people with arteriosclerosis.
2. The site of obstruction is just behind the lamina cribrosa where artery compresses the vein or due to thrombus formation.
3. Hypertension, DM, hyperlipidemia, hyper-coagulable states, vasculitis and oral contraceptives are known risk factors.
4. CRVO is associated with POAG in about 33% of cases.
5. Patients with periphlebitis retinae, sarcoi-dosis, Behçet's disease and orbital cellulitis may suffer from occlusion of the vein.

### Symptoms

The main symptom is unilateral painless loss of vision. Floaters and red vision may be other symptoms.

### Types

CRVO manifests in two forms:
1. Ischemic
2. Nonischemic.

### Signs

1. *Ischemic CRVO*
   - The features of ischemic CRVO include dilated and tortuous retinal veins, optic disk hyperemia, edema and macular edema.
   - Extensive dot-blot and flame-shaped hemorrhages in all four quadrants of the retina (Fig. 8.6) and cotton-wool spots are often seen.

8

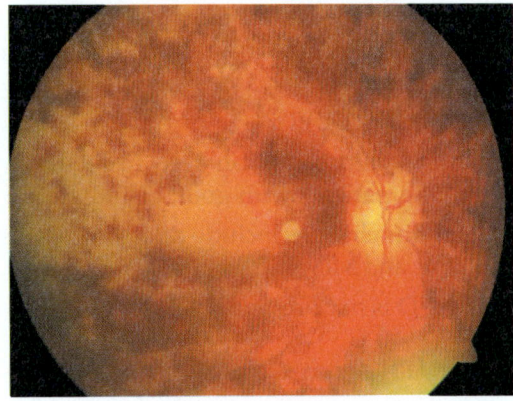

**Fig. 8.6:** Extensive hemorrhages all over the fundus in central retinal vein occlusion (*Courtesy:* Dr Dhananjay Shukla, Aravind Eye Hospital, Madurai)

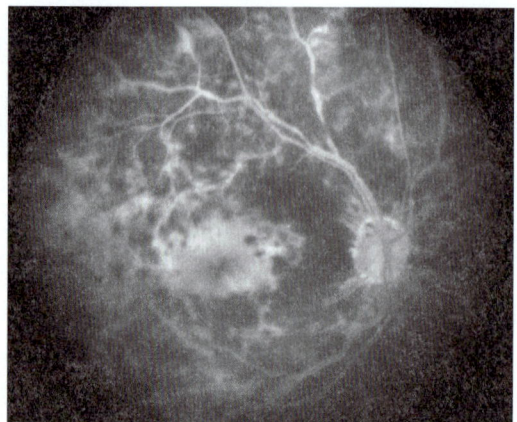

**Fig. 8.7:** Areas of nonperfusion on FA (*Courtesy:* Dr Dhananjay Shukla, Aravind Eye Hospital, Madurai)

- FA shows extensive areas of capillary non-perfusion (Fig. 8.7).
- Later, neovascularization of optic disk, retina, iris and the angle of anterior chamber can develop.
- Recurrent vitreous hemorrhages may occur due to neovascularization.
- Cystoid macular edema, pigmentary degeneration of retina, optic atrophy and neovascular glaucoma are likely to supervene.
- There occurs relative afferent pupillary defect (RAPD) in the affected eye.
- The visual prognosis is poor due to retinal capillary nonperfusion, neovascular glaucoma and macular ischemia.

2. *Nonischemic CRVO*
   - It is a mild condition seen in relatively young patients with good visual acuity.
   - Fundus changes include dilated tortuous veins and a few intraretinal hemorrhages.
   - RAPD is not present.

### Differential Diagnosis

1. DR
2. Ocular ischemic syndrome
3. Radiation retinopathy.

### Diagnosis

1. Check for history of hypertension, DM, use of contraceptive pills and hypercoagulable state.
2. Vision, clinical features and FA can distinguish between ischemic and nonischemic CRVO.
3. Slit-lamp examination can detect the presence of neovascularization of iris and angle of the anterior chamber while tonometry helps to diagnose increased intraocular pressure (IOP).
4. Dilated fundus examination reveals the clinical evidence of CRVO.
5. OCT is advised to find the macular edema and its extent.
6. Electroretinogram (ERG) helps to monitor the progress of disease. The ratio of b-wave to a-wave on ERG should normally be more than 1. If it is less than 0.50, it is indicative of poor inner retinal function and suggestive of ischemic CRVO.

### Treatment

1. Control and treat risk factors especially hypertension, dyslipidemia, DM and open-angle glaucoma.
2. Ischemic CRVO with neovascularization is managed with panretinal photocoagulation.
3. If media are hazy, anterior retinal cryopexy is considered.
4. Macular edema may be treated by:
   - Intravitreal triamcinolone (1–4 mg/0.1 mL)
   - Ozurdex implant (0.7 mg dexamethasone)
   - Intravitreal ranibizumab (0.5 mg/0.1 mL), bevacizumab or aflibercept (anti-VEGF agents)
   - Grid laser photocoagulation in the absence of macular nonperfusion.
5. Retinal vein cannulation with tissue plasminogen activator (tPA) infusion and

decompression of central retinal vein by radial optic neurotomy or sheathotomy remain controversial.

### Follow-up

1. Follow-up examination at an interval of 2–4 weeks is necessary to assess visual acuity, IOP and residual or active neovascularization. The neovascularization should be treated with prompt PRP and/or anti-VEGF therapy.
2. Examination of the fellow eye is important because there is about 10% chance of development of CRVO in the eye.

## 8.4 BRANCH RETINAL VEIN OCCLUSION

### Etiology

1. BRVO is usually associated with hypertension, cardiovascular disease and POAG.
2. Causes and risk factors mentioned in the etiology of CRVO also apply to it.
3. The superotemporal branch is prone for occlusion due to several crossing by the artery.

### Symptoms

1. The patient remains symptom-free unless macula is involved.
2. Patients may complain of loss of vision in one sector of field of vision.

### Signs

1. Flame-shaped hemorrhages along the vein are seen in the area drained by the vein and they do not cross the horizontal raphe.
2. Hemorrhages, tortuous and dilated veins, attenuated and sheathed arteries, cotton-wool spots, retinal edema and neovascularization of optic disk or retina are found (Fig. 8.8).
3. Macular edema or hemorrhage and perifoveal capillary occlusion can cause visual loss.
4. Sectorial or hemifield visual field defects are common.

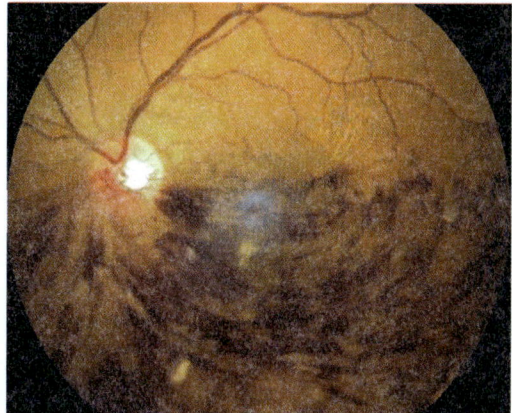

**Fig. 8.8:** Branch retinal vein occlusion: Occlusion of the lower temporal branch causing extensive hemorrhages

### Diagnosis

1. Dilated fundus examination by indirect ophthalmoscopy and 78 or 90 diopter slit-lamp biomicroscopy.
2. Procedures mentioned for CRVO may be carried out if and when indicated.

### Treatment

1. The risk factors must be managed meticulously.
2. Spontaneous resolution of edema and hemorrhages may occur within 3 months.
3. Nonischemic BRVO with macular edema is usually managed with anti-VEGF therapy.
4. Paramacular vascular leaks require grid laser photocoagulation.
5. Patients with ischemic BRVO with macular edema and retinal neovascularization are managed with laser photocoagulation.
6. Pars plana vitrectomy is required for nonclearing vitreous hemorrhage.

## 8.5 CENTRAL RETINAL ARTERY OCCLUSION

### Etiology

1. Arteriosclerosis and hypertension are common causes of central retinal artery occlusion (CRAO).
2. An embolic occlusion may also occur.

**8**

3. Emboli are of three types: (1) cholesterol, (2) calcium and (3) fibrin-platelet.

4. Cholesterol and fibrin platelet emboli originate from atheroma of carotid arteries and calcium from diseased cardiac valves.

5. CRAO in young people may be associated with systemic lupus erythematosus, polyarteritis nodosa and hypercoagulable and hematological disorders.

6. CRAO is seen in toxemia of pregnancy, giant cell arteritis, quinine toxicity, acute angle-closure glaucoma and during retinal reattachment surgery and neurosurgery.

## Symptoms

1. Sudden painless profound loss of vision (vision is usually reduced to counting fingers or less).

2. Central vision is retained in the presence of perfused cilioretinal artery.

3. Patient may give history of black-outs or transient ischemic attacks preceding CRAO.

## Signs

1. Fundus examination reveals thread-like retinal arteries.

2. Retina looks edematous and milky-white.

3. *Cherry-red spot* is seen at the posterior pole (Fig. 8.9).

4. RAPD is seen in the involved eye.

5. Movements of blood column (cattle-truck phenomenon) may be noticed by putting some pressure on the eyeball in patient with incomplete CRAO.

6. Later, the retina regains its transparency and sheen.

7. Visual recovery is invariably poor due to macular ischemia or vascular optic atrophy.

8. Rubeosis iridis and neovascular glaucoma may develop in a small percentage of cases.

## Differential Diagnosis

1. Exclude other causes of cherry-red spot.

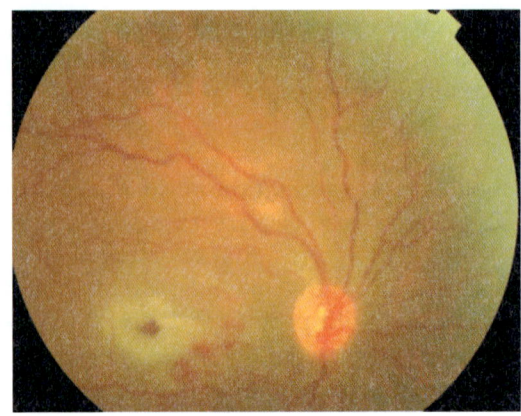

**Fig. 8.9:** Dull white edematous posterior pole with cherry-red spot (not prominent) in CRAO (*Courtesy:* Dr Meena Chakrabarti, Sr Consultant, Chakrabarti Eye Care Center, Trivandrum)

2. Commotio retinae: A positive history of blunt trauma and the condition resolves without any treatment.

3. Retinal detachment: Rhegmatogenous retinal detachment that is of recent origin, shallow and with macula off has to be differentiated from CRVO because it may also give a cherry-red spot appearance.

## Diagnosis

1. *Blood tests:* Fasting blood sugar, glycosylated hemoglobin, sedimentation rate, prothrombin time, lipid profile and antinuclear antibody.

2. BP, electrocardiography (ECG) and echocardiography and a complete cardiac evaluation by a cardiologist.

3. Dilated funduscopy can diagnose majority of cases.

4. FA shows a delayed arm to retina time and prolonged transit time.

5. ERG shows decrease in amplitude of b-wave.

6. Duplex Doppler ultrasonography for evaluation of carotid artery.

## Treatment

1. There is no rational treatment for CRAO; however, some empirical measures are recommended.

2. Massaging the globe intermittently to dislodge the embolus from the central circulation to a peripheral location.
3. Lower the IOP by intravenous acetazolamide or anterior chamber paracentesis to improve the arterial perfusion.
4. Inhalation of amyl nitrate may be tried.
5. CRAO caused by giant cell arteritis needs high doses of corticosteroids.
6. Neovascularization of iris is managed with PRP and anti-VEGF agents.

## 8.6 BRANCH RETINAL ARTERY OCCLUSION

### Etiology

1. The most important cause of BRAO is thromboembolism.
2. The most common site is the bifurcation of superotemporal artery.
3. Like CRAO, the emboli may originate from atheroma of carotid arteries (cholesterol and fibrin platelet) or cardiac valvular diseases (calcium).
4. Emboli may come from fracture of bone and infective endocarditis.

### Symptoms

Painless partial loss of vision and scotomatous visual field defects.

### Signs

1. The retinal area supplied by the artery appears white and opaque due to edema.
2. The artery becomes narrow and an embolus consisting of cholesterol crystal may be seen at the bifurcation of artery (Hollenhorst plaque).
3. White calcium emboli cause infarcts in the retinal periphery.
4. Cotton-wool spots may be found in the affected area.
5. Movements of segmented blood column in the artery (cattle-truck phenomenon) may be elicited by pressure on the globe.

### Diagnosis

1. Dilated fundus examination can diagnose almost all cases.
2. Associated systemic disorders may require investigations (*See* CRAO).

### Treatment

1. The management of BRAO needs treatment of the underlying systemic cause.
2. A digital ocular massage.

## 8.7 SICKLE CELL RETINOPATHY

### Etiology

1. Sickle cell (SC) disease is an autosomal recessive disease. A single point mutation occurs in the beta chain of hemoglobin (glutamic acid is replaced by valine) in the short arm of chromosome 6 resulting in sickle hemoglobin (Hb-S).
2. In sickle cell (SS) disease, there are two alleles of Hb-S. When one allele is Hb-S and another is abnormal like Hb-C, it is called sickle cell trait (AS).
3. Presence of abnormal Hb causes red blood cells (RBCs) to become more rigid and take anomalous shape and obstruct small blood vessels.

### Symptoms

1. Initially, it is a symptom-free condition but later flashes of light, floaters, color vision defects and loss of vision may occur.
2. Acute pain can develop in any part of the body that remains for hours to days.
3. Painful cries and acute chest syndrome, fever and tachycardia are not uncommon.

### Signs

Goldberg classified SC disease into following five stages:
1. Peripheral arteriolar occlusion and ischemia
2. Peripheral arteriovenous anastomoses
3. Neovascular proliferation from anastomoses

8

4. Vitreous hemorrhage
5. Fibrovascular proliferation and retinal detachment
   - The disease can produce both nonproliferative and proliferative retinopathy.
   - The nonproliferative retinopathy may present tortuosity of retinal veins, marked narrowing of arterioles, preretinal or intraretinal hemorrhages at the equator (Salmon patches), patches of hyperplasia of retinal pigment epithelium (sunbursts), retinal vascular occlusion and angioid streaks.
   - The characteristic lesion of proliferative SC retinopathy is a sea-fan-shaped peripheral retinal vascularization fed by a single artery and drained by a vein.
   - Avascular and vascular areas in the periphery of retina are seen.
   - Fibrovascular proliferation can lead to macular edema, macular hole, epiretinal membrane, retinoschisis and RD.
   - Other ocular changes are sausage-like dilation of conjunctival vessels, iris atrophy and secondary glaucoma.
   - Patients with SC disease suffer from hemolytic anemia.
   - Intermittent vascular occlusion of musculoskeletal system and internal organs cause painful autosplenectomy, aseptic necrosis of bones, hand-feet syndrome and acute chest syndrome.

### Differential Diagnosis

1. DR
2. Eales' disease
3. Retinopathy of prematurity
4. Sarcoidosis.

### Diagnosis

1. Positive family history of SC disease
2. Dilated fundus examination reveals characteristic changes.

3. FA demonstrates areas of filling of sea-fans and nonperfusion in the periphery of retina and leakage from new formed vessels.
4. The characteristic morphology of RBSs in blood smear.
5. Presence of sickle hemoglobin can be demonstrated as it is reduced by sodium metabisulfite.
6. Electrophoresis of hemoglobin can demonstrate slow moving hemoglobin as well as genotype.
7. Polymerase chain reaction to detect SC mutation for genotyping.

### Treatment

1. Hydroxyurea, omega-3 fatty acid and nifedipine decrease disease severity.
2. Sector laser photocoagulation or PRP checks neovascularization.
3. Intravitreal injections of anti-VEGF agents
4. Vitrectomy is indicated for nonclearing vitreous hemorrhage, rhegmatogenous retinal detachment, macular hole and pucker. Scleral buckling surgery and vitrectomy in these patients carry a risk of developing anterior segment ischemia.
5. Gene therapy and stem cell transplantation may be considered.

## 8.8 CENTRAL SEROUS CHORIORETINOPATHY

### Etiology

1. It is characterized by a central serous detachment of neurosensory retina. The central serous chorioretinopathy is seen more in young males than females.
2. There is a breakdown of blood-retinal barrier resulting in leakage of fluid from choriocapillaris. The RPE fails to pump out subretinal fluid.
3. Psychological stress, hypertension, abuse of alcohol, systemic lupus erythematosus (SLE), organ transplantation and elevated blood level of cortisol have been implicated in the etiology of CSC.

4. Topical use of corticosteroid drops, ointments, nasal or oral spray or skin cream may precipitate CSC.

## Symptoms

Unilateral or bilateral (30–40%) blurring of vision, metamorphopsia, washed-out colors of objects, black shadow or scotoma and headache are common symptoms.

## Signs

1. Macula appears edematous and foveal reflex is lost (Fig. 8.10).
2. The retina shows a shallow detachment at the posterior pole.
3. Deposition of yellowish lipid-rich sub-retinal fluid gives a leopard-spot appearance.
4. Healed CSC may leave RPE irregularities and deposition of subretinal fibrin.
5. Some patients may develop choroidal neovascularization (CNV).

## Differential Diagnosis

1. Macula off retinal detachment (RD)
2. Age-related macular degeneration
3. Choroidal tumor
4. RPE detachment.

## Diagnosis

1. Amsler grid test reveals the extent of scotoma and distortion of both horizontal and vertical straight lines.
2. Slit-lamp examination with 78 or 90 D lens to exclude optic pit and CNV.
3. Dilated fundus examination using an indirect ophthalmoscope to rule out RD and choroidal tumor.
4. Fluorescein angiography is of great diagnostic importance. Initially, a small hyperfluorescent spot (ink-blot appearance) appears (Fig. 8.11) that may expand and ascend vertically in a *smoke-stack* manner. It can also spread laterally to present a *mushroom* or *umbrella pattern*.
5. OCT shows neurosensory detachment of retina, subretinal fluid and choroidal thickening.
6. Estimation of cortisol in blood and urine.

## Treatment

1. Stop use of steroids in any form.
2. CSC is often transient and resolve spontaneously.
3. Laser photocoagulation should be done in patients with recurrent attacks. To avoid CNV, low intensity laser photocoagulation should be done.

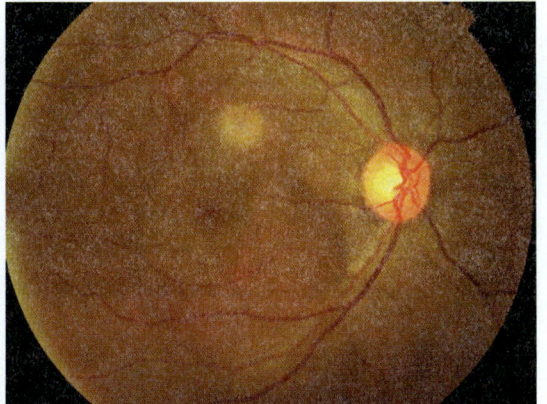

**Fig. 8.10:** Central serous chorioretinopathy (*Courtesy:* Dr Meena Chakrabarti, Sr Consultant, Chakrabarti Eye Care Center, Trivandrum)

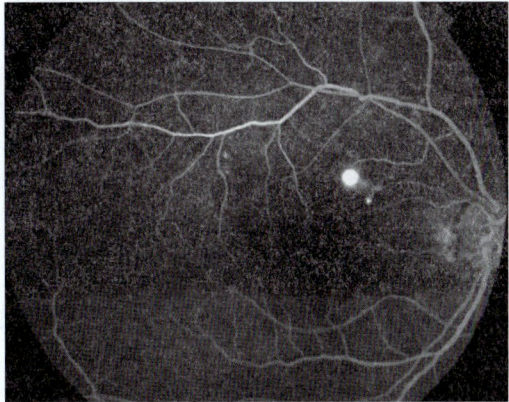

**Fig. 8.11:** FFA in central serous choroidopathy showing a fluorescent spot (*Courtesy:* Dr Meena Chakrabarti, Sr Consultant, Chakrabarti Eye Care Center, Trivandrum)

8

4. Photodynamic therapy is recommended for chronic CSC.

5. Use anti-VEGF in the presence of CNV.

### Follow-up

1. Recurrence of CSC is common and may lead to permanent visual loss. Therefore, a periodic follow-up at 2 monthly intervals is recommended.

2. Examination of contralateral eye of the patient must be done as it may also get involved.

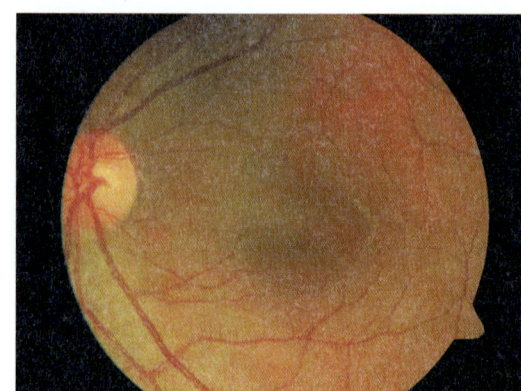

**Fig. 8.12:** Cystoid macular edema (*Courtesy:* Dr Meena Chakrabarti, Sr Consultant, Chakrabarti Eye Care Center, Trivandrum)

### 8.9 CYSTOID MACULAR EDEMA

### Etiology

1. Cystoid macular edema (CME) is often seen following intraocular surgery.

2. The incidence of CME increases with surgical complications like vitreous prolapse and incarceration of vitreous or iris in the wound. It is also seen after glaucoma and retinal detachment surgeries, vitrectomy and photocoagulation.

3. Other causes of CME include pars planitis, retinal vasculitis, DR, CRVO, RP, age-related macular degeneration and intra-ocular tumors.

4. Topical use of epinephrine can induce CME in aphakic or iridocyclitis patients.

### Symptoms

To start with decrease vision may be the only symptom; later profound visual loss may occur.

### Signs

1. CME classically presents multiple cystoid spaces (Fig. 8.12).

2. The macula looks like a honeycomb. Severe cases develop retinal hemorrhages, cells in vitreous, edema of optic disk and lamellar macular hole.

### Diagnosis

1. History of recent intraocular surgery, inflammation or medication.

2. Slit-lamp biomicroscopy of macula with 90 D lens may show macular edema with multiple cystoid spaces or a lamellar hole.

3. Definitive diagnosis is made on FA. During the late phase, the macular area presents hyperfluorescence showing a flower petal appearance (Fig. 8.13).

4. OCT (Fig. 8.14) is helpful in the diagnosis of CME as well as in monitoring its treatment.

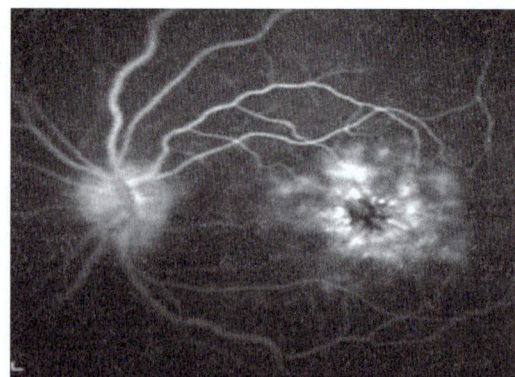

**Fig. 8.13:** FA of cystoid macular edema showing flower-petal appearance (*Courtesy:* Dr Meena Chakrabarti, Sr Consultant, Chakrabarti Eye Care Center, Trivandrum)

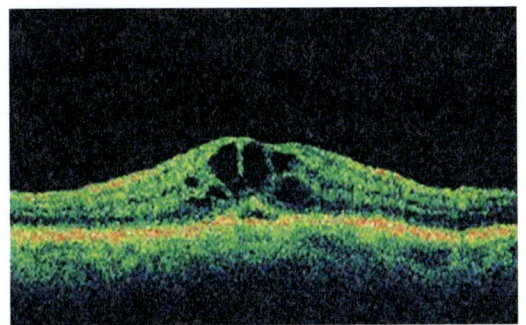

**Fig. 8.14:** OCT showing presence of large cystoid cylindrical cavities involving the central fovea indicating chronic edema in cystoid macular edema (*Courtesy:* Dr Meena Chakrabarti, Sr Consultant, Chakrabarti Eye Care Center, Trivandrum)

## Treatment

1. Development of CME must be prevented by proper management of complication of intraocular surgery.
2. All CME-related diseases must be controlled prior to surgery.
3. Topical nonsteroidal anti-inflammatory drug [like ketorolac (0.5%), nepafenac (0.1%), bromfenac (0.1%)] should be used preoperatively for 2–3 days, then post-operatively for 3 months.
4. Periocular and systemic steroids or carbonic anhydrase inhibitors are given for early resolution. Anti-VEGF agents have been tried especially in non-pseudophakic CME.
5. Grid photocoagulation may be tried for chronic CME.

## 8.10 HISTOPLASMOSIS

### Etiology

1. Histoplasmosis is caused by *Histoplasma capsulatum*.
2. *H. capsulatum* has two forms, yeast and filamentous. The former is responsible for both ocular and systemic infections.
3. The disease has a high incidence in the Mississippi-Missouri river valley.

4. A high prevalence of HLA-B7 (human leukocyte antigen-B7) and HLA-DR2 has been found in patients with primary ocular histoplasmosis syndrome.

### Symptoms

Almost all patients (99%) are asymptomatic if macula is involved, distortion of objects and impairment of vision can occur.

### Signs

1. The classical signs of ocular histoplasmosis is punched-out, round, depigmented spots (histo spots) (Fig. 8.15). The spots are about 200 microns in size and yellow in color and often seen in the peripheral retina.
2. Histo spots that appear during adolescence probably represent the lesions of childhood. The spots are associated with pigment clumps at the margins.
3. An exudative maculopathy or hemorrhagic retinochoroiditis is a late manifestation occurring between 20 and 50 years of age usually at the site of histo spot situated between optic disk and macula. It appears as a gray-green patch associated with exudates and hemorrhages.
4. CNV may be associated with old macular lesion that causes recurrent hemorrhages and subsequently disciform scarring.

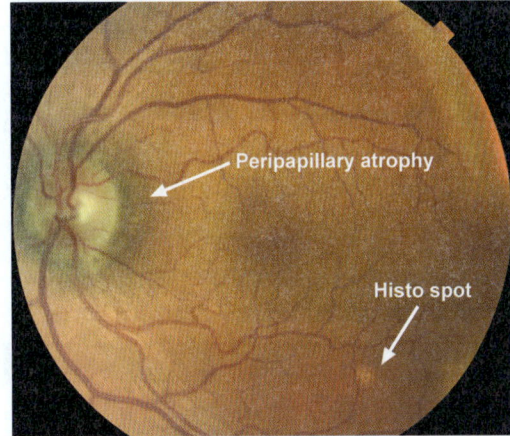

**Fig. 8.15:** Histo spots and peripapillary atrophy in histoplasmosis (*Courtesy:* Prof. Suresh Chandra, University of Wisconsin, Madison)

5. Circumpapillary atrophy and linear streaks at the equator are found.
6. Vitreous cells are usually not seen in POHS.

## Differential Diagnosis

1. Toxoplasmosis
2. Age-related macular degeneration
3. Pathological myopic degeneration and maculopathy.

## Diagnosis

1. Typical triad of peripheral histo spots, peripapillary atrophy and macular CNV or disciform scarring clinch the diagnosis of POHS.
2. High prevalence of HLA-B7 and HLA-DR2 in POHS patients.
3. FA to detect active macular lesion and choroidal neovascular membrane or macular scar.
4. OCT shows subretinal fluid, CNV and/or disciform scarring in the macula.

## Treatment

1. Oral corticosteroids (80 mg/day for 8–10 days then gradually tapered), periocular corticosteroids or intravitreal steroids can be given.
2. Destruction of the CNV situated in the juxtafoveal zone by thermal laser photocoagulation has been tried with limited success.
3. Photodynamic therapy for CNV related to POHS is safe and beneficial.
4. Anti-VEGF therapy is effective against POHS-related choroidal neovascular membrane.
5. Antifungal drugs have no effect on POHS.

## 8.11 CANDIDIASIS

### Etiology

1. Candidiasis is caused by *Candida albicans*.
2. Ocular candidiasis is not common. It may be seen in patients with AIDS or diabetes.

## Symptoms

Floaters and decreased vision are common symptoms.

## Signs

1. The posterior uvea is more frequently involved.
2. Multiple yellow white, fluffy lesions develop at the posterior pole. The vitreous above these lesions shows haziness.
3. The lesions originate in the retina and involve the choroid with associated retinal hemorrhages and perivascular sheathing.
4. Over a period of time lesions spread into the vitreous and appear "cotton-ball-like". Multiple cotton-ball opacities may give a "string of pearls" appearance.
5. The central lesions resemble with toxoplasmic choroiditis, whereas the peripheral lesions with intermediate uveitis.
6. If anterior uveitis occurs, it is associated with hypopyon which may progress to severe panuveitis and vitreous abscess.

## Diagnosis

1. Characteristic fundus findings
2. Positive blood culture
3. Culture and smear examination of vitreous tap.

## Treatment

1. Topical atropine 1%, three times a day.
2. Oral or intravenous fluconazole (400–600 mg/daily) may be useful.
3. Voriconazole 200 mg twice daily is found to be effective in controlling the infection.
4. In severe infection, patients may need intravenous or intravitreal amphotericin B (5 µg/0.1 mL) or intravitreal voriconazole (50–100 µg/0.1 mL); the latter is preferred.
5. Pars plana vitrectomy in recalcitrant cases is often needed.

## 8.12 RETINAL LESIONS IN AIDS

### Etiology

1. The human immunodeficiency virus causes AIDS.

2. There is a marked decrease in the CD4 lymphocytes and immune system is practically paralyzed.

**Symptoms**

Patients complain of blurred vision and black spots in the field of vision.

**Signs**

1. Discrete and fluffy lesions are found at the posterior pole.
2. Focal infarctions give multiple cotton-wool spots in the fundus.
3. Retinal vasculitis, flame-shaped and dot-blot hemorrhages, Roth spots and micro-aneurysms are commonly seen.
4. Cytomegalovirus retinitis is the most common ocular opportunistic infection seen in patients with AIDS. It is marked by intraretinal hemorrhages, exudates, vitritis, periphlebitis and retinal necrosis.
5. Progressive outer retinal necrosis (PORN) results from opportunistic herpetic infection. It is characterized by a large area of peripheral retinal whitening, optic neuritis, vascular occlusion and retinal breaks and rhegmatogenous RD.
6. Other secondary infections in patients with AIDS are syphilis, toxoplasmosis and mycosis of the retina.

**Diagnosis**

1. History
2. Serological tests like enzyme-linked immunosorbent assay (ELISA) and Western blot
3. Assessment of ratio between T-helper and T-suppressor lymphocytes
4. Culture and isolation of virus.

**Treatment**

1. The prevalence of HIV retinopathy has decreased due to early initiation of highly active antiretroviral therapy (HAART).
2. Ganciclovir (5 mg/kg twice daily) or foscarnet (90 mg/kg twice daily) should be administered for 2 weeks as an induction dose and then reduced.
3. Intravitreal ganciclovir implant is available.
4. Systemic or intravitreal ganciclovir is effective in PORN.

## 8.13 EALES' DISEASE

**Etiology**

1. Eales' disease (periphlebitis retinae) is inflammation of the vessels of the peripheral retina.
2. It affects healthy young males.
3. The disease has an obscure etiology. However, septic lesions elsewhere in the body are implicated.

**Symptoms**

Floaters and decreased vision are common. The left eye is usually affected first but the fellow eye may get involved within a short period.

**Signs**

1. The disease starts in the periphery of the retina as sheathing of veins with tiny hemorrhages.
2. Clinical features of the disease depend on vasculitis and obliteration of capillaries.
3. The retinal hypoxia leads to upregulation of vasoproliferative substances causing neovascularization, sheathing and hemorrhages (Fig. 8.16).
4. Vitreous haze and retinal neovascularization are important signs.
5. The patient suffers from sudden loss of vision due to hemorrhage in the vitreous. Recurrent vitreous hemorrhages can cause retinitis proliferans.
6. Rubeosis iridis, neovascular glaucoma and TRD are complications of the disease.

**Differential Diagnosis**

Other causes of vitreous hemorrhage (*Refer* 8.29).

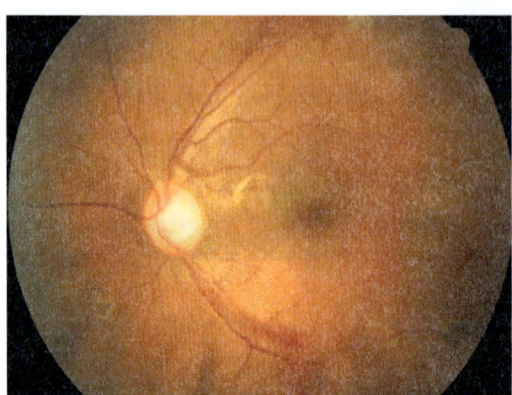

**Fig. 8.16:** Sheathing of vessels and hemorrhages in Eales' disease

## Diagnosis

1. Dilated fundus examination shows signs of retinal vasculitis, vascular obliteration and/or retinal neovascularization.
2. Fluorescein angiography may show areas of capillary dropouts, shunt vessels and retinal neovascularization (Fig. 8.17).

## Treatment

1. Periocular and systemic corticosteroids may control periphlebitis retinae.
2. Photocoagulation of neovascularized area is the most preferred treatment.
3. Long-standing and nonclearing vitreous hemorrhage is dealt with pars plana vitrectomy.

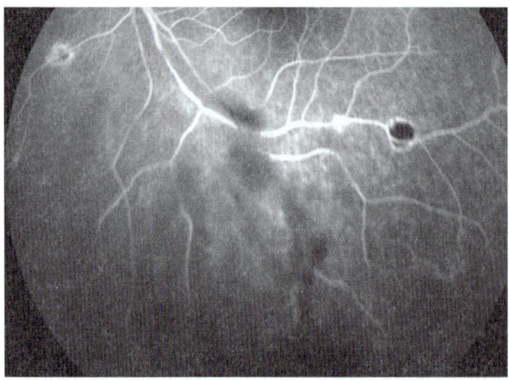

**Fig. 8.17:** FFA of patient with Eales' disease

## 8.14 SOLAR RETINOPATHY

### Etiology

1. Solar retinopathy or sun retinal damage develops after seeing a solar eclipse directly or indirectly.
2. The visible light causes photochemical retinal damage.
3. It may be found in persons engaged in astronomy, aviation and military services and in psychiatric patients.
4. Young emmetropic persons are at a higher risk of solar retinopathy.

### Symptoms

Photophobia, decreased vision, a persistence of after image phenomenon, positive scotoma, metamorphopsia, defective color vision and headache are common symptoms.

### Signs

1. In mild burn, funduscopy is unremarkable except pigmentary disturbance in the macular area. These cases have normal vision.
2. An acute burn often presents a small yellow-white spot at macula and subsequent bull's eye maculopathy. It gets replaced by a red dot surrounded by a granular pigmented halo.
3. A red cyst or lamellar macular hole develops within 2–3 weeks.
4. The vision is significantly reduced.
5. Visual field charting demonstrates central or paracentral scotoma.

### Differential Diagnosis

1. Macular hole
2. Macular cyst
3. Foveomacular dystrophy.

### Diagnosis

1. History of viewing solar eclipse
2. Amsler grid test shows scotoma

3. Central or paracentral scotoma on visual field charting

4. Slit-lamp examination with 60 or 90 D lens

5. FFA reveals window defect

6. OCT can differentiate between acute and chronic disease as well as between a macular cyst and a hole.

## Treatment

1. Prevention by education and protection by goggles is recommended.

2. Majority of cases do not need treatment as vision recovers.

3. Management of macular hole is surgical.

## 8.15 CHLOROQUINE MACULOPATHY

### Etiology

1. Chloroquine and hydroxychloroquine are used in the treatment of malaria, rheumatoid arthritis and SLE.

2. Safe dose of chloroquine is 3 mg/kg body weight and hydroxychloroquine 6.5 mg/kg body weight per day.

3. The long-term use of these drugs or use in higher doses causes maculopathy.

4. It is presumed that chloroquine causes impairment of ganglion cells and RPE functions.

### Symptoms

Patient may remain symptom-free or complain of decreased vision, color vision defects and inconvenience in low illumination.

### Signs

Chloroquine retinopathy is divided into two forms: (1) mild and (2) advanced.

1. Mild form is a premaculopathy stage and presents as irregularity of macular pigmentation giving it a granular appearance with loss of foveal reflex.

2. The characteristic lesion of advanced form is "bull's eye" maculopathy. It is marked by a perimacular ring of depigmentation surrounded by increased pigmentation.

3. Arteries are attenuated and sheathed.

4. Visual acuity is subnormal.

5. Bilateral central or paracentral scotoma is seen on visual field charting.

6. Corneal deposits (verticillata) may be found.

### Differential Diagnosis

1. Age-related macular degeneration

2. Stargardt disease

3. Cone dystrophy.

### Diagnosis

1. History of drug use.

2. Color vision becomes abnormal only in late stage of disease.

3. Amsler grid testing detects paracentral scotomas. Amsler grid is generally given to the patient for self-monitoring of the disease.

4. Slit-lamp examination for corneal deposits.

5. Dilated fundus examination to look for "bull's eye" maculopathy.

6. FA reveals atrophy of the RPE (transmission defect).

7. Visual field charting is done for confirming Amsler test finding and detecting scotoma, that are mostly in central region in chloroquine toxicity.

8. OCT shows peripapillary retinal nerve fiber layer thinning.

9. EOG becomes abnormal in advanced disease and multifocal ERG shows depression.

### Treatment

1. Six monthly eye screening is recommended in patients who are on long-term chloroquine or hydroxychloroquine.

2. The drug should be stopped, if signs of toxicity manifest.

8

## 8.16 AGE-RELATED MACULAR DEGENERATION

### Etiology

1. Age-related macular degeneration (AMD) is more common in people over the age of 60 years and is one of the leading causes of blindness.
2. Besides old age, smoking, family history, blue eyes, hypermetropia, hypertension, and malnutrition are important risk factors.

### Types

AMD is classified into two types:
1. Nonexudative (dry) AMD
2. Exudative (neovascular) AMD.

#### Nonexudative AMD

##### Symptoms

Patients remain symptom-free for a long period and then may notice decrease in vision.

##### Signs

1. Multiple small, yellowish round drusen at the posterior pole are seen.
2. Drusen may be small, intermediate or large.
3. Presence of intermediate and large drusen is diagnostic of dry AMD (Fig. 8.18).

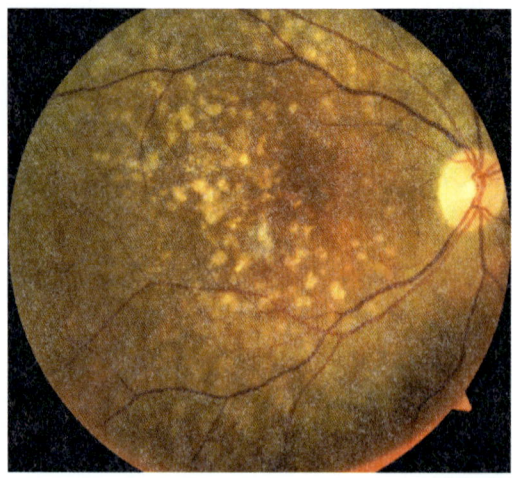

**Fig. 8.18:** Nonexudative AMD (*Courtesy:* Dr A Bhargava, Retina Hospital, Indore)

4. Histopathologically, drusen consists of thickening of Bruch's membrane and deposition of lipid rich material.
5. Clumping of pigments and hypopigmentation occur and RPE atrophy exposes choroidal vessels.

#### Differential Diagnosis

1. Central serous choroidopathy
2. Macular dystrophy
3. Myopic degeneration
4. Macular detachment.

#### Diagnosis

1. Family history of AMD.
2. Amsler grid test to detect central scotoma and to monitor the disease progression by the patient.
3. Slit-lamp biomicroscopy with 60 or 90 D lens.
4. Dilated funduscopy.
5. FA shows staining of drusen in late phase of angiogram or pooling of dye in areas of diffuse thickening. RPE window defect is seen in the early phase of FA corresponding to the areas of pigment atropy.
6. OCT is useful for both diagnostic and therapeutic purposes.

#### Treatment

1. The patient should be advised to quit smoking.
2. They may be educated to recognize symptoms of disease progression.
3. Patients with multiple intermediate (more than 20) to large drusen and geographic atrophy are likely to progress to exudative AMD.
4. Nutritional supplementation with high dose combination of vitamins and essential minerals [(500 mg vitamin C, 400 IU vitamin E), 10 mg lutein, 2 mg zeaxanthin and zinc (80 mg zinc oxide and 2 mg cupric oxide)] is recommended by Age Related Eye Disease Study 2 (AREDS) to decrease

8

disease progression and visual loss. This supplement is also known as AREDS 2 formulation.

### Exudative AMD

#### Symptoms

A sudden diminution of vision, distortion of objects, flashes of light and a positive scotoma may occur.

#### Signs

1. Drusen, subretinal exudates and retinal hemorrhages are common.
2. Retinal telangiectasia, retinochoroidal angiomatosis, superficial retinal hemorrhages and detachment of RPE may precede or follow CNV (Fig. 8.19).
3. CNV is the hallmark of the disease. A grayish neovascular membrane may be seen.
4. Ultimately, proliferation of fibrovascular complex results in a disciform scar with gross loss of vision (Fig. 8.20).
5. Occasionally, vitreous hemorrhage may be found.

#### Differential Diagnosis

1. Ocular histoplasmosis
2. Idiopathic polypoidal choroidopathy
3. High myopia

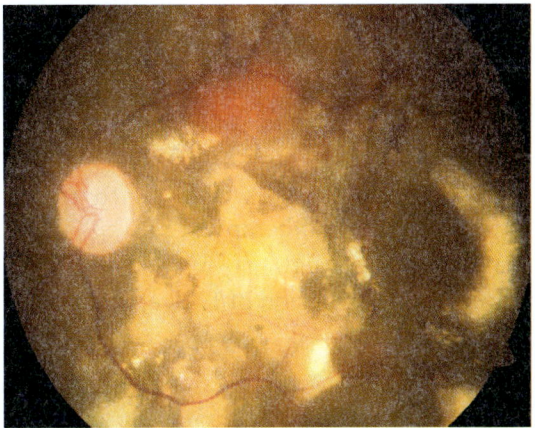

**Fig. 8.20:** Advanced AMD with scars and marked loss of vision (*Courtesy:* Prof Ravindran, AEH, Madurai)

4. Angioid streaks: Angioid streaks appear as brown irregular lines radiating from the disk, deeper to the retinal vessels and are irregular in distribution. They may be seen in patients with pseudoxanthoma elasticum, Ehlers-Danlos syndrome, sickle cell anemia and Paget's disease.

#### Diagnosis

1. Family history of AMD and associated risk factors.
2. Amsler grid test
3. Slit-lamp examination with 60 or 90 D lens
4. FA can show drusen and retinal pigment atrophy distinctly. FA of classic CNV presents a characteristic picture. In the early phase it shows a uniform hyperfluorescence which increases in the late phase.
5. Indocyanine green angiography images the occult CNV much better than FA. Three morphological types of CNV, namely a small hyperfluorescent hot spot, a plaque-like lesion, or a combination of two may be found. The plaque-like lesion is more common.
6. OCT is helpful in the diagnosis and assessing the thickness of CNV membrane, RPE detachment and macular edema. It is also useful in monitoring the treatment.

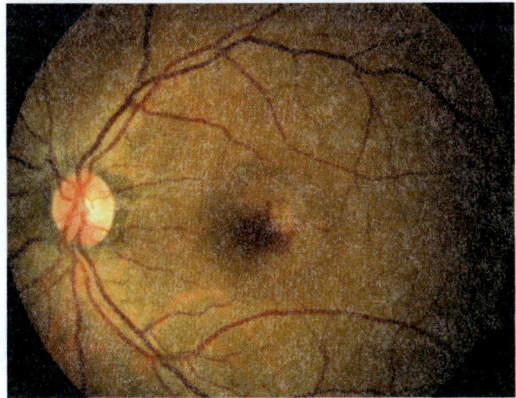

**Fig. 8.19:** Exudative AMD

8

### Treatment

1. Subfoveal CNV is mainly treated with anti-VEGF. Intravitreal injections of anti-VEGF (bevacizumab, pegaptanib, aflibercept) are approved by Food and Drug Administration.
2. Extrafoveal CNV is dealt with trans-pupillary thermotherapy (TTT).
3. Photodynamic therapy, at 3-monthly intervals for a period of 1–2 years, is found to be effective.

### Follow-up

All cases of exudative AMD should be followed on monthly basis till CNV disappears.

## 8.17 RETINITIS PIGMENTOSA

### Etiology

1. RP is inherited in all three modes: (1) autosomal dominant, (2) recessive and (3) sex-linked.
2. Autosomal recessive trait is the most common and manifests early in life while dominant type is seen in adult life.
3. Sex-linked inheritance is most severe and has an early onset.
4. About 20% of patients have history of consanguinity.
5. Retinal degeneration slow (RDS) gene causes RP.
6. The site of gene mutation affects the severity of RP.

### Symptoms

1. Night-blindness is the main symptom of the disease.
2. Later, progressive decrease in vision and marked contraction in visual fields handicap the patient even in ambulation especially at night.

### Signs

1. Irregular pigment mottling in the equatorial zone and attenuation of arterioles are early changes in the retina.

2. Pigments from equator spread both anteriorly and posteriorly.
3. Later pigments become jet-black and assume shape of bone spicules with spidery outlines.
4. Pigments appear in the entire retina mostly along with the course of the retinal veins and hide the vessels (Fig. 8.21).
5. The choroidal vessels are visible due to migration of pigments.
6. Areas of depigmentation and atrophy of the RPE are also seen.
7. Cystoid maculopathy is common (70%).
8. Complicated posterior subcapsular cataract, epiretinal membrane and consecutive optic atrophy are frequent sequelae.
9. Ring scotoma and progressive concentric contraction leaving a small central field of tubular vision are common visual field defects.

### Atypical Retinitis Pigmentosa

RP can manifest in the following atypical forms:

1. *RP sine pigmento* does not show any pigments in the fundus.
2. *Retinitis punctata albescens* shows presence of multiple white dots all over the fundus.
3. *Inverse RP* is confined to the macular region. It is also known as the central RP.

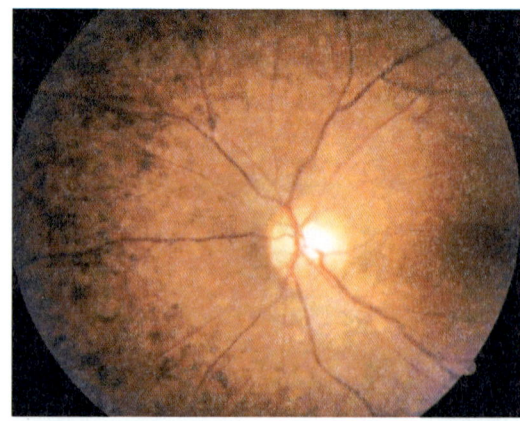

**Fig. 8.21:** Retinitis pigmentosa

4. *Sectorial RP* shows classical changes of RP in one or two sectors of the fundus.
5. *Unilateral RP* affects only one eye.

### Differential Diagnosis

1. Syphilitic disseminated chorioretinitis
2. Rubella retinopathy
3. Ophthalmic artery occlusion
4. Spontaneously reattached retina.

### Retinitis Pigmentosa Associated Syndromes

1. *Bardet-Biedl syndrome* is characterized by retinitis pigmentosa, mental retardation, obesity syndactyly and hypogenitalism.
2. *Laurence-Moon syndrome* has features of Bardet-Biedl syndrome with spastic paraplegia but without obesity and polydactyly.
3. *Usher syndrome* has RP with congenital sensorineural hearing loss.
4. *Refsum's syndrome* is characterized by RP, deafness, ataxia and polyneuropathy.
5. *Bassen-Kornzweig syndrome or abetalipoproteinemia* presents RP, acanthocytosis, and fat soluble vitamin deficiency.
6. *Kearns-Sayre syndrome* is marked by progressive ophthalmoplegia and cardiac conduction defects.

### Diagnosis

1. Dilated fundus examination shows a characteristic picture of pigmentary degeneration of retina.
2. If fundus examination in initial stage of RP is inconclusive, diagnosis can be made with the help of ERG; β-wave is subnormal and later extinguishes. EOG shows an absence of light rise.
3. The dark adaptation time is significantly increased.
4. Visual field shows ring scotoma.

### Treatment

1. There is no rational treatment for RP. However, empirically high doses of vitamin A were recommended in the past.

2. Genetic counseling should be done. Currently, the possibility of gene therapy is being explored.
3. Attempts are being made to improve visual acuity by transplantation of epiretinal microchips in patients with RP (Bionic eye or Argus II retinal implant).

### Follow-up

1. The patients must be followed at yearly interval.
2. The progression of the disease is monitored by recording of visual field and electroretinography.
3. Patients with RP may retain some vision.

## 8.18 RETINOSCHISIS

### Etiology

Retinoschisis is of two types:
1. Juvenile retinoschisis is a sex-linked recessive hereditary disease.
2. Age-related retinoschisis is a degenerative disease.

### Symptoms

Usually, the patients of age-related retinoschisis are symptom-free. Juvenile retinoschisis causes diminution of vision.

### Signs

1. Juvenile retinoschisis
   - Juvenile retinoschisis is characterized by poor visual acuity, nystagmus and cartwheel appearance of macula.
   - Foveal changes are also known as stellate maculopathy due to edema and radiating folds from the center of the macula.
   - The nerve fiber layer splits from the outer layers of the retina in the inferotemporal quadrant.
   - Retinal breaks may be seen with RD, vitreous hemorrhage and pigmentary changes in the retina.
2. Age-related degenerative retinoschisis

- Age-related retinoschisis is a bilateral condition, more common in hyperopic eyes and manifests as dome-shaped schisis (due to splitting of retina at the level of outer plexiform layer) in the inferotemporal quadrant.
- It may be associated with frosting on the inner layer of retina and sheathing of retinal vessels.
- The split layer of retina is immobile. It is not associated with pigmentary changes in the retina or vitreous hemorrhage, but RD may occur.

## Differential Diagnosis

Rhegmatogenus RD

## Diagnosis

1. Slit-lamp examination with 60 or 78 D lens to confirm the cart-wheel appearance of macula in juvenile retinoschisis.
2. Dilated funduscopy to rule out RD.
3. Visual field charting shows a scotoma in the quadrant of schisis.
4. B-scan ultrasonography (USG) reveals split of a thin layer of retina in the inferotemporal quadrant.
5. Indocyanine green angiography can visualize cystoid foveal changes.
6. OCT is useful in knowing the site of split in the retina.

## Treatment

1. Keep the patient under follow-up with sufficient education about symptoms of RD.
2. If patient develops RD, it must be repaired surgically.

## 8.19 MACULAR HOLE

### Etiology

1. The etiology of macular hole is multi-factorial

2. Approximately, 80% of cases are idiopathic
3. Ocular trauma contributes to less than 10% of cases
4. Patients with high myopia may develop foveal schisis that can progress to macular hole
5. Vitroretinal traction plays an important role in the pathogenesis
6. Common after the age of 55 years
7. Increased axial length of eyeball, retinal reattachment surgery and chorioretinal atrophy are known risk factors.

### Staging of Macular Hole

Gass classified macular hole in four stages:

- Stage 1a: Foveal detachment with presence of yellow spot at the center of fovea
- Stage 1b: Yellow spot changes to a donut-shaped yellow ring
- Stage 2: Full-thickness hole of macula of less than 400 μ size with or without operculum
- Stage 3: Full-thickness macular hole of more than 400 μ size
- Stage 4: Full-thickness macular hole with complete separation of vitreous from the macula and optic disk

### Symptoms

1. Initially, the patient is asymptomatic especially if the hole is partial
2. Later, blurred vision and distortion of objects (metamorphopsia) are common
3. Difficulty in reading and driving develop
4. A central scotoma may be noticed by the patient with gross reduction of vision.

### Signs

1. Visual acuity may vary between 2/60 and 6/24.
2. In early stage, fundus examination shows a partial thickness hole with yellow dots; the dots represent lipofuscin laden macrophages with eosinophilic material.

3. Later, it becomes a full-thickness hole (Fig. 8.22).

4. Biomicroscopic examination of the hole presents a round excavation with well-defined margins and the slit-lamp beam is interrupted (dipped in the hole). The hole is covered by a semitranslucent pseudo-operculum.

5. Over time chronic changes like hyperplasia or atrophy of RPE and epiretinal membrane may be seen.

### Differential Diagnosis

1. Cystoid macular edema
2. Pseudomacular hole
3. Macular cyst
4. Macular hemorrhage.

### Diagnosis

1. Amsler chart may show central scotoma (hole) and bowing of lines (macular cyst).

2. Microperimetry

3. Biomicroscopic examination of macula with 60 or 90 D contact lens on slit lamp

4. FFA can differentiate macular hole from CME

5. B-scan USG may reveal vitreous traction

6. OCT can detect macular hole, its stage, changes in the surrounding retina and vitreoretinal interface (Fig. 8.23). Fellow eye examination and OCT reveal macular hole in about 12% of patients.

7. Multifocal ERG may show loss of function corresponding to the hole.

### Treatment

1. Approximately 50% of stage 1 macular holes may resolve spontaneously. Occasionally, a full-thickness macular hole may also close with visual recovery.

2. The surgical management of macular hole includes vitrectomy, internal limiting membrane peeling and long-acting gas (C3F8) tamponade.

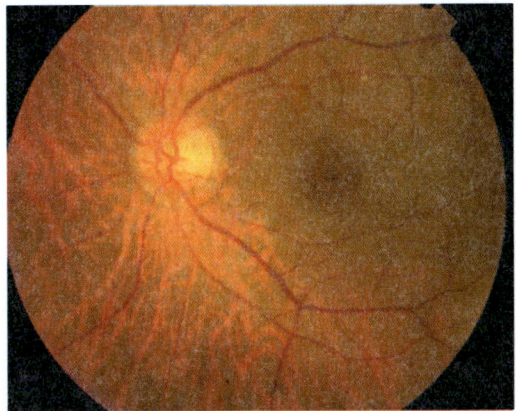

**Fig. 8.22:** Macular hole (*Courtesy:* Dr Meena Chakrabarti, Sr Consultant, Chakrabarti Eye Care Center, Thiruvananthapuram)

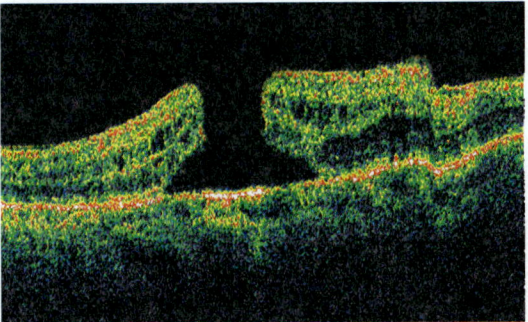

**Fig. 8.23:** OCT of macular hole (*Courtesy:* Dr Meena Chakrabarti, Sr Consultant, Chakrabarti Eye Care Center, Trivandrum)

3. Adjuvants such as transforming growth factor-beta (TGF-beta), recombinant TGF-beta, autologous serum and plasmin have been recommended in traumatic or myopic holes, ruptured cyst and recurrent holes.

## 8.20 RHEGMATOGENOUS RETINAL DETACHMENT

### Etiology

1. Rhegmatogenous retinal detachment (RD) is caused by a break in the retina.

2. The liquefied vitreous enters through the break between RPE and neuroretinal layers causing separation.

8

3. High degenerative myopia, aphakia, trauma, age-related degenerative changes in the peripheral retina (lattice degeneration) and liquefied vitreous are considered as potential risk factors for RD.

## Symptoms

1. Patient may complain of transient flashes of light, distortion of objects, black spots and foggy or cloudy vision.
2. Typically, the patient describes that a curtain has come down in front of the eye and the objects are partially visible.

## Signs

1. Elevated retina with subretinal fluid (Fig. 8.24) and presence of full-thickness tear or break are the most characteristic signs. The coursing blood vessels over the detached retina appear more darker than normal.
2. More than one break may be found. Breaks may be round, horseshoe or dialysis. Size of breaks may vary; some are very small while others may be large [giant retinal tear (GRT)].
3. Slit-lamp examination reveals fine pigmented cells or tobacco-dust on the anterior face of vitreous (*Shafer's sign*) and in the anterior chamber.
4. RAPD may be present.

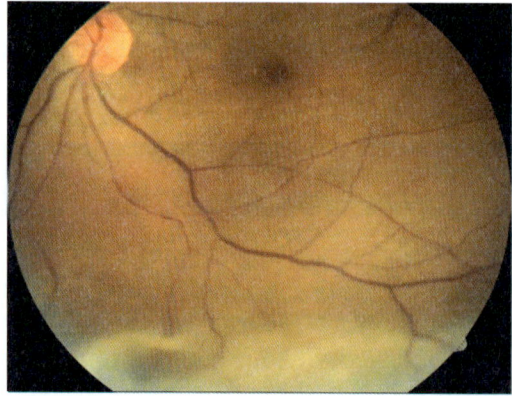

**Fig. 8.24:** Inferior rhegmatogenous retinal detachment

5. IOP is decreased in the affected eye.
6. Subretinal fluid is nonshifting type.
7. Shallow detachment presents a normal sheen but gradually it shows gray discoloration with folds. The folds may oscilate during ocular movements.
8. Old RD presents with fixed folds and other signs of proliferative vitreoretinopathy (PVR). A pigmented demarcation line between the detached and the attached retina may be seen in old RD.
9. Macular involvement causes a gross visual loss.
10. Cataract may develop as a complication.

## Differential Diagnosis

Retinoschisis.

## Diagnosis

1. Dilated fundus examination using an indirect ophthalmoscope with scleral depression to locate the retinal break and chart the extent of RD with accompanied changes.
2. Slit-lamp biomicroscopy with 60 or 90 D lens to look for macular changes and find small breaks.
3. If ocular refracting media are hazy, B-scan USG is helpful.
4. OCT is used to know the status of macula.
5. Visual field charting may be done which shows an absolute scotoma corresponding to the sector of the RD.

## Treatment

1. Prophylactic laser photocoagulation is recommended in patients with lattice degeneration and retinal breaks.
2. The principle of treatment for rhegmatogenous RD is to seal and support the retinal break. A scleral buckle reduces the dynamic vitreoretinal traction and supports the break.
3. Primary vitrectomy to repair the detachment is commonly practiced nowadays. Patients with GRT or PVR are usually managed by vitrectomy.

## 8.21 EXUDATIVE RETINAL DETACHMENT

### Etiology

1. The exudative RD is not common.
2. The etiology of exudative RD may be congenital, transudative, inflammatory, neoplastic and iatrogenic
   - Congenital anomalies include optic pit, morning glory syndrome and Coats' disease.
   - Transudative conditions are idiopathic central serous chorioretinopathy, toxemia pregnancy, renal hypertension and uveal effusion syndrome.
   - Inflammatory causes comprise posterior scleritis, Vogt-Koyanagi-Harada syndrome and orbital cellulitis.
   - Neoplastic conditions include choroidal hemangioma, malignant melanoma, retinoblastoma exophytum and metastases in choroid.
   - CNV and laser photocoagulation can also cause exudative RD.

### Symptoms

Decreased vision that shows fluctuation with the change in the position of head.

### Signs

1. RD that is smooth; it may become bullous but lacks folds.
2. The shifting of subretinal fluid with the change in head position is the hallmark of the disease.
3. Extension of RD is gravity dependent.
4. Absence of a retinal tear and PVR changes.
5. RAPD may be seen
6. Exudative RD may settle spontaneously or with treatment and results in RPE atrophy with exaggerated red fundal glow.

### Diagnosis

1. Dilated funduscopy in different postures reveals shifting of subretinal fluid and absence of any retinal break.
2. FA confirms the presence of subretinal fluid and its source.
3. B-scan USG can exclude neoplastic lesions.
4. OCT can identify the cause of exudative detachment if it is located in the posterior pole.

### Treatment

1. Exudative RD may undergo spontaneous regression.
2. Inflammatory diseases causing exudative RD are treated with a combination of steroids and antibiotics.
3. Surgery or chemotherapy is often needed to manage neoplasms.

## 8.22 TRACTIONAL RETINAL DETACHMENT

### Etiology

1. Recurrent hemorrhages in the vitreous stimulate proliferation of fibroblasts. The contraction of fibroblastic band pulls and detaches the retina. Similarly, an epiretinal membrane may also contract and cause tractional retinal detachment (TRD).
2. Proliferative diabetic retinopathy, Eales disease, penetrating injury, retinopathy of prematurity (ROP) and proliferative SC retinopathy are important causes of TRD.

### Symptoms

Patient complains initially of metamorphopsia or impairment of vision and subsequently of loss of vision.

### Signs

1. Presence of traction band on retina may be visible (Fig. 8.25).
2. Detached retina is immobile and appears concave.
3. If tear develops, the detached retina takes a convex bullous configuration (combined mechanism RD).
4. Hemorrhage and pigment dispersion may be seen in the vitreous.

8

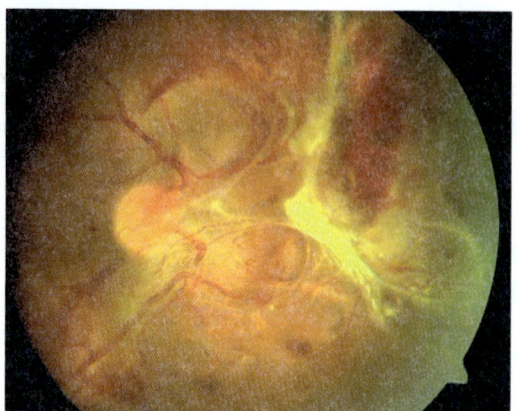

**Fig. 8.25:** Tractional retinal detachment (*Courtesy:* Dr Meena Chakrabarti, Sr Consultant, Chakrabarti Eye Care Center, Trivandrum)

5. TRD generally does not extend to ora serrata.
6. RAPD may be seen in patients with extensive TRD.

### Diagnosis

1. Dilated fundus examination for identifying the extent of RD and vitreoretinal traction bands.
2. Slit-lamp biomicroscopy with 90 D lens for locating small tears.
3. B-scan USG if media are hazy.
4. OCT can help to locate the tractional band and identify the nature of TRD.

### Treatment

1. The tractional pull is surgically managed by segmentation or delamination.
2. The epiretinal membrane needs peeling.
3. Prophylactic circumferential buckle may be considered.
4. Complicated cases are dealt with photo-endocoagulation or injection of silicone oil.

### 8.23 STARGARDT'S MACULAR DYSTROPHY FUNDUS FLAVIMACULATUS

Both dystrophies are variants of a single disorder.

### Etiology

1. Stargardt's macular dystrophy is inherited as autosomal recessively.
2. ABCA4 gene abnormality is implicated in in the etiology of the disease. The dystrophy manifests in the first or second decade of life.

### Symptoms

1. Patients may remain initially symptom-free.
2. Later, they complain of bilateral progressive impairment of vision that is often out of proportion to the macular lesion.

### Signs

1. Heavily pigmented RPE may be the only sign in some cases.
2. Bilateral elliptical atrophic maculopathy having a beaten-bronze appearance.
3. Macula develops a "bull's eye" appearance due to atrophy of RPE (Fig. 8.26A).
4. Fundus flavimaculatus manifests later than Stargardt's disease. It is marked by the presence of oval or pisciform white flakes all over the posterior pole.

### Differential Diagnosis

1. Bull's eye maculopathy:
   - Cone dystrophy
   - Chloroquine retinopathy
   - Batten disease
2. White retinal spots or dots:
   - Retinitis punctata albicans
   - Fundus albipunctatus
   - Familial dominant drusen: They are yellow dots or flecks arranged in a honeycomb pattern.

### Diagnosis

1. Dilated fundus examination
2. FA may show blockage of choroidal fluorescence (dark choroidals or silence

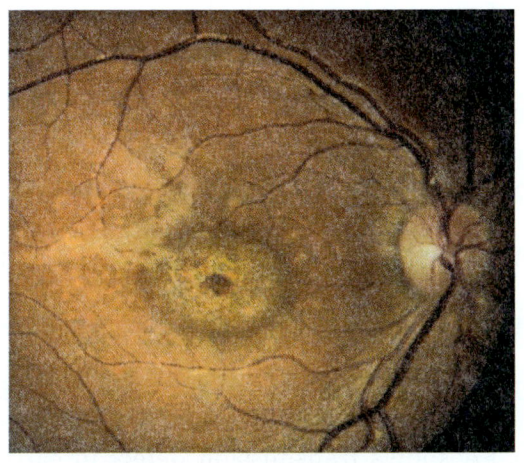

Fig. 8.26A: Stargardt disease

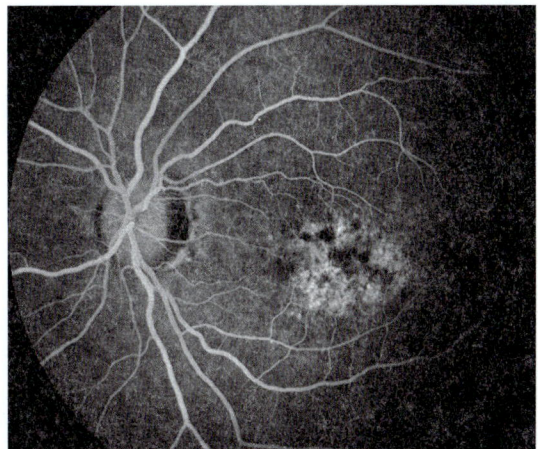

Fig. 8.26B: FFA of Stargardt disease

choroidals) or midnight fundus due to increased lipofuscin in the RPE. Bull's eye maculopathy shows window defect and mottled hyperfluorescence in the late phase of FA (Fig. 8.26B).

3. Fundus autofluorescence can detect altered RPEs even before the appearance of ophthalmoscopically visible changes.
4. Visual field defects.
5. ERG and electro-oculogram (EOG) are subnormal.

### Treatment

1. Refract, reassure and give dark glasses
2. Low vision aids.

## 8.24 BEST VITELLIFORM DYSTROPHY

### Etiology

Best vitelliform dystrophy is inherited as an autosomal dominant condition with variable penetrance often present at birth or may have a juvenile-onset.

### Symptoms

Bilateral, gradual visual impairment.

### Signs

1. Best macular dystrophy is bilateral and its fundus features may be divided into following five stages:

- *Previtelliform stage:* Fundus is normal
- *Vitelliform stage:* Bilateral egg-yolk lesions are found at macula
- *Pseudohypopyon stage:* Disintegrated egg-yolk with cyst formation
- *Vitelliruptive stage:* It presents scrambled egg appearance
- *End stage:* Macular scar or macular CNV and hemorrhage can develop.

2. Some patients show hyperopia and strabismus.

### Differential Diagnosis

1. AMD
2. Pattern dystrophy.

### Diagnosis

1. *Dilated funduscopy:* Classical clinical picture.
2. Slit-lamp biomicroscopy with 60 or 78 D lens.
3. EOG is confirmatory.
4. FA and OCT are useful in the end stage disease to detect CNV.

### Treatment

1. CNV may be treated with anti-VEGF therapy or photodynamic therapy (PDT).
2. Correct the refractive error and may give low vision aids in advance disease.

8

## 8.25 CONE DYSTROPHY

### Etiology

1. Hereditary cone dystrophy is transmitted in autosomal dominant or sex-linked manner but majority of cases are sporadic.
2. It manifests between 1 and 30 years of age.

### Symptoms

Light intolerance, decreased vision, color deficiency and nystagmus.

### Signs

1. Fundus may be normal in childhood.
2. Later a classical *"bull's eye" maculopathy* develops (Fig. 8.27).
3. Pigment clumping occurs in the macular area as well as elsewhere in the retina due to rod-cone degeneration.
4. Optic disk is pale.
5. Nystagmus is an important sign.

### Differential Diagnosis

1. Stargardt's disease
2. Chloroquine maculopathy
3. Age-related macular degeneration (non-exudative)
4. Central areolar choroidal dystrophy

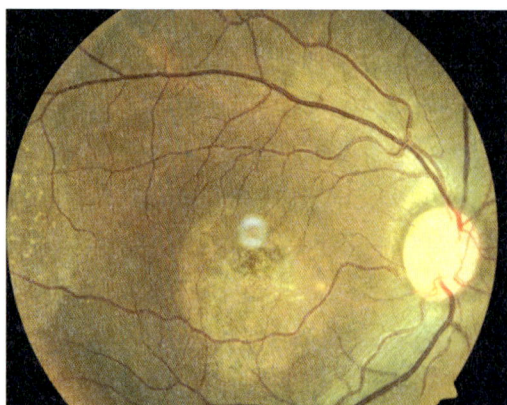

**Fig. 8.27:** Cone dystrophy (*Courtesy:* Dr Arun Bhargav, Retina Hospital, Indore)

5. Long-standing macular hole
6. Batten disease.

### Diagnosis

1. Family history is positive.
2. Test for color vision defect (Farnsworth-Munsell 100 hue test).
3. Visual field testing for central/paracentral scotoma.
4. ERG is markedly reduced especially the photopic component.
5. Fundus autofluorescence detects altered RPEs.
6. FA shows transmission defect in early phase of angiogram.

### Treatment

1. No definitive treatment is available
2. Tinted glasses or contact lenses can be used for photophobia
3. Low vision aid should be given to the patient.

## 8.26 IDIOPATHIC POLYPOIDAL CHOROIDAL VASCULOPATHY

### Etiology

1. Idiopathic polypoidal choroidal vasculo-pathy (PCV) or posterior uveal bleeding syndrome is a disease of old age (50–65 years) predominantly occurring in males.
2. It affects the pigmented races about four times more than the white.
3. The incidence of PCV is high in patients with neovascular AMD.

### Symptoms

Sudden or gradual decrease in vision.

### Signs

1. Classical presentation is a bilateral sub-retinal hemorrhages (Fig. 8.28) with hemorrhagic detachment of RPE.
2. The choroidal vascular channels terminate in red-orange, polyp-like dilatations.

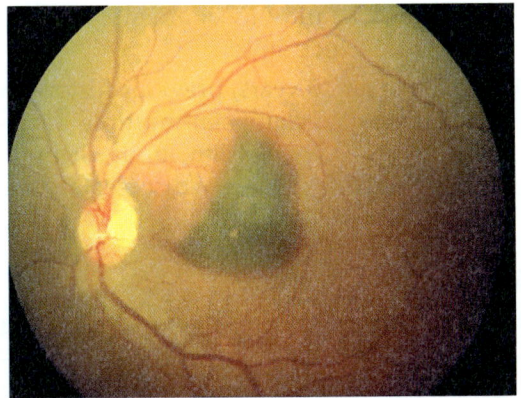

**Fig. 8.28:** Idiopathic polypoidal choroidal vasculopathy (*Courtesy:* Dr Dhananjay Shukla, AEH, Madurai)

3. Polypoidal lesions are of two types:
   i. A large solitary round aneurysmal dilatation
   ii. Cluster of small aneurysmal dilatations, that are more prone for hemorrhages.
4. Central lesion can be located in the macular or peripapillary area.
5. Mid-periphery lesions are often associated with recurrent hemorrhages.
6. Rarely, massive choroidal hemorrhage may occur that has a grave prognosis.
7. Circinate subretinal exudates and CNV without any drusen may develop.
8. Fibrous proliferation with disciform macular scar is less common.

**Differential Diagnosis**

1. AMD
2. Retinal arterial macroaneurysm
3. Other causes of CNV.

**Diagnosis**

1. Slit-lamp examination with 60 or 78 D lens.
2. Dilated funduscopy shows orange polypoid lesions.
3. OCT shows thickening of retina over polyps, macular edema and subretinal fluid.
4. FA shows an early staining network of vessels which fades away in late phase.

CNV is seen as diffuse staining plaque in late phase of the angiogram.
5. Indocyanine green angiography is the best tool to delineate CNV lesion. It demonstrates terminal dilatation of choroidal vessels as popcorn-like lesions as well as occult CNV.

**Treatment**

1. Some cases may resolve spontaneously, just follow them.
2. Intravitreal injections of steroid and anti-VEGF agents can control recurrent exudation and hemorrhages.
3. Photocoagulation and PDT of feeder vessels are effective procedures.
4. Autologous RPE transplantation is a relatively newer treatment option that looks promising.

## 8.27 OCULAR ISCHEMIC SYNDROME

**Etiology**

1. Ocular ischemic syndrome (OIS) is caused by atheroma of the carotid artery and embolization in retinal arteries.
2. The embolus may be composed of cholesterol or fibrin-platelet; the latter is more common. OIS often occurs in advance age and predominantly affects male gender.

**Symptoms**

The patient complains of transient attacks of blackouts, decreased vision, especially after exposure to light and ocular pain.

**Signs**

1. Retinal arteries are narrow.
2. Retinal veins are not tortuous in spite of their dilatation and irregular caliber.
3. Retinal hemorrhages are seen in retinal midperiphery.
4. Microaneurysms, cotton-wool spots and neovascularization are found in the retina.
5. An embolus may be seen at the bifurcation of retinal artery.

8

6. Pulsation or occlusion of central retinal artery may be found.
7. Anterior segment changes include corneal edema, iris neovascularization (80%), iris atrophy, anterior uveitis, increased IOP (neovascular glaucoma) and cataract.

## Differential Diagnosis

1. DR
2. CRVO
3. Takayasu arteritis.

## Diagnosis

1. History of transient attacks of blindness.
2. Slit-lamp examination to find neovascularization of iris and chamber angle, and to measure IOP.
3. Medical evaluation for hypertension, diabetes, atherosclerosis and carotid artery disease.
4. FFA to compare fluorescein appearance time in the retinal arteries of two eyes (arm to retina time).
5. Duplex Doppler USG.
6. MRI arteriography of carotid artery should be considered if surgery is planned.

## Treatment

1. Treat the associated systemic diseases.
2. Raised IOP is managed on the lines of neovascular glaucoma.
3. A combination of intravitreal injection of anti-VEGF and PRP can control neovascularization.
4. Stenosis of carotid artery is dealt with endarterectomy.

## 8.28 RETINOPATHY OF ECLAMPSIA

### Etiology

1. The cause of preeclampsia and eclampsia is not known.
2. Preeclampsia and eclampsia occur after 20 weeks of gestation. Abnormalities of the placenta have been described to coexist.

3. Both genetic and environmental factors contribute to eclampsia.
4. Women over 40 years, previous history of preeclampsia/eclampsia, multiple gestation, obesity, hypertension, lupus, rheumatoid arthritis and kidney diseases are the risk factors.

### Symptoms

1. Transient blurring of vision, decreased vision, difficulty in near vision, photophobia, occasional diplopia and swelling of lower eyelids in the morning may occur.
2. Headache and edema of face and feet are common. Rarely, seizures may develop.

### Signs

1. Eclampsia presents a classical triad of hypertension, proteinuria and generalized edema.
2. Retinopathy of eclampsia may develop in some cases; in fact, it is a manifestation of pregnancy induced hypertension.
3. The earliest change is focal spasm and narrowing of nasal retinal arterioles. Gradually, narrowing may involve the other arterioles.
4. Cotton-wool spots due to retinal ischemia, retinal hemorrhages and focal retinal edema may be seen.
5. Persistent ischemia leads to neovascularization of retina, detachment of macula, disk edema and ischemic optic neuropathy resulting in serious visual loss.
6. Bilateral serous bullous detachment of retina may develop in some patients with eclampsia.
7. Hypertensive encephalopathy, occipital lobe infarcts, renal failure and liver dysfunction are systemic features of eclampsia.

### Differential Diagnosis

Hypertensive retinopathy.

## Diagnosis

1. History of pregnancy
2. Clinical evidence of hypertension and gene-ralized edema of the body
3. Dilated fundus examination shows arterio-lar spasm and picture of advanced hyper-tension
4. Urinalysis demonstrates proteinuria
5. MRI is advised to exclude CNS compli-cations.

## Treatment

1. Proper control of hypertension and electrolyte imbalance is essential to prevent eclampsia.
2. If fundus examination shows the presence of optic disk edema and exudative RD, termination of pregnancy is recommended; otherwise, it may cause maternal and fetal mortality.

## 8.29 VITREOUS HEMORRHAGE

### Etiology

1. The most common cause of vitreous hemor-rhage (VH) is blunt or penetrating trauma.
2. It can also occur in a number of other condi-tions such as proliferative DR, ischemic CRVO, Eales disease, blood dyscrasia, SC disease and complicated posterior vitreous detachment (PVD). Other causes are neo-vascular AMD, intraocular tumors (mela-noma), hypertension, Terson syndrome and ROP.

### Symptoms

Sudden onset of floaters or cobwebs, hazy vision, decreased vision or loss of vision may occur.

### Signs

1. Red fundus reflex may be dull (partial VH) or completely lost (massive VH).
2. VH may occur in the subhyaloid space or in the vitreous cavity (Fig. 8.29).

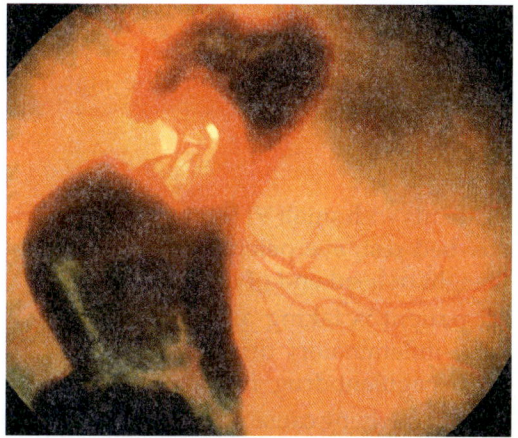

**Fig. 8.29:** Vitreous hemorrhage

3. The subhyaloid blood remains unclotted for a long period. It then gravitates and takes the shape of a boat.
4. VH on clotting forms a white opaque mass in the vitreous.
5. RAPD may be seen in massive VH.
6. Tractional RD, ghost cell glaucoma and hemosiderosis bulbi may develop following recurrent nonclearing vitreous hemor-rhages.
7. Additional retinal and systemic changes may occur depending on the etiology of VH.

### Differential Diagnosis

1. RD
2. Vitritis.

### Diagnosis

1. History of trauma or systemic diseases.
2. Slit-lamp examination for neovasculari-zation of iris and gonioscopy to look for angle neovascularization.
3. Dilated fundus examination for PVD, retinal tears, RD and intraocular tumors.
4. FA of both eyes to find the etiology of hemorrhage, if fundus reflex in one eye is lost, useful information may be obtained from the fellow eye.

8

5. B-scan USG, in the eye where retinal details are obscured due to dense VH, can provide useful information about the status of vitreous and retina.

## Treatment

1. Patients with small VH show improvement by bed rest, eye patching and raising the height of head end of the bed.
2. If patient is taking aspirin, nonsteroidal anti-inflammatory drugs (NSAIDs) or any anticoagulant drug, it must be stopped.
3. The underlying cause of VH must be treated as early as possible.
4. Increased IOP should be managed medically.
5. Patients with mild to moderate VH may take 1–3 months for clearing.
6. If VH is associated with neovascularization of iris, retinal tears, RD, or DR, early vitrectomy is indicated.

## 8.30 POSTERIOR VITREOUS DETACHMENT

### Etiology

1. Posterior vitreous detachment (PVD) is the separation of cortical vitreous from the retina; it may occur with or without vitreous liquefaction and collapse.
2. The causes of PVD include old age, VH, posterior uveitis and proliferative diabetic retinopathy.
3. Liquefaction of vitreous, high myopia, aphakia, defect in the posterior lens capsule and recurrent vitritis are known risk factors for PVD.

### Types

PVD can be either partial or complete. It may be simple or complicated that is associated with VH, retinal tear, macular hole, vitreomacular traction or RD.

### Symptoms

Floaters, flashes of light and blurred vision.

### Signs

1. Gray to black opacities in vitreous.
2. A condensed vitreous may be seen behind the lens.
3. Optically empty spaces develop in the vitreous cavity that are best seen with contact lens on slit-lamp examination.
4. A characteristic fine ring of tissue (Weiss ring) may be seen on the detached posterior hyaloid membrane anterior to the optic disk (Fig. 8.30).
5. Hemorrhages may occur on the optic disk margin or in the retinal periphery. Sometime vitreous hemorrhage may result due to avulsion of retinal blood vessel.
6. Tobacco dust-like cells liberated from the RPE may be deposited on the anterior vitreous when PVD is complicated by a retinal tear (Shafer sign).
7. Focal vitreous traction on peripheral retina causes retinal breaks and detachment; retinal breaks are often found in acute PVD.
8. Persistent attachment of vitreous to the macula results in vitreomacular traction (VMT).
9. Mechanical traction on the macula may cause CME.

### Differential Diagnosis

Vitritis.

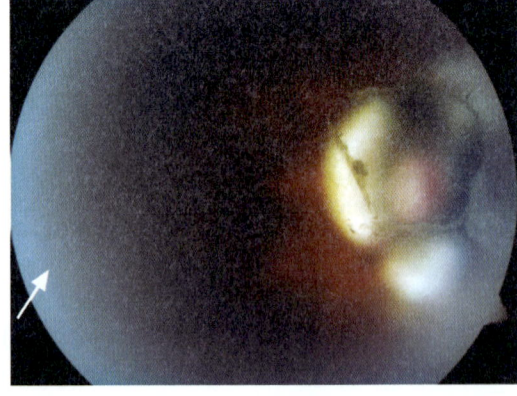

Fig. 8.30: Posterior vitreous detachment (*Courtesy:* AEH, Madurai)

## Diagnosis

1. History of retinal disease, trauma or intraocular surgery.
2. Slit-lamp examination with 60 or 90 D lens can identify Weiss ring over optic disk.
3. Dilated fundus examination for retinal tears, vitreous traction, RD and extent of PVD.
4. If media are hazy, B-scan USG can diagnose the extent of PVD and exclude RD and intraocular tumor.
5. OCT can demonstrate an initial PVD over macular region and its radial extension. It is also helpful in diagnosing VMT and CME.

## Treatment

1. PVD does not need any treatment.

2. Treatment is needed for associated complications. Retinal breaks must be sealed with photocoagulation before development of RD.
3. Surgical reattachment is necessary once RD occurs.
4. VMT and CME are managed by relieving the traction on the macula.

## Follow-up

1. All cases with PVD must be followed on 1–2 monthly intervals to check for increase in symptoms and to look for any retinal break, RD and VH.
2. The patient should be educated about the presenting symptoms of RD and in the event of fresh symptoms like loss of vision in the upper or lower half of visual field, an early consultation is warranted.

8

# CHAPTER
# 9

# Lids, Lacrimal Apparatus and Orbit

## 9.1 ACQUIRED PTOSIS

### Etiology

1. The acquired ptosis or blepharoptosis may be caused by aponeurotic, neurogenic, mechanical, traumatic and myogenic causes.
2. Aponeurotic ptosis is caused by dehiscence of the aponeurosis of levator palpebrae superioris (LPS) as a result of traction in ocular surgery or rubbing of the eye.
3. Neurogenic ptosis is due to oculomotor nerve palsy and Horner's syndrome.
4. Mechanical ptosis is due to multiple chalazia, trachoma and upper lid tumors.
5. Trauma to LPS and its aponeurosis also causes ptosis.
6. Acquired myogenic ptosis is uncommon and seen in patients with myasthenia gravis or muscular dystrophy.
7. Ptosis is a feature of chronic progressive ophthalmoplegia.

### Symptoms

Drooping of upper lid is main symptom, occasionally, decrease in vision and diplopia may occur.

### Signs

1. Drooping of the upper lid may be mild (Fig. 9.1) or moderate (Fig. 9.2).

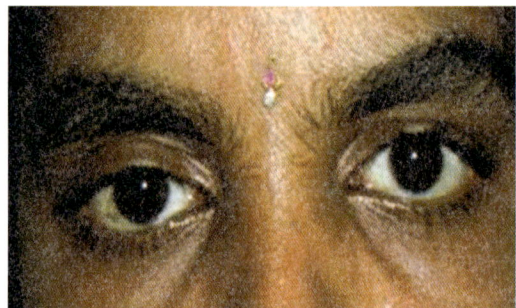

Fig. 9.1: Ptosis right eye

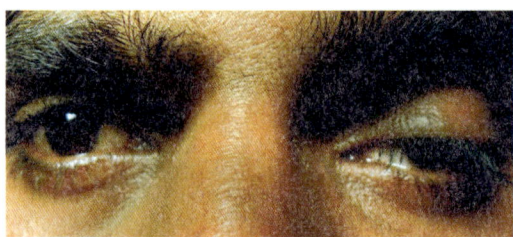

Fig. 9.2: Moderate ptosis

2. Aponeurotic ptosis is worse in down gaze.
3. Unilateral ptotic lid may be raised on jaw movements or mastication (Marcus Gunn jaw winking phenomenon) due to abnormal nerve connection.
4. The cornea may be covered partially or completely depending on degree of ptosis.
5. Absence of upper eyelid crease.
6. Partial or complete third nerve palsy presents exotropia, limitation of ocular

174

movements, diplopia on elevation of ptotic lid and dilated nonreacting pupil.

7. Hordeolum or growth in upper lid may be found in mechanical ptosis.

8. Fluctuating ptosis and diplopia is a sign of myasthenia gravis.

### Differential Diagnosis

Pseudoptosis is seen in the following conditions:

1. Anophthalmos and microphthalmos
2. Enophthalmos
3. Phthisis bulbi
4. Dermatochalasis
5. Congenital ptosis.

### Diagnosis

1. History and old photographs can differentiate between acquired and congenital ptosis.
2. Clinical examination can exclude myasthenia, lid growth, third cranial nerve palsy, chronic progressive external ophthalmoplegia and Horner syndrome.
3. In case of doubt, ice or sleep test for myasthenia and cocaine or apraclonidine for Horner syndrome may be performed.
4. Computed tomography (CT) or magnetic resonance imaging (MRI) can delineate superior orbital mass.
5. Magnetic resonance angiography is useful in the diagnosis of intracranial aneurysm and carotid artery dissection.

### Treatment

1. Manage the underlying etiology; excision of chalazion or lid growth, treatment of myasthenia gravis.
2. Conservative treatment is recommended for isolated third cranial nerve palsy.
3. Ptotic lid can be elevated with the help of crutches attached to frame of glasses if it is not associated with diplopia.
4. New growth in the orbit requires surgery.

5. More often acquired ptosis needs surgical correction by levator resection either through transconjunctival or transcutaneous approach.
6. Unilateral ptosis with Marcus Gunn jaw-winking phenomenon is corrected by bilateral sling operation with disinsertion of LPS.

## 9.2 BLEPHARITIS

Blepharitis is a chronic inflammatory disease of the margin of eyelid which may be classified into anterior and posterior forms.

### Anterior Blepharitis

#### Etiology

1. The anterior blepharitis primarily involves the bases of eyelashes.
2. It may be a seborrheic and infective in types.
3. Seborrheic blepharitis is associated with seborrhea of scalp and skin of face.
4. Infective blepharitis is caused by *Staphylococcus aureus.*
5. Blepharitis caused by crab louse and *Demodex folliculorum* is not rare.
6. Chronic conjunctivitis, dacryocystitis, eyestrain and refractive errors are risk factors.

#### Symptoms

Irritation, grittiness, watering, intense itching, burning, photophobia and falling of eyelashes are common.

#### Signs

1. Seborrheic blepharitis
   - Lid margins are glossy and hyperemic.
   - Dandruff is deposited at the root of eyelashes.
   - Soft scales appear on lid margins and lashes may be matted.
   - Dandruff of scalp is often present.
2. Staphylococcal blepharitis
   - Eyelid margins are swollen and hyperemic.

9

- Crusting or scaling on the margins are found.
- Meibomitis with inspissated glands are often seen at the lid margin.
- Chronic papillary conjunctivitis is always present.
- Eyelashes are sparse.
- Chronic blepharitis distorts the lid margin and leads to madarosis, trichiasis, tylosis and ectopion.
- Chronic blepharitis may be associated with dry eye, recurrent styes, angular conjunctivitis, punctate epithelial erosions predominantly in the lower part of the cornea, catarrhal marginal corneal ulcers, acne rosacea and phlyctenulosis.

## Diagnosis

1. It is mostly clinical.
2. Presence of nits at the roots of eyelashes indicates parasitic blepharitis.
3. Smear and culture examination reveals the etiology.

## Treatment

1. Hot compresses, cleaning of lid margin and mechanical expression of the meibomian glands relieve symptoms.
2. Removal of the crust, application of the antibiotic-corticosteroid ointment and massage of the lid margin are beneficial.
3. Frequent use of preservative-free tear substitutes prevents dry eye.
4. Oral tetracycline 250 mg four times a day, for 2–3 weeks is effective in nonresponsive cases. It is contraindicated in children below 8 years and pregnant mothers. Erythromycin may be given.

## Posterior Blepharitis

### Etiology

Chronic posterior blepharitis is caused by meibomian gland dysfunction associated with its vicarious secretion.

### Symptoms

Symptoms are same as seen in the chronic anterior blepharitis.

### Signs

1. Opening of the meibomian ducts are plugged with oil globules.
2. Telangiectasia of the posterior lid margin is seen.
3. Squeezing of lid margin results in expression of white toothpaste-like material.
4. Yellowish streaks of dilated meibomian glands may be found in the upper palpebral conjunctiva.
5. Deposition of foamy and frothy secretion may be found on the inner canthus and the lid margin.
6. Chronic posterior blepharitis may be associated with dry eye, atopic keratoconjunctivitis, ocular rosacea, chalazion and contact lens (CL) intolerance.

### Diagnosis

It is mostly clinical.

### Treatment

1. Dandruff can be managed by medicated shampoo.
2. Warm compression and lid massage may prevent the blockade of meibomian glands.
3. Tetracycline (250 mg 2–4 times a day for 6 weeks) is the drug of choice.
4. Erythromycin (250 mg twice a day) should be used in children.
5. Preservative-free tear substitute is used 3–4 times in a day to prevent dry eye.
6. Topical antibiotic and steroids (for short period) are also recommended for comfort and prevention of secondary infection.
7. Cyclosporine (0.05%) eye drops twice a day can control meibomitis.

## 9.3 ENTROPION

### Etiology

Entropion or inward rolling of lid margin is of following types:

9

1. Involutional entropion is seen in old age due to horizontal laxity of the eyelid.
2. Spastic entropion is caused by spasm of orbicularis oculi and seen in acute conjunctivitis, corneal ulcer, tight bandaging of eye, blephrospasm, microphthalmos, etc.
3. Cicatricial entropion is found in trachoma, membranous conjunctivitis, ocular burns, cicatricial pemphigoid, Stevens-Johnson syndrome, etc.
4. Congenital entropion is seen in microphthalmos.

## Symptoms

Mild entropion does not give any symptoms but moderate to severe entropion causes foreign body (FB) sensation, irritation, redness, watering and photophobia.

## Signs

1. Entropion may be mild when only posterior lid margin is turned inside.
2. In moderate entropion intermarginal strip rotates inward (Fig. 9.3).
3. The entire lid margin rolls inwards in severe entropion.
4. Rubbing of eyelashes against conjunctiva and cornea may lead to injection of conjunctiva, corneal infiltrations and multiple corneal erosions.
5. Corneal ulcer, corneal vascularization and corneal thinning may be seen in patients with severe entropion.

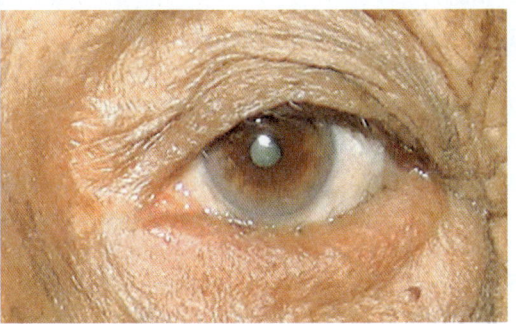

**Fig. 9.3:** Entropion lower lid

## Diagnosis

1. History of ocular infection, burn and drug reaction
2. Clinical evidence of turning inside of lid margin
3. Examination of conjunctiva and cornea is important for complication and sequelae.

## Treatment

1. Treat the cause and corneal lesions
2. Discard the tight bandage and apply antibiotic ointment
3. Severe spastic entropion may need skin-muscle operation
4. Almost all cicatricial entropions require surgical correction. Jaesche-Arlt and Snellen's partial tarsectomy may be performed.
5. Involutional entropion can be corrected by horizontal tightening of eyelid with repair of retractors.

## 9.4 ECTROPION

### Etiology

1. Outward rolling of the lid margin is known as ectropion. Ectropion is usually seen in the lower eyelids.
2. Ectropion is of the following types:
   - Senile ectropion is caused by laxity of orbicularis oculi in old age.
   - Spastic ectropion develops due to contraction of orbicularis oculi during photophobia.
   - Cicatricial ectropion can occur following trauma, burn, ulcers, dermatitis.
   - Paralytic ectropion results from seventh nerve palsy.
   - Mechanical ectropion occurs as a result of a growth of the lower eyelid.
   - Congenital ectropion is developmental in origin.

### Symptoms

Watering due to eversion of lower punctum is the main symptom.

9

## Signs

1. Outward turning of the lower lid with visible lower punctum may be the only sign of mild ectropion.
2. Lower palpebral conjunctiva is usually visible in moderate ectropion.
3. The lower fornix is seen in severe ectropion (Fig. 9.4).
4. A part of the lower conjunctiva remains exposed.
5. Initially, the exposed conjunctiva is congested and later, becomes dry, thickened and keratinized.
6. The lower part of cornea may develop superficial punctate keratitis (SPK) or exposure keratitis in severe ectropion.
7. Cicatricial ectropion may be associated with scarring of lid or conjunctiva and damage to cornea.
8. Lagophthalmos and features of facial palsy may be found.

## Diagnosis

1. Diagnosis is mainly based on clinical signs.
2. History of trauma, burn or palsy is helpful.

## Treatment

1. Protect cornea from exposure keratitis by frequent use of lubricants.
2. Measures like taping the lids or temporary tarsorrhaphy can be adopted.
3. Patients with facial palsy may resolve spontaneously.

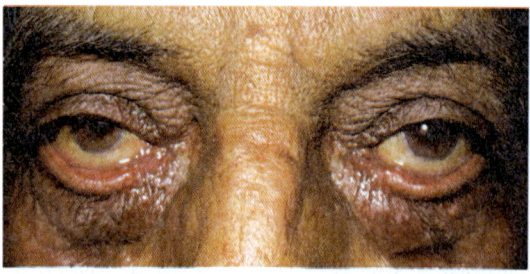

**Fig. 9.4:** Bilateral ectropion lower eyelids

4. SPK or exposure keratitis should be treated with topical cycloplegic drops and antibiotics.
5. Corrective surgery may be needed in some patients. Depending on the type of ectropion, one of the following procedures should be performed:
   - Medial conjunctivoplasty for epiphora
   - Bick's procedure for moderate ectropion
   - Lateral strip and conjunctivoplasty for senile ectropion
   - V-Y plasty or Z-plasty for cicatricial ectropion.

## 9.5 ESSENTIAL BLEPHAROSPASM

### Etiology

1. Essential blepharospasm is an involuntary closure of one or both eyes.
2. It predominantly affects women in the age group of 45–65.
3. Etiology of blepharospasm is not known and considered idiopathic. It may be due to involvement of the basal ganglion.

### Symptoms

1. Initially, a bilateral uncontrolled increased blinking and mild twitching of the lids may be noticed.
2. Frequent forceful closures of eyes adversely affect vision and the patient becomes handicapped in his routine activities.

### Signs

1. Forced contractions and closure of the eyelids (Fig. 9.5).
2. The patient cannot open the eyes.
3. Blephrospasm disappears during sleep.
4. It may be associated with uncontrollable movements of face, neck and head known as Meige syndrome.
5. Essential blepharospasm can cause ectropion in children while elderly women develop entropion.

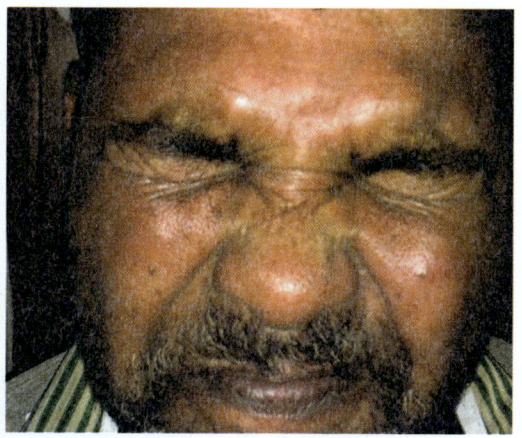

Fig. 9.5: Essential blepharospasm

## Differential Diagnosis

1. Corneal ulcer or FB
2. Trigeminal neuralgia
3. Hemifacial spasm: It is unilateral and does not disappear during sleep.
4. Apraxia of eyelid: It is a sign of Parkinson disease.

## Diagnosis

1. History of central nervous system (CNS) or mental disease or intake of medicine
2. Exclude ocular irritation or FB
3. MRI of brain may exclude suspected lesions of posterior fossa.

## Treatment

1. Muscle relaxants or sedatives may help in some cases.
2. Botulinum toxin is injected into the orbicularis oculi at different sites in small doses.
3. Mymectomy of orbicularis may be effective.
4. Ablation of facial nerve.

## 9.6 FLOPPY EYELID SYNDROME

### Etiology

1. Etiology of floppy eyelid syndrome (spontaneous eversion of upper lid) is not known.
2. It is considered as idiopathic. The defect lies in the collagen and elastin fibers of the lids.
3. Frequent rubbing of eyes may be a risk factor.
4. It is more common in males than females, and in obese people.
5. Floppy eyelid syndrome is associated with obstructive sleep apnea, hyperglycemia and keratoconus.

### Symptoms

Irritation, redness, mucous or ropy discharge in the morning, headache and blurring of vision may occur.

### Signs

1. Eversion of upper lids during sleep is the hallmark of the syndrome.
2. Flaccid upper lid
3. The upper tarsus is soft, rubbery, loose, lax and easily everted by just pulling the lid upward (Fig. 9.6).
4. Eye is red with chronic papillary conjunctivitis of palpebral conjunctiva due to exposure.
5. Mild ptosis, SPK, dry eye disease, corneal erosion or ulcer, bacterial keratitis and vascularization may be found.
6. Chronic sleep apnea may be associated with raised intracranial pressure, papilledema, optic neuropathy, pulmonary hypertension and cardiopathy.

### Differential Diagnosis

1. Giant papillary conjunctivitis: History of use of CL or prosthesis.
2. Vernal keratoconjunctivitis.

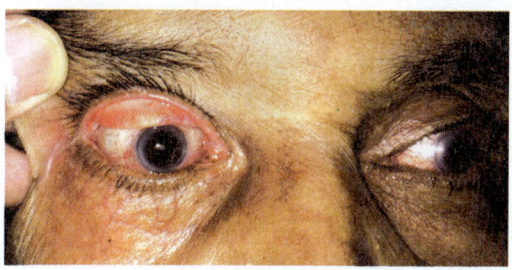

Fig. 9.6: Floppy eye syndrome

## Diagnosis

1. History of obstructive sleep apnea
2. See for spontaneous eversion by pulling the upper lid upward
3. Slit-lamp examination for corneal signs.

## Treatment

1. Advice the patient to sleep on side position and avoid the face down position.
2. Refer the patient to physician for the treatment of obstructive sleep apnea.
3. Tape the eyelids before sleep or use eye shields.
4. Definitive treatment is surgical horizontal tightening of the upper lid.

## 9.7 MALIGNANT TUMORS OF EYELIDS

### Etiology

1. The malignant tumors of lid often affect males above the age of 50 years.
2. Carcinoma of lid is common and manifests as: *Basal cell carcinoma, squamous cell carcinoma and sebaceous gland carcinoma.*
3. About 90% of malignant tumors of eyelid are basal cell carcinoma.
4. Most of squamous carcinomas arise from solar keratosis or actinic keratosis and affect people with fair-colored skin.
5. Patients give history of systemic malignancy in the family.

### Basal Cell Carcinoma

#### Symptoms

Most patients of basal cell carcinoma remain symptom-free initially.

#### Signs

1. A nodule with a pearly surface and telangiectatic vessels develops on the lower lid or on the medial canthus (Fig. 9.7).
2. It is a firm growth with raised margin and superficial vascularization.
3. Later it ulcerates, bleeds and forms a central crater often referred to as rodent ulcer.

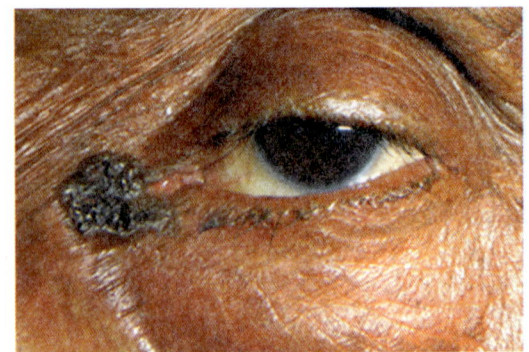

**Fig. 9.7:** Basal cell carcinoma (*Courtesy:* Dr SCL Chandravansi, SS Medical College, Rewa)

4. It is locally invasive and does not metastasize; however, it can invade the orbit.
5. The less common fibrosing basal cell carcinoma has an aggressive course than the nodular type.

#### Diagnosis

1. Clinical evidence can diagnose the carcinoma in majority of cases.
2. Biopsy confirms the diagnosis (Fig. 9.8).

#### Treatment

1. Surgical excision is the most preferred treatment.

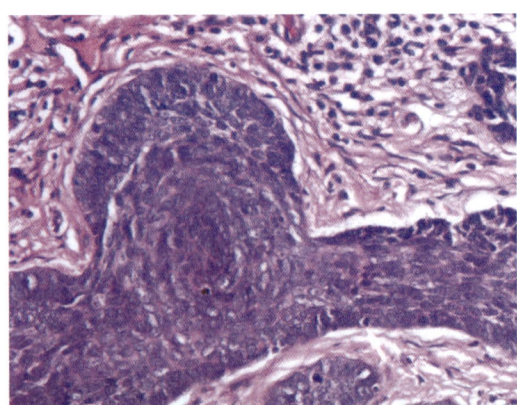

**Fig. 9.8:** Microphotograph of basal cell carcinoma showing basal cells infiltrating in the subepithelial tissue with palisading of nuclei (*Courtesy:* Dr Amit Verma, Department of Pathology, SAIMS, Indore)

2. Radiotherapy is the other modality of treatment but should not be used for canthal carcinoma because of damage to lacrimal drainage system.

## Squamous Cell Carcinoma

### Symptoms

Swelling on the lid margin, watering and disfigurement are common complaints.

### Signs

1. Squamous cell carcinoma arises from the lid margin.
2. It starts as a small nodule on the lid margin.
3. It is painless and grows slowly.
4. The nodule ulcerates and its base is indurated.
5. Gradually, the growth enlarges in size.
6. If infected, it presents as a fungating mass.
7. Squamous carcinoma has tendency to involve preauricular and submandibular lymph glands and remote metastases.

### Diagnosis

Biopsy is confirmatory (Fig. 9.9).

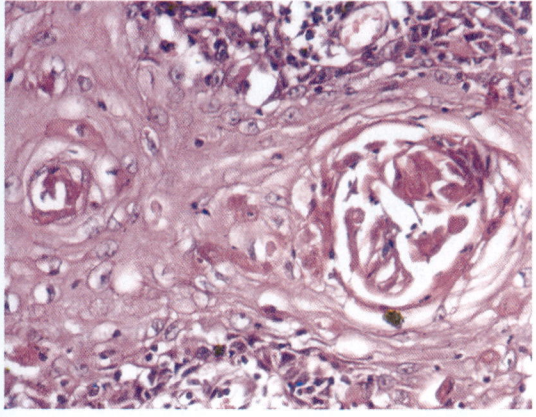

**Fig. 9.9:** Microphotograph of squamous cell carcinoma showing lobules of sebaceous cells infiltrating in the stroma (*Courtesy:* Dr Amit Verma, Department of Pathology, SAIMS, Indore)

### Treatment

Squamous carcinoma requires a wide excision of the growth followed by radiotherapy.

## Sebaceous Gland Carcinoma

### Etiology

Sebaceous gland carcinoma arises from the meibomian glands or sebaceous glands of the eyelashes.

### Symptoms

Presents a painless swelling of the upper lid.

### Signs

1. A firm painless nodule appears in the upper eyelid and looks like a chalazion.
2. The skin over it is free but the nodule is fixed with underlying tissue.
3. Gradually, it destroys the meibomian gland. It is a highly malignant tumor.
4. It metastasis into the regional lymph glands.

### Diagnosis

A full-thickness biopsy helps in the diagnosis.

### Treatment

Wide surgical excision is the treatment of choice.

## 9.8 DACRYOCYSTITIS IN ADULTS

The dacryocystitis in adults manifests either as an acute or a chronic form.

### Acute Dacryocystitis

#### Etiology

1. An acute inflammation of the lacrimal sac is caused by *S. pneumoniae*, *S. pyogenes*, *S. aureus*, *Actinomyces*, etc.
2. Obstruction of nasolacrimal duct, a pre-existing chronic dacryocystitis, diabetes, infective conjunctivitis and immuno-compromised status are considered as risk factors.

### Symptoms

1. Severe pain, discharge, swelling and redness of the sac region and the eyelids are common symptoms.
2. Constitutional symptoms like fever and malaise may develop.

### Signs

1. The sac region is usually swollen, red, tense and tender (Fig. 9.10).
2. The swelling spreads to the cheek and the regional lymph glands are tender and enlarged.
3. The distended sac forms a lacrimal abscess. It bursts on the skin surface forming a lacrimal fistula with oozing pus.
4. Mismanaged cases of acute dacryocystitis may suffer from corneal ulcer, osteomyelitis and orbital cellulitis.

### Differential Diagnosis

1. Facial cellulitis: Sac is free
2. Frontal mucocele: The site is different and sac is not involved.
3. Acute ethmoid sinusitis: Sac region is tender but sac is free.

### Diagnosis

1. History of watering and concurrent acute conjunctivitis.
2. Characteristic clinical features help in diagnosis.
3. Lacrimal syringing is contraindicated.

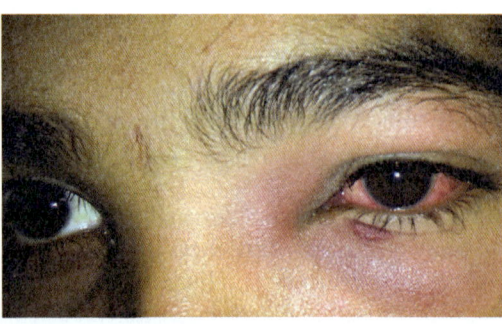

**Fig. 9.10:** Acute dacryocystitis

4. Discharge should be cultured for infective organism.
5. CT scan of paranasal sinuses excludes ethmoid sinusitis and mucocele of the frontal sinus.

### Treatment

1. Pain can be relieved by local hot compresses and systemic nonsteroidal anti-inflammatory drugs (NSAIDs).
2. Infection can be controlled by topical moxifloxacin (0.5%) or gatifloxacin (0.3%) drops, six times a day.
3. The patients should be treated with cefazolin (1 g IV three times a day).
4. Mild cases may be treated with cefalexin (500 mg, four times a day).
5. In case pus point is formed evacuate it.
6. When acute infection is controlled, a combined fistulectomy with dacryocystorhinostomy (DCR) operation is performed.

## Chronic Dacryocystitis

### Etiology

1. Chronic dacryocystitis is more common.
2. Chronic dacryocystitis is often unilateral and affects females (80%).
3. It is usually caused by obstruction of the nasolacrimal duct.
4. *S. aureus, S. pneumoniae, Enterobacter, E. coli* and *P. aeruginosa* may infect the sac following obstruction.
5. The tuberculous lesion of bones can involve the sac.
6. Tertiary syphilis and *Rhinosporidium seeberi* can also involve the lacrimal sac.
7. Risk factors for chronic dacryocystitis include nasal polyp, deviation of the septum, rhinitis and hypertrophied inferior turbinate.

### Symptoms

Mucopus discharge is the most common symptom. A painless cystic swelling in the sac region may be noticed.

## Signs

1. Partial obstruction of nasolacrimal duct with low grade infection causes a mucocele.
2. Mucocele is a round, nontender, cystic swelling in the sac region (Fig. 9.11).
3. If pressure is applied on sac, mucous regurgitates through the lower punctum and rarely, mucous passes into the nose.
4. More commonly, there is no swelling but only persistent watering and discharge.
5. Lacrimal fistula may be present. It indicates that patient had an acute dacryocystitis in the past.
6. An acute dacryocystitis can supervene on a chronic one.

## Differential Diagnosis

Cyst or tumor of the lacrimal sac.

## Diagnosis

1. Regurgitation test: Pressure on sac causes regurgitation of mucous.
2. Syringing may locate the site of block in the lacrimal passage.
3. Dacryocystography may be performed to confirm the site of obstruction.
4. Discharge should be cultured to know the type of infection.

## Treatment

1. Infection is controlled by topical antibiotic.

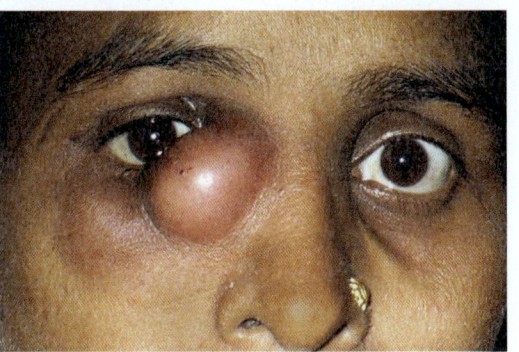

**Fig. 9.11:** Chronic dacryocystitis: Mucocele

2. Dacryocystectomy is advised in tuberculosis of sac or osteomyelitis of nasal bones.
3. Dacryocystorhinostomy (DCR) is a preferred surgical procedure.
4. If DCR fails, a silicone tube intubation is performed.
5. Conjunctivo DCR can be performed in patients with blockage of both canaliculi.

## 9.9 DRY EYE DISEASE

### Etiology

1. Dry eye disease (DED), a disorder of tear film is caused by deficiency of aqueous, mucin or lipid component of tears.
2. The aqueous tear deficiency is seen in keratoconjunctivitis sicca.
3. Mucin deficiency is caused by destruction of goblet cells due to trachoma, membranous conjunctivitis, ocular cicatricial pemphigoid, Stevens-Johnson syndrome, chemical burns and injuries.
4. Chronic blepharitis and acne rosecea can cause lipid deficiency.
5. DED can also occur as a result of impaired blinking and irregularity of the corneal surface.
6. Use of drugs like antihistaminics, antispasmodics, antipsychotics, antidepressants oral contraceptive, beta blockers, diuretic, etc. can cause DED.
7. Deficiency of vitamin A and androgen may lead to dryness.
8. Laser-assisted *in situ* keratomileusis (LASIK) and other keratorefractive procedures, connective tissue disorders, radiation and chemotherapy are considered important causes.
9. Dry, dusty, smoky and windy atmosphere, working on computer or watching TV for long period, old age and menopause in women are known risk factors.

9

## Symptoms

Symptoms include ocular discomfort, FB sensation, itching, discharge, heaviness of lids, dryness of eyes, redness and photophobia.

## Signs

1. Signs of dryness vary depending on the severity (mild, moderate and severe) of the disease.
2. Discharge is scanty.
3. Meibomitis with blocked opening of ducts of the glands.
4. Dry conjunctiva
5. Palpebral conjunctiva may show papillary hypertrophy.
6. Cornea may look dry with SPK, filamentary keratitis, keratinization (Fig. 9.12), mucous plaque, corneal ulcer, and band keratopathy.

## Diagnosis

1. The height of tear miniscus on slit-lamp is diminished (less than 1 mm).
2. Mucin deficiency can be assessed by tear film break-up time (BUT). After touching the fluorescein strip to the lower palpebral conjunctiva, the patient is asked to blink several times and examined on the slit-lamp. The time is measured between last blink and development of a dry spot. A time of less than 10 seconds is considered abnormal.

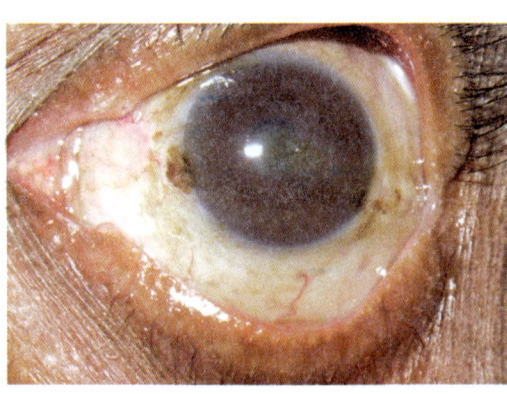

**Fig. 9.12:** Dry eye: Corneal changes

3. Eyes are examined on the slit-lamp after staining with fluorescein dye. Punctate or blotchy staining may be seen in dry eyes; it is more obvious in the cornea than in conjunctiva.
4. Rose Bengal stains the dead epithelial cells. A triangular staining of the interpalpebral conjunctiva is often seen in kerato-conjunctivitis sicca.
5. Lissamine green-staining causes less irritation and can be used in place of rose Bengal.
6. Schirmer test measures the tear production but gives variable results. A 5 mm bent part of 5 × 35 strip of Whatman paper strip is kept in the lower fornix. A less than 10 mm strip wetting from bent part, after 5 minutes is suggestive of dry eye.
7. Conjunctival impression cytology provides information about density of goblet cells.
8. Conjunctival biopsy may be considered in rare cases.

## Treatment

1. As far as possible risk factors should be eliminated.
2. The treatment of DED will differ according to severity of the disease:
   - *Mild DED:* Preservative-free tear substitutes are used 3–4 times in a day.
   - *Moderate DED:* Discourage the use of CLs and avoid LASIK surgery.
     - Preservative-free tear substitutes are instilled hourly or two hourly and use lubricating gel 3–4 times. As an alternative, a lacrisert can be inserted in the lower fornix to supply lubrication continuously.
     - Associated eye and systemic diseases should be treated adequately. Blepharitis must be treated aggressively with massage, topical antibiotic ointment and oral tetracycline.
     - Dry eye with mild ocular inflammation responds to topical corticosteroids

[loteprednol (0.5%)] two to three times in a day.

- Topical cyclosporine (0.05%, two times a day) should be tried in nonresponding patients.
- Punctal block can preserve the scanty tears.

■ *Severe DED:*

- Use lubricating gel (four to six times a day) and cyclosporine (0.05%, twice daily). A permanent punctal block may be done by argon laser punctoplasty or cauterization.
- Autologous serum (20% in sterile saline used six times/day) acts as a lubricant and inhibits cytokines and metallo-proteinases.
- Use of acetylcystein (10%) drops reduces formation of mucous strands.
- Hydrophilic CLs with artificial tears and moist chamber goggles may provide comfort.
- Lateral tarsorrhaphy is performed to decrease the tear evaporation. Correction of trichiasis or entropion is essential for protection of cornea.
- Stem cell and amniotic membrane transplantation may correct ocular surface disorder.

## 9.10 LACRIMAL GLAND TUMOR

### Types

1. Tumors of the lacrimal gland are benign and malignant.
2. The most common benign tumor is mixed-cell tumor (pleomorphic).
3. The adenoid cystic carcinoma is the most common malignant tumor of lacrimal gland.
4. Other malignancies of lacrimal gland are adenocarcinoma, squamous cell carcinoma and lymphoma.

### Symptoms

Symptoms include swelling of upper lid, watering, diplopia, dryness and bulging of eye and pain.

### Signs

1. The upper lid assumes S-shaped contour.
2. Swelling develops in the upper lateral orbit.
3. A nontender mass appears in the lacrimal fossa.
4. Mixed-cell tumor is a slow-growing mass; it can give proptosis and dislodge the eye downward and medially.
5. Proptosis may cause exposure keratitis.
6. Adenoid cystic carcinoma grows rapidly. It presents a tender mass which extends posteriorly and restricts ocular motility.
7. Intraocular pressure (IOP) is often increased.
8. The tumor can cause papilledema and choroidal folds.
9. Preauricular lymph nodes are enlarged.

### Differential Diagnosis

1. Sarcoidosis
2. Dacryoadenitis
3. Dermoid cyst
4. Idiopathic orbital inflammatory syndrome (pseudo tumor of orbit)
5. Inflammatory granuloma of lacrimal gland.

### Diagnosis

1. Exclude sarcoidosis.
2. CT scan shows general enlargement of orbit in mixed-cell tumor.
3. CT scans in malignant tumors reveal bony erosion and calcification.
4. MRI of orbit can assess intracranial extension.
5. CT of chest for sarcoidosis, tuberculosis and primary malignancy
6. Lacrimal biopsy to confirm the diagnosis.

### Treatment

1. Surgical excision is needed for mixed-cell tumor.

2. Chemotherapy with intra-arterial *cis* platinum followed by radical excision is recommended for adenoid cystic carcinoma.

3. Patients may be treated by exentration followed by radiotherapy.

4. Malignant lymphoma responds to irradiation.

## 9.11 ORBITAL CELLULITIS

### Etiology

1. Orbital cellulitis is most commonly caused by spread of infection from paranasal sinuses.

2. It can also develop following dental infection, dacyocystitis, blow-out fracture, trauma and facial erysipelas.

3. *S. pyogenes, S. pneumoniae, S. aureus, P. aeruginosa, Aspergillus, Mucor* and parasitic infestation can cause orbital cellulitis.

4. Diabetes, human immunodeficiency virus (HIV) infection and malignancy are considered as predisposing factors.

### Symptoms

1. Supraorbital pain, diplopia, decrease in vision, swelling of the eyelids and red eye are common.

2. Nasal congestion or discharge, fever, dental pain, headache and bulging of eyes are other complaints.

### Signs

1. Lids are swollen and red (Fig. 9.13).

2. Chemosis of conjunctiva is marked; the conjunctiva may protrude through the palpebral aperture in severe cases.

3. Proptosis is an important feature of orbital cellulitis.

4. Ocular motility is restricted and movements are painful.

5. Displacement of the eyeball and increase in proptosis may occur due to abscess formation in one of the orbital spaces.

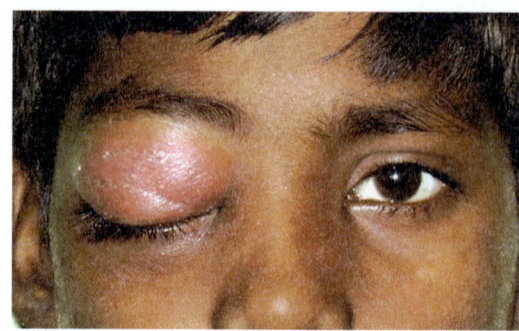

Fig. 9.13: Orbital cellulitis

6. Engorgement of the veins, papilledema and optic neuritis may be seen.

7. Visual loss, abnormal pupillary reactions and multiple cranial nerve palsies indicate involvement of the orbital apex.

8. Orbital cellulitis may cause cavernous sinus thrombosis resulting in a rapid increase in proptosis.

9. Septic meningitis and cerebral abscess may supervene.

### Differential Diagnosis

1. Orbital abscess

2. Cavernous sinus thrombosis

3. Idiopathic orbital inflammation.

### Diagnosis

1. History of sinusitis with mucous discharge from nose or obstruction of nose.

2. Complete blood picture (CBP) shows leukocytosis.

3. Discharge from eye and nose should be cultured for bacteria and fungus.

4. CT of paranasal sinuses may show blocked sinus or its destruction.

5. CT scan can reveal fracture of orbit or FB.

6. Biopsy of the necrotic tissue for fungus infection.

### Treatment

1. Protect the cornea from exposure by frequent use of lubricants, cycloplegic (once a day) and antibiotic.

2. Ampicillin (300 mg in four divided doses, IV per day) should be administered in children.
3. A combination of ceftriaxone (2 g IV twice a day) and metronidazole (500 mg four times a day) is used in adult patients.
4. The associated meningitis can be managed with IV vancomycin in consultation with neurologist.
5. Corticosteroid therapy may be considered after 1–2 days of antibiotic therapy.
6. Excision of the nasal mass and administration of amphotericin B (5 mg/kg, IV) may benefit patients with fungal orbital cellulitis.
7. If the condition does not improve within 3 days of medical therapy, a surgical drainage of sinus or orbital abscess should be considered.

## 9.12 IDIOPATHIC ORBITAL INFLAMMATORY SYNDROME

### Etiology

1. The idiopathic orbital inflammatory syndrome (IOIS) was earlier known as pseudotumor of the orbit.
2. It is not a neoplastic condition but a nonspecific inflammation of the orbit.
3. Idiopathic orbital inflammatory syndrome is unilateral in adults and bilateral in children.

### Symptoms

1. Symptoms are variable. IOIS may have an acute painful onset. Orbital pain, swelling of lids, redness, diplopia and decrease in vision are common.
2. Headache, fever, malaise, nausea, vomiting and abdominal pain can occur in 50% of children.

### Signs

1. Clinically, it may manifest as dacryoadenitis, myositis of extraocular muscles, and superior orbital fissuritis.

2. Eyelids are red and edematous.
3. Conjunctiva is chemotic.
4. Proptosis occurs due to increase in orbital fat and thickening of the extraocular muscles.
5. Ocular movements are usually restricted.
6. Increased IOP, iritis, optic neuropathy and enlarged lacrimal gland are uncommon features.
7. Idiopathic sclerosing inflammation of the orbit presents minimal inflammatory signs.

### Differential Diagnosis

1. Graves' ophthalmopathy
2. Myositis of extraocular muscles.
3. Orbital cellulitis
4. *Tolosa-Hunt syndrome:* An idiopathic granuloma at the apex of the orbit.
5. Sarcoidosis.

### Diagnosis

1. History of smoking or systemic ailment.
2. Idiopathic orbital inflammation is a diagnosis of exclusion.
3. Blood examination for leucocytosis, eosinophilia, raised erythrocyte sedimentation rate (ESR) and antinuclear antibody (ANA) level.
4. CT scan and B-scan ultrasonography can help in the diagnosis of myositis as the extraocular muscle tendons show thickening at the insertion.
5. CT scan or MRI of orbit reveals enlargement of lacrimal gland in dacryoadenitis.
6. Biopsy for idiopathic sclerosing inflammation of the orbit.

### Treatment

1. Systemic corticosteroids therapy (adult dose 80–100 mg of prednisolone) is the main stay of treatment. It should be tapered more slowly.
2. Bilateral cases need prolonged therapy.
3. Ranitidine (150 mg twice a day) is given to avoid acidity.

9

4. Immunosuppressant methotrexate (5–15 per week, IV, IM or oral) or cyclophosphamide (200 mg/day) may be effective.
5. Orbital irradiation (13,000c Gys) is recommended for steroid-nonresponders. However, radiation is contraindicated in diabetic subject because it can exacerbate diabetic retinopathy.

## 9.13 GRAVES' OPHTHALMOPATHY

### Etiology

1. The Graves' ophthalmopathy has an obscure etiology; it may be caused by an autoimmune reaction.
2. The ophthalmopathy occurs in 30–70% cases of the Graves' disease and affects women more frequently than men.
3. Graves' disease is caused by anti-TSHR (thyroid stimulating hormone receptor) gene and the ophthalmopathy by the orbital fibroblasts.
4. Smoking is an important risk factor.
5. Ophthalmopathy may be seen 6% cases of euthyroid.

### Symptoms

1. Initial symptoms are ocular discomfort, irritation, dry eyes, lacrimation, photophobia and blurred vision.
2. Late symptoms include prominent eyes with staring look, retraction of upper lid, swelling of lids, diplopia and decrease vision.
3. Weight loss, anxiety, nervousness, fatigue, sweating, tachycardia and tremors are constitutional symptoms.

### Signs

1. The retraction of the upper eyelid is the most common sign (90%).
2. A number of other lid signs like von Graefe sign (upper eyelid lags on down gaze), Gifford sign (eversion of upper eyelid is difficult), Stellwag sign (infrequent and incomplete blinking) and Kocher sign (spasmodic retraction of upper lid during fixation), may be found.
3. Convergence deficiency (Mobius sign) and inability to maintain fixation on extreme lateral gaze (Suker's sign) may also be present.
4. Periorbital edema and engorgement of vessels at the site of insertion of horizontal rectus muscles are often seen.
5. Proptosis and lid retraction are characteristic signs (Fig. 9.14).
6. SPK, keratoconjunctivitis sicca and keratitis due to exposure may be found.
7. Proptosis with restrictive extraocular myopathy occurs as a result of enlargement of extraocular muscles.
8. Thickened extraocular muscles at the apex of orbit may cause pupillary defect due to compressive optic neuropathy.
9. IOP may be increased.
10. Hyperthyroidism, tremors, wasting of muscles and cardiac arrhythmia are systemic features.

### Differential Diagnosis

Myasthenia gravis.

### Diagnosis

1. Classical evidences of the Graves' disease are eyelid retraction, proptosis and restriction of ocular movements.
2. Thyroid function tests like tri-iodo-thyronine (T3), tetra-iodothyronine (T4)

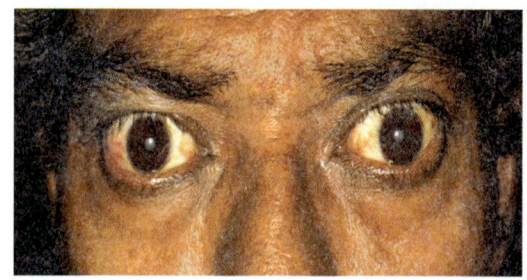

**Fig. 9.14:** Graves' disease: Bilateral exophthalmos

and thyroid stimulating hormone (TSH) should be estimated.

3. Compression of optic nerve must be diagnosed early with the help of visual acuity (VA), visual field examination, funduscopy and MRI to prevent loss of vision.

4. CT shows enlargement of extraocular muscles with sparing of the tendons (Fig. 9.15). The involvement of the extraocular rectus muscles is in following order: Inferior, medial, superior and lateral.

### Treatment

1. Abstinence from smoking
2. Correct abnormal thyroid function
3. Tear substitutes, lubricants and sunglasses can protect the cornea from dryness and exposure.
4. Pulse intravenous prednisolone is administered to arrest the progress of ophthalmopathy. Oral steroid is recommended for a long-term but it carries risk of increasing the IOP.
5. The orbital radiotherapy is questionable. It is not recommended.

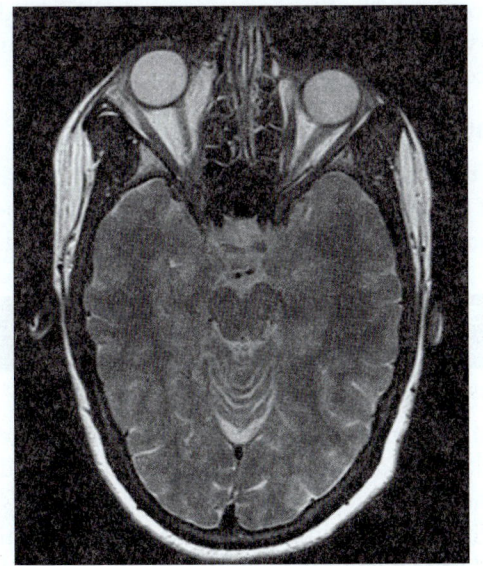

**Fig. 9.15:** CT shows enlargement of extraocular muscles

6. The use of biologic agents like rituximab and infliximab has shown promise in progressive ophthalmopathy. However, the agents are still in experimental stage.

7. Orbital decompression is indicated for preventing the compressive optic neuropathy.

8. Strabismus surgery may correct the diplopia.

9. Correction of eyelid retraction.

### 9.14 PROPTOSIS

### Etiology

1. Causes of proptosis or exophthalmos are different in childhood and adults.

2. Common causes of proptosis in children are trauma, dermoid, capillary hemangioma and developmental shallowing of orbit. Proptosis is a feature of neoplastic conditions like retinoblastoma optic glioma, rhabdomyosarcoma and leukemia.

3. Causes of proptosis in adults include thyroid disorder, thrombosis of cavernous sinus, mucocele of the frontal sinus, meningioma and tumors of the orbit including secondaries.

4. A severe blow or fall upon the head can cause pulsating proptosis. An establishment of a communication between cavernous sinus and internal carotid artery causes pulsation. It may also be seen in patients with meningoencephalocele.

5. Intermittent proptosis is a feature of orbital varices and polycythemia vera.

### Symptoms

Pain, prominent eyes or bulging of eyes, impairment of vision and diplopia may occur.

### Signs

1. Direction of displacement of the globe is important; it may be axial or nonaxial; mass lesion in the muscle cone produces axial (Fig. 9.16) and outside the cone nonaxial proptosis (Fig. 9.17).

9

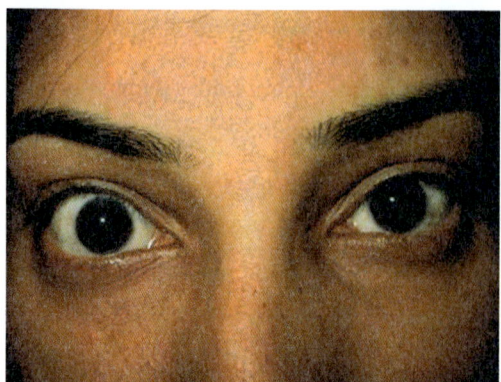

**Fig. 9.16:** Axial proptosis of right eye

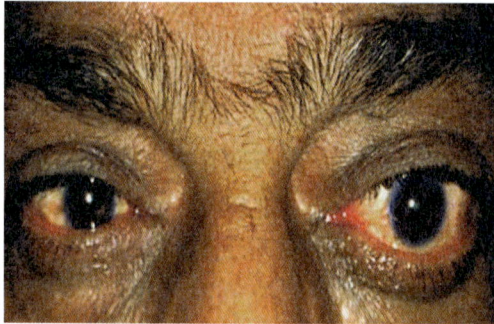

**Fig. 9.17:** Nonaxial proptosis of left eye

2. Ocular movements are restricted by an orbital mass.
3. Graves' ophthalmopathy restricts the ocular movements markedly.
4. Different types of abnormalities may be present on the eyelid. They may be suggestive of the etiology of proptosis, for example, strawberry birthmark suggests capillary hemangioma, S-shaped curve, neurofibromatosis, etc.
5. Lid signs can help to diagnose Graves' disease.
6. Slow or nonreactive pupil is seen in compressive optic neuropathy.
7. IOP may be increased.
8. Funduscopy reveals papilledema or optic atrophy (meningioma) or retinal striae (cavernous hemangioma).
9. Cranial nerve palsies may be found.

10. Intermittent proptosis of varying degrees can occur on bending or crying in patients with orbital varices.

**Differential Diagnosis**

1. Pseudoproptosis
2. Buphthalmos
3. Axial high myopia.

**Diagnosis**

1. History of head injury, thyroid disorder, leukemia, sinus diseases, congenital malformations or malignancy.
2. CT scan can diagnose any defect in bony orbit, enlargement of the extraocular muscles and IOFB.
3. Spiral CT is preferred in children.
4. MRI provides better view of the orbital apex.
5. B-scan ultrasonography can define the site, size and shape of the lesion.
6. MR arteriography can diagnose aneurysm and arteriovenous malformation.
7. Patients with suspected thyroid disorder should be investigated for serum T3, T4 and TSH levels.
8. Diagnosis of an orbital mass lesion can be confirmed by biopsy; tissue can be obtained by fine needle aspiration biopsy or excisional biopsy.

**Treatment**

1. Treat the cause.
2. If there is a risk of compressive optic neuropathy, orbital decompression is warranted.

## 9.15 MALIGNANT ORBITAL TUMORS IN ADULTS

**Classification**

1. Malignant orbital tumors in adults may be classified as primary, secondary and metastatic.
2. The primary tumor may arise from lacrimal gland, vascular element and lymphoid tissues.

3. Lymphoma appears as a painless, firm mass in the anterior orbit in old female.
4. The secondary tumors involve orbit from eyelids, conjunctiva and sinuses.
5. Carcinoma of breast and lungs and malignant melanoma of skin can cause metastatic deposits in the orbits.

### Primary Malignant Lymphoma

1. Most malignant lymphomas are of the non-Hodgkin low-grade B-cell type.
2. A chronic infection from *Chlamydia psittaci* or *Helicobacter pylori* may play a role in the etiology of lymphoma.
3. Orbital lymphoma presents a painless, progressive, palpable subconjunctival mass in the anterior orbit in elderly female above 50 years of age.
4. It can produce ectropion of the lower lid.
5. About 50% of patients may develop systemic disease.
6. CT scan, tissue biopsy and immunohisto-chemical studies can establish the diagnosis.
7. External beam radiation therapy (EBRT) is a treatment of choice.
8. EBRT with chemotherapy is recommended for systemic lymphomas.
9. Rituximab alone or in combination with ibritumomab is effective.
10. Anti-*H. pylori* triple therapy successfully controls the infection.

### Secondary Orbital Tumors

1. Secondary orbital tumors invade the orbit from adjacent structures such as the eyeball, eyelids, nasal cavity, sinuses and brain.

2. Retinoblastoma and malignant melanoma often spread to orbit.
3. Squamous cell carcinoma, adenocarcinoma and basal cell carcinoma can involve the orbit through direct extension.
4. Maxillary sinus tumors most frequently involve orbit.
5. Orbital involvement is also seen in the primary tumor of the nasopharynx.

### Metastatic Orbital Tumors

1. Acute lymphoblastic leukemia can give deposits in the orbit.
2. Chloroma, a collection of malignant cells, may be seen in the orbit in acute myeloid leukemia.
3. Bronchogenic carcinoma and operated or unoperated cancer of breast have a tendency to metastasize in orbit.
4. Malignant melanoma of skin can invade the orbit.
5. Proptosis, ocular discomfort, watering, pain, bony destruction and limitation of ocular movements are modes of manifestations of metastatic orbital tumors.
6. CT scan and estimation of embryonic antigen level may help in diagnosis. Biopsy of the orbital mass is confirmatory.
7. Treatment includes local radiation and chemotherapy for metastatic orbital tumors.
8. Metastasis from breast tumors needs hormonal therapy.

9

# Pediatric Ophthalmology

## 10.1 CONGENITAL/DEVELOPMENTAL CATARACT

### Etiology

1. The most common cause of congenital cataracts is genetic mutation.
2. They are inherited usually as autosomal dominant but autosomal recessive and sex-link inheritances can also occur.
3. Unilateral congenital cataracts are sporadic.
4. Congenital cataracts may be caused by chromosomal anomalies and present as a part of syndrome.
5. Congenital cataracts may present at birth.
6. Rubella, cytomegalic inclusion disease, toxoplasmosis and syphilis can cause developmental cataract.
7. Exposure to radiation during pregnancy, administration of corticosteroids or thalidomide, and nutritional deficiency are risk factors for cataract formation.

### Types

Developmental or congenital cataracts are of several types, only common ones are described below.

#### Zonular Cataract

1. The most common congenital cataract is zonular (Fig. 10.1).

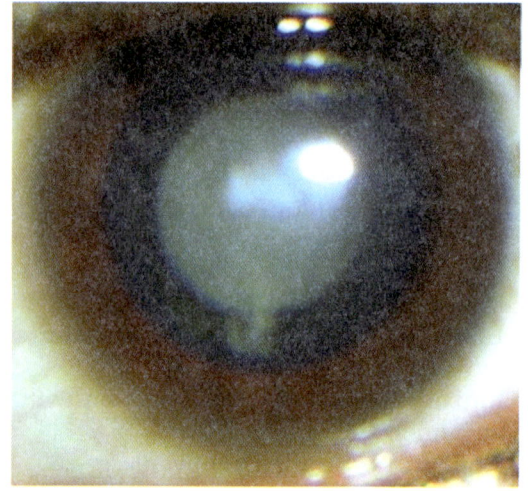

**Fig. 10.1:** Zonular cataract

2. Bilateral zonular cataract is inherited as autosomal dominant.
3. Pregnant mother with hypoparathyroidism may deliver a newborn with zonular cataract.
4. Zonular cataract may be associated with disorder of calcium metabolism, deficiency of vitamin D and dental defect.
5. It decreases visual acuity.
6. The opacities are confined to particular lamellae and encircle the nucleus.
7. It appears disk-shaped and the surrounding cortex is clear.
8. The opacity is heterogenous and consists of both dense and translucent areas.

9. Cataract shows characteristic radial projections known as riders.

### Posterior Polar Cataract

1. The posterior polar cataract confines to the posterior pole and posterior capsule.
2. It is characterized by concentric rings of opacities (Fig. 10.2).
3. It may be associated with an occult posterior capsular defect, anterior tunica vasculosa lentis, and Mittendorf dot on the posterior capsule.
4. The dot may remain stationary or progress.

### Central Nuclear Cataract

1. The central nuclear cataract or embryonic nuclear cataract is caused by failure of development of lens during first three months of embryogenesis.
2. The cataract is bilateral and confined to the embryonic nucleus.
3. It has a dominant inheritance.
4. The lens opacity is small and does not cause gross visual impairment.

### Galactosemic Cataract

1. Galactosemia is an inborn error of metabolism due to the deficiency of galactose-1-phosphate uridyltransferase (GPUT).

2. Accumulation of dulcitol in the lens causes opacity.
3. The dust-like lenticular opacities develop in the lens soon after birth.
4. It may or may not present a classical oil-droplet appearance.
5. Opacities are initially lamellar.
6. Avoid giving food containing galactose and lactose to the child during first 3 years of life for the prevention of galactosemic cataract.
7. Systemic manifestations of galactosemia include mental retardation, splenohepato-megaly, jaundice and ascites.

### Lowe's Syndrome

1. Lowe's syndrome is an inborn error of amino acid metabolism.
2. It is a sex-linked disorder caused by mutation in OCRL gene, locus Xq26.1.
3. Patients with Lowe's syndrome develop congenital cataract and glaucoma.
4. The cataract is often found but glaucoma is seen in two-thirds of patients.
5. The lens opacities may be nuclear or cortical.
6. Other less common ocular features are strabismus, nystagmus, microphthalmos, iris atrophy and miosis.
7. The systemic manifestations are mental retardation, aminoaciduria, renal rickets, muscular hypotonia and osteomalacia.

### Rubella Cataract

1. A progressive nuclear cataract may develop in an infant born to a mother who had German measles infection.
2. The entire lens may become opaque and pearly-white. The Rubella virus causes necrosis of lens and colobomatous defects (Fig. 10.3).
3. Other associated anomalies are rigid pupil, chronic uveitis, and pigmentary retinopathy (salt-and-pepper fundus).

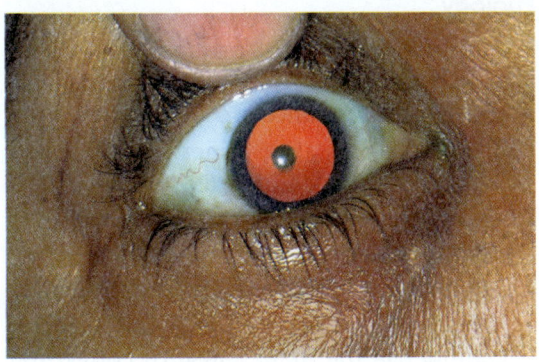

**Fig. 10.2:** Posterior polar cataract

10

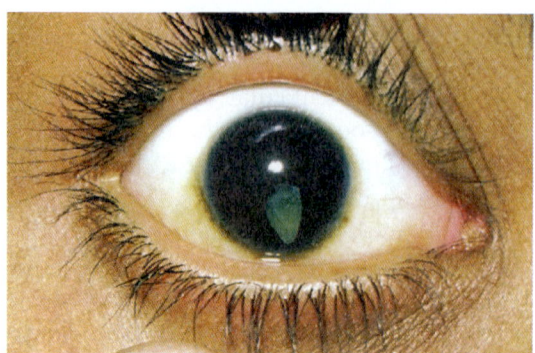

**Fig. 10.3:** Rubella cataract with coloboma of iris

4. Rubella can cause microphthalmos, microcephaly, mental retardation and deafness.

### Differential Diagnosis

All causes of leukocoria.

### Diagnosis of Cataract

1. History of maternal infection and type of delivery
2. A dull reflex on retinoscopy; assess the refractive error
3. Slit-lamp examination to ascertain the type of cataract and associated ocular anomalies
4. Dilated funduscopy often presents a dull fundus glow.
5. If cataract is dense and obscures the fundus view, B-scan ultrasonography should be advised.
6. Consult a pediatrician and exclude inborn errors of metabolism.
7. Look for the signs of rubella and its antibody titers.

### Treatment

1. Small size of the eyeball, visual impairment, development of amblyopia and late complications should be taken into consideration while planning the management of developmental cataract.
2. Stationary cataracts with good vision need not be operated.
3. The use of mydriatics may be considered in suitable cases for short-time.

4. In bilateral congenital cataract, surgery must be performed on one eye before the age of 3 months. The fellow eye may be taken for operation after a gap of 4 weeks.
5. Operation on unilateral cataract is preferred before the age of 6 weeks.
6. Phacoaspiration and pars plana lensectomy are common surgical techniques for developmental cataract.
7. Prompt correction of postoperative aphakia is necessary to prevent amblyopia.
8. Bilateral aphakic children over the age of one year can tolerate the aphakic spectacles correction.
9. Silicone soft contact lenses can be fitted and removed on weekly interval.
10. Primary IOL implantation is preferred in older children to avoid limitations of aphakia.

### Follow-up

1. Periodic follow-up of all operated and unoperated cases of developmental cataract is necessary for correction of refractive errors and management of surgical complications.
2. The visual prognosis of unilateral congenital cataract is poor because visual deprivation causes irreversible amblyopia.

## 10.2 GLAUCOMA OF INFANCY (BUPHTHALMOS) AND CHILDHOOD

### Etiology

1. Majority of cases of primary congenital glaucoma are sporadic. An autosomal recessive inheritance is seen in only 10%.
2. Two main causative genes: DYP1B1 and LTBP2 have been identified.
3. Glaucoma of infancy is bilateral in 65–80% cases.
4. Male infants are affected more frequently.
5. Dysgenesis of the angle of the anterior chamber is the main cause of congenital glaucoma.

10

6. The gonioscopy shows open angle with the presence of a membrane, anterior insertion of the root of iris and collapse of the canal of Schlemm.

## Symptoms

1. The classical triad of buphthalmos includes photophobia, lacimation and photophobia.
2. Later decreased vision or loss of vision may occur.

## Signs

1. If the intraocular pressure (IOP) is elevated before the age of 2 years, it results in enlargement of the globe. The enlarged eye is termed *buphthalmos* (Fig. 10.4).
2. The enlarged eye is slightly proptosed.
3. IOP remains high.
4. The corneal diameter is larger than normal diameter.
5. Cornea is edematous, hazy and shows breaks in the Descemet's membrane in the form of horizontal and circumferential stromal opacities (Habb striae).
6. The anterior chamber is irregularly deep and iris is tremulous due to luxation of the lens.
7. Gonioscopy reveals picture of angle dysgenesis or trabeculodysgenesis.
8. Funduscopy under general anesthesia reveals pale-white optic disk and cupping of the optic nerve head.

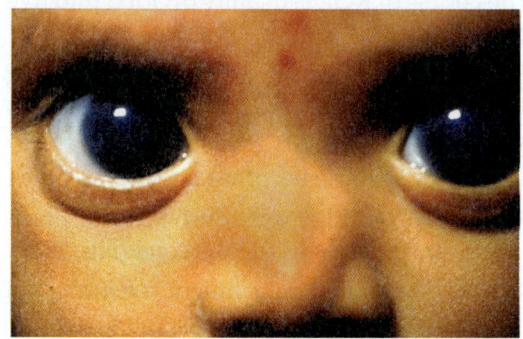

**Fig. 10.4:** Bilateral buphthalmos (*Courtesy:* Dr Rajul Parikh, Director, Shreeji Eye Clinic, Mumbai)

9. Later, bluish discoloration of sclera, iris atrophy, myopic shift in refraction and gross enlargement of eye may be found.

## Differential Diagnosis

1. Keratoglobus
2. Megalocornea
3. Retinoblastoma
4. Congenital hereditary corneal dystrophy
5. Mucopolysaccharidosis.

## Diagnosis

The infant/child should be examined under general anesthesia.

1. More than 12 mm of corneal diameter before 1 year of age with high IOP suggests the presence of congenital glaucoma.
2. High IOP
3. Gonioscopy to find anterior chamber angle dysgenesis, Barkan's membrane and abnormally high insertion of iris seen.
4. Funduscopy shows vertically increased cup/disk ratio and damaged neuroretinal rim.
5. Periodic ultrasonography for recording the changes in the axial length.
6. Optical coherence tomography (OCT) is helpful in assessing retinal nerve fiber loss.

## Treatment

1. Use topical beta-blockers and systemic acetazolamide (15 mg/kg/day in three divided doses) to reduce IOP and to clear cloudy cornea before surgery.
2. Brimonidine is avoided in children below the age of 10 years as it may cause hypotension, hypotonia and apnea.
3. Goniotomy or trabeculotomy is performed if cornea is clear.
4. Trabeculotomy *ab externo* is performed in patients with opaque cornea.
5. In failed cases, trabeculectomy with or without mitomycin C is recommended.

10

## 10.3 JUVENILE OR CHILDHOOD GLAUCOMA

### Etiology

1. Primary juvenile glaucoma or late-onset primary congenital glaucoma develops between the ages of 3 and 10 years.
2. The angle of the anterior chamber is poorly differentiated resulting in decreased aqueous outflow.
3. Myocilin (MYOC) gene is associated with juvenile open-angle glaucoma.

### Symptoms

The child remains symptom-free or may complain of decreased vision.

### Signs

1. IOP remains moderately increased without enlargement of the eye and corneal changes.
2. Fundus examination shows cupping of the optic disk and neuroretinal rim thinning.
3. Glaucomatous visual field defects may be found.

### Diagnosis

1. Age of the child
2. Moderately increased IOP
3. Gonioscopy shows poorly differentiated structures of the angle of the anterior chamber
4. OCT to assess the damage to optic nerve head (ONH) and retinal nerve fiber loss
5. Typical visual field defects.

### Treatment

Trabeculotomy or trabeculectomy provides satisfactory results.

## 10.4 RETINOPATHY OF PREMATURITY

### Etiology

1. Retinopathy of prematurity (ROP) is a bilateral proliferative retinopathy of premature infants.

2. Prematurity of less than 32 weeks of gestational age and low birth weight of less than 1,250 g are important risk factors.
3. Premature infants may be exposed to high concentration of oxygen therapy.
4. Concurrent respiratory disorders, patent ductus arteriosus, apnea and sepsis may be other contributors.

### Symptoms

1. Parents of the infant may complain of white reflex in the pupil.
2. Older children and adults may report with visual impairment or loss of vision.
3. Most of the children are, however, asymptomatic and diagnosed during screening for ROP.

### Signs

Signs largely depend on the location and the stage of ROP.

### Location

The location of ROP is documented in three zones:

1. Zone I includes the posterior pole within a 30° circle centered on the optic nerve
2. Zone II extends between nasal border or zone I and the nasal ora serrata
3. Zone III includes the retina outside zone II.

### Stages

The course of ROP is usually divided into five stages:

1. *Stage 1:* It presents a gray line demarcating between vascular and nonvascular retina in the periphery.
2. *Stage 2:* The line becomes a vascular ridge.
3. *Stage 3:* The ridge with fibrovascular proliferation extends in the vitreous (Fig. 10.5).
4. *Stage 4A:* Retinal detachment is extrafoveal and in *stage 4B:* RD involves the fovea.
5. *Stage 5:* Retinal detachment is total taking a funnel shape.

10

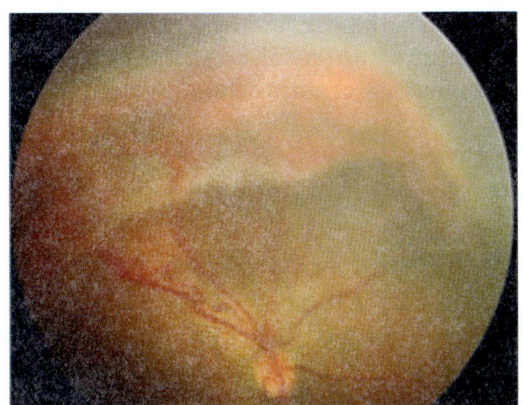

**Fig. 10.5:** Retinopathy of prematurity

## Other Features

Other features of ROP are plus disease, rush disease and threshold disease.

## Plus Disease

1. It is characterized by engorged and tortuous blood vessels at least in two quadrants of posterior pole, iris vascular engorgement, poor dilatation of pupil and vitreous haze.
2. If clinical evidence is insufficient, it is called pre-plus disease.

## Rush Disease

Zone 1 ROP with aggressive plus disease is known as rush disease. It rapidly progresses to stage 5 escaping other stages. It shows hemorrhages between vascular and avascular retina.

## Threshold Disease

Stage 3 ROP with plus disease seen in zone I or II. It involves five contiguous clock hours or eight cumulative clock hours.

## Differential Diagnosis

1. All causes of leukocoria:
   - Retinoblastoma
   - Cataract
   - Retinal detachment
   - Taxocariasis
   - Posterior choroiditis
   - Persistent hyperplastic primary vitreous
   - Coats' disease.
2. Familial exudative vitreoretinopathy: Familial disease presents peripheral neovascularization but no history of prematurity and oxygen therapy.

## Diagnosis

1. Birth weight less than 1,500 g
2. Gestational age less than 32 weeks
3. High risk newborns of more than 1,500 g weight or 32 weeks gestational age must be screened.
4. Two dilated fundus examinations are essential for low weight premature children.
5. Critical analysis of fundus photographs.

## Treatment

1. ROP may show spontaneous regression.
2. Prethreshold disease needs close follow-up.
3. Early treatment is needed for plus disease.
4. Laser photocoagulation of the avascular retina for threshold disease. Use of anti-VEGF agents intravitreally is becoming popular and looks promising.
5. Stage 4: ROP is managed with scleral buckling.
6. Stage 5: ROP may need bimanual vitrectomy with sectioning of the bands and peeling of the membrane.

## 10.5 OPHTHALMIA NEONATORUM

### Etiology

1. Ophthalmia neonatorum is a severe conjunctivitis of newborn. The infection is usually contacted during birth. The infection may come from the genitourinary tract of the mother, soiled linen or fingers of the nurse.
2. The ophthalmia is caused by *Neisseria gonorrhoeae, Staphylococcus aureus, Strepto-*

10

*coccus pneumoniae, Staphylococcus hemolyticus, E. coli*. Chlamydia, herpes and adenoviruses can also cause the disease.

## Symptoms

Copious discharge from both the eyes, red eyes, pain, swelling and inability to open the eyes.

## Signs

1. Both eyes are involved.
2. Lacrimation starts in the first week of birth; it becomes mucopurulent and ultimately purulent.
3. The lids are swollen and brawny.
4. The conjunctiva is intensely inflamed, red, chemotic and may bulge through the lids.
5. The flakes of discharge are deposited over the medial canthi, lid margins and conjunctiva.
6. In untreated cases, a corneal ulceration may develop that is prone to perforation.
7. A mild to severe degree of iridocyclitis may accompany the ulcer.
8. The perforation of ulcer may lead to blinding sequelae.

## Differential Diagnosis

1. Chemical or toxic conjunctivitis
2. Acute viral conjunctivitis
3. Acute congenital dacryocystitis.

## Diagnosis

1. A bilateral purulent conjunctivitis with stormy course in an infant is highly suggestive.
2. History of venereal disease in the mother.
3. Conjunctival smear/scrap examination after Gram and Giemsa-stain for bacteria and Chlamydia inclusion bodies.
4. Conjunctival smear for culture and sensitivity tests.
5. Herpes or Chlamydia infection can be confirmed by virus culture.

6. Chlamydia can also be confirmed by immunofluorescent antibody test or polymerase chain reaction (PCR).

## Prophylaxis

1. Ophthalmia neonatorum can be prevented easily by treatment of mother's birth canal infection before delivery and by adopting aseptic measures during delivery.
2. Soon after birth, prophylactic topical erythromycin eye drops or a combination of bacitracin and polymyxin B should be used.
3. Povidone-iodine 5% drops can also be used as it does not cause any toxic reaction like *Crede's method* (1% silver nitrate).

## Treatment

1. The eye should be frequently irrigated with saline.
2. No treatment is required for chemical conjunctivitis induced by Crede's prophylaxis except use of preservative-free artificial tears.
3. *Neisseria gonorrhoeae* infection is treated with intensive antibiotic therapy. Earlier the standard regimen was instillation of penicillin drops.
4. Considering resistance to penicillin, the drug is seldom used. The topical therapy with tetracycline, bacitracin or fluoroquinolone is recommended.
5. The most effective treatment is ceftriaxone 25–50 mg/kg IV, 12 hourly or cefotaxime 100 mg/kg IV or IM as a single dose.
6. Topical tetracycline, erythromycin and systemic azithromycin (1 g single adult dose) are very effective.
7. Gram-positive infection (*Staphylococcus aureus*) responds to topical 25–50 mg/mL or systemic 100 mg cefazoline therapy.
8. Gram-negative microorganism infection is controlled by topical tobramycin (14 mg/mL) or ceftriaxone (50 mg/mL).

9. If smear and culture reports are incon-clusive, topical and systemic erythromycin should be administered.
10. Herpes infection requires acyclovir (45–60 mg/kg IV in divided 3–4 doses for 14 days) therapy.
11. Topical atropine with intensive antibiotic therapy is necessary in the presence of corneal ulcer but eye should not be patched.

## 10.6 CONGENITAL DACRYOCYSTITIS

### Etiology

1. The congenital dacryocystitis is usually caused by obstruction of the lower opening of the nasolacrimal duct.
2. Blockage may occur due to anomalous development.
3. The blockage causes infection of the lacrimal sac.

### Symptoms

Recurrent watering or discharge, localized redness and swelling of the sac region and pain may occur.

### Signs

1. The nasolacrimal duct obstruction is common at birth but patency may be restored spontaneously later.
2. A pressure over sac causes regurgitation of mucopus from the lower punctum.
3. A localized erythema and swelling of the skin is seen below the medial canthal tendon.
4. The swelling increases in size, it becomes red, tense and tender and extends around the periorbital region (Fig. 10.6).
5. It may progress to lacrimal sac abscess or fistula formation and rarely, lead to orbital cellulitis or facial cellulitis.

### Differential Diagnosis

Acute conjunctivitis.

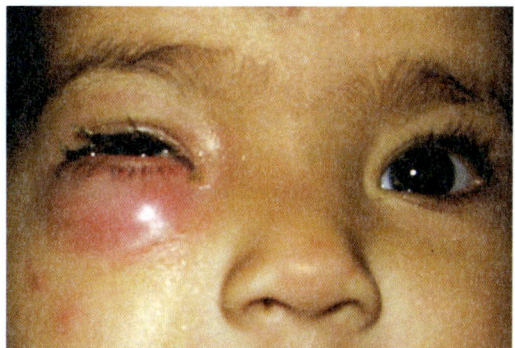

Fig. 10.6: Congenital dacryocystitis

### Diagnosis

1. Exclude conjunctivitis and other causes of watering.
2. Mucous/mucopurulent discharge from the lower punctum when pressure is applied (regurgitation test) is confirmatory.
3. Place fluorescein dye in both eyes, retaining the dye after 10 minutes is highly suggestive of the obstruction.

### Treatment

1. Frequent massaging of sac region and topical use of antibiotic drops usually relieve the condition in majority of infants, and the duct becomes patent.
2. Probing of the lacrimal passage is performed if massage fails and infant is older than 6 months. Probing is done under general anesthesia.
3. Repeat probing may be necessary if watering persists.
4. Failed probing cases need treatment with balloon dacryoplasty at a later age.
5. Turbinate in fracture and intubation with silicone tube for 6 months is another option.
6. Dacryocystorhinostomy (DCR) is the last resort in recalcitrant cases.

## 10.7 CONGENITAL PTOSIS

### Etiology

1. Congenital ptosis is usually caused by defective functioning of levator palpebrae

10

superioris (LPS) and Müller muscles due to neuromyogenic abnormality.

2. Myogenic ptosis is due to maldevelopment of LPS. A fibrous tissue replaces the muscle.

3. Neurogenic ptosis is due to innervational defects resulting from the IIIrd cranial nerve palsy.

## Symptoms

Symptoms include inability to open one or both eyes, unequal width of the palpebral aperture and diminished visual acuity.

## Signs

1. Drooping of lid may be unilateral or bilateral.

2. The cornea may be covered partially or completely depending on severity of ptosis (Fig. 10.7).

3. The child with bilateral congenital ptosis tries to raise the lids by frontalis overaction.

4. Absence of upper eyelid crease.

5. Unilateral ptotic lid may be raised on jaw-winking or mastication (Marcus Gunn jaw-winking syndrome) in some cases.

6. Mild unilateral ptosis may be associated with anisocoria, heterochromia and anhydrosis (Horner syndrome).

7. Ptosis may be seen with other congenital anomalies like epicanthal folds, telecanthus, blepharophimosis syndrome (Fig. 10.8).

## Differential Diagnosis

1. Pseudoptosis is an apparent drooping of the upper eyelid often seen in anophthalmos,

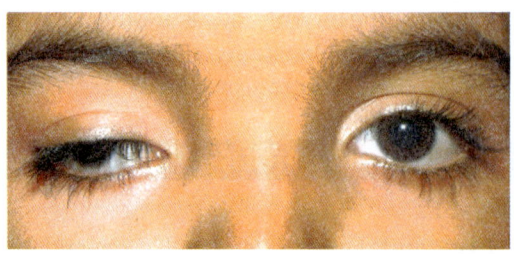

Fig. 10.7: Congenital unilateral ptosis (right eye)

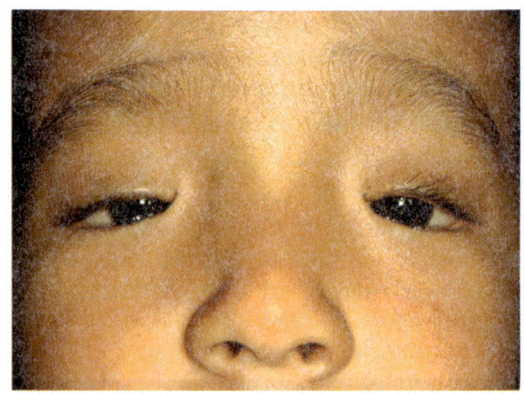

Fig. 10.8: Congenital ptosis with blepharophimosis syndrome

microphthalmos, enophthalmos and phthisis bulbi.

2. Traumatic ptosis: History of trauma
3. Horner syndrome
4. Blepharophimosis syndrome.

## Diagnosis

1. Congenital ptosis is present from birth and remains stationary.

2. The vertical height of interpalpebral fissure is reduced.

3. The marginal reflex distance (MRD) is used to know the degree of ptosis. Difference of MRD between two eyes determines the grade in unilateral ptosis, while scale measurements are required in bilateral ptosis.

4. Levator action can be measured by a scale. Levator palpebrae superioris (LPS) function in children with ptosis is less than normal (15 mm normal).

5. The presence of wrinkling on the forehead indicates frontalis overaction that may mask the ptosis.

6. An upper-eyelid crease (high, duplicated or asymmetric crease) suggests abnormal insertion of the levator aponeurosis.

7. See for Bell's phenomenon (presence of upward and outward rolling of the eyeball on forced closure of the eyelids) and

10

chances of corneal exposure after ptosis correction.

8. Exclude the presence of Marcus Gunn jaw-winking phenomenon.

9. Visual functions and refractive errors to exclude amblyopia.

10. Pupillary examination and pharmacological testing to diagnose Horner's syndrome [*Cocaine drop test*: Pupil in Horner's syndrome fails to dilate with topical cocaine (4%) due to absence of norepinephrine].

11. Exclude the presence of the IIIrd cranial nerve palsy.

### Treatment

1. In the presence of IIIrd nerve paralysis, ptosis operation is contraindicated due to postoperative diplopia.

2. When the levator action is weak, its resection can correct a mild to moderate degree of ptosis. Fasanella-Servat operation provides good cosmetic result.

3. The frontalis sling operation (Hess operation) is preferred if there is no levator action.

4. Bilateral Hess operation should be performed in ptotic patients with jaw-winking phenomenon after the disinsertion of the LPS.

### 10.8 ESODEVIATION IN CHILDHOOD

### Etiology

The esodeviation is common in hyperopes and starts in childhood (Fig. 10.9). An attack of a debilitating disease can precipitate it.

### Types

Two main types of esodeviation are: (1) *comitant* and (2) *incomitant*.

### Comitant Esodeviation

Comitant esodeviation is further divided into three subtypes:

1. *Congenital or infantile esotropia* starts at birth or manifests by the age of 6 months.

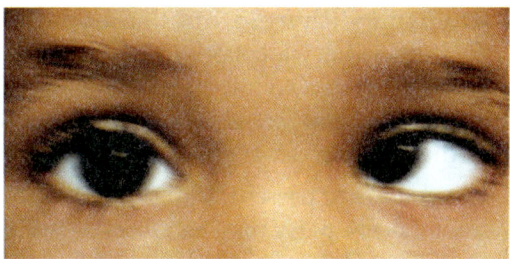

**Fig. 10.9:** Esodeviation left eye

The angle of esodeviation is larger than 30° and remains constant for near and distant fixations. Later, it may be associated with latent nystagmus, overaction of inferior oblique, dissociated vertical deviation, and neurological disorders like hydrocephalus, cerebral palsy, etc.

2. *Accommodative esotropia* manifests around the age of 2 years. It is further divided into 3 types:

   - *Refractive accommodative esotropia* is due to uncorrected hyperopia of about +5D and deficiency of fusional divergence. The angle of esotropia is about 20–30 degree.

   - *Nonrefractive accommodative esotropia* is due to abnormal AC/A ratio; excessive convergence and occurs during accommodation.

   - *Partial or decompensated accommodative esotropia* is a residual esotropia after full hyperopic correction. It is nonaccommodational component of esotropia that can be corrected by surgery.

3. *Nonaccommodative esotropia:* It may manifest as monocular or binocular condition. Sensory deprivation, divergence insufficiency and paralysis are important factors. Divergence insufficiency has a sudden onset and is greater at distance than at near fixation.

### Incomitant Esodeviation

1. Incomitant esodeviation may be caused by the VIth cranial nerve palsy due to central nervous system (CNS) disorders, restrictive

10

strabismus (thyroid ophthalmopathy, fracture medial wall of orbit, etc), weakness of lateral rectus following trauma, contracture of medial rectus or over resection of medial rectus.

2. The child may present with diplopia. VIth cranial nerve palsy may be associated with nystagmus, headache and clinical features of neurological disease. The esodeviation is greater in lateral gaze at distance fixation than at near fixation.

### Diagnosis

1. History of congenital or infantile onset.
2. Ocular movements are restricted and old children present overaction of inferior oblique.
3. Measure esodeviation in different directions of gaze and at distance and at near fixation to find the type of esodeviation.
4. Assess refractive errors under cycloplegia.
5. Children with palsy or paralysis of VIth cranial nerve may be subjected to a head computed tomography (CT) or magnetic resonance imaging (MRI) for finding CNS lesions.
6. In restricted esodeviation, forced duction and force generation tests under anesthesia should be performed.

### Treatment

1. Congenital esotropia
   - Almost all cases of congenital esotropia need strabismus surgery.
   - Surgical approaches include: (i) recession of bilateral medial rectus muscles, (ii) recession of medial rectus muscle combined with resection of the lateral rectus muscle.
2. Accommodative esodeviation
   - In children below 6 years a full hyperopic correction is provided after cycloplegic refraction.

- Children above 6 years may not tolerate full correction; they should be corrected as possible as close to hyperopic correction.
- In spite of full correction, eyes of some children are straight at distance fixation but still show esodeviation at near fixation; they can be corrected by prescription of bifocal lenses (add + 2.5D for near over full distance correction) or by surgery on extraocular muscle with posterior fixation suture.

3. Nonaccommodative esodeviation
   - Refractive correction should be prescribed.
   - Residual esodeviation should be corrected by muscle surgery.
4. Sensory deprivation esodeviation
   - Prescribe full cycloplegic correction
   - Correct esodeviation by extraocular muscle surgery
   - Children with monocular poor vision need amblyopia therapy with occlusion of better eye and exercises.

### Follow-up

1. Periodic follow-up examination of child should be carried out to assess visual acuity with glasses, cycloplegic refraction for change of glasses and degree of esodevation at distance and at near fixation.
2. Hyperopia gradually decreases with increase in age of the child, and therefore, power of glasses should be reduced to improve vision.

### 10.9 EXODEVIATION IN CHILDHOOD

1. The exodeviation is less common and seen at later age than the esodeviation.
2. When the sound eye fixates, the eye with poor vision diverges.

10

## Types

Exodeviation can be divided into 3 types: (1) exophoria, (2) intermittent exotropia and (3) constant exotropia.

1. Exophoria
   - It is usually controlled by fusional reflex.
   - It may cause asthenopia.
2. Intermittent exotropia
   - It is common and manifests before the age of 5 years. The eye deviates larger for distance than for near (Fig. 10.10).
   - It may be associated with hyperopia.
   - Intermittent exotropia presents three forms of deviations:
     - Constant deviation at distance and at near fixation
     - More frequent exotropia at distance and
     - Sudden exotropia of one eye spontaneously or if covered.
   - Intermittent exotropia is of four types:
     - *Basic exotropia* is almost same at distance and near fixations
     - *True divergence excess* is more for at distance fixation than near.
     - *Simulated divergence excess* presents initially more deviation for distance but it becomes almost same for distance and near fixations after monocular occlusion.
     - *Convergence insufficiency* shows greater deviation at near fixation.

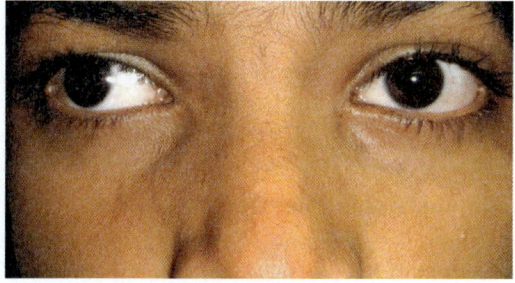

Fig. 10.10: Exodeviation right eye

3. Constant exotropia
   - Constant exotropia is congenital or consecutive in origin. It may be associated with craniofacial anomalies.
4. Other conditions: A number of other conditions such as isolated IIIrd cranial nerve palsy, convergence paralysis, idiopathic orbital inflammation, internuclear ophthalmoplegia, dissociated horizontal deviation, etc may also cause exodeviation.

### Differential Diagnosis

1. Retinopathy of prematurity
2. Positive angle kappa
3. Wide interpupillary distance.

### Diagnosis

1. Test visual acuity and evaluate amblyopia.
2. Refraction should be performed under cycloplegia in young children.
3. Test ocular movements in different directions of gaze.
4. Measure exodeviation in all cardinal directions of gaze and at distance and near fixations using prisms.
5. Perform detail ocular examination including dilated funduscopy to know the cause of amblyopia.
6. Patients with CNS or orbital diseases may be subjected to CT or MRI scans.

### Treatment

1. Exophoria does not need any treatment unless it is progressing.
2. Optical correction should be given for mild-moderate myopic and more than +4.0D hyperopic refractive errors.
3. Long-term success may be obtained by antisuppression therapy, fusional convergence training, and periodic patching.
4. Base-in prisms are used to promote fusion in intermittent exotropia.
5. Base-in prisms are also prescribed to prevent diplopia in convergence paralysis.
6. Majority of patients with intermittent exotropia require surgery. Surgery is also

10

needed for congenital exotropia, consecutive exotropia and dissociated horizontal deviation.

7. The most common surgery for intermittent exotropia is bilateral recession of lateral rectus muscles.

8. Recession of lateral rectus muscle combined with resection of medial rectus muscle of the same eye can be performed in basic type of intermittent exotropia.

## 10.10 COMMON SYNDROMES ASSOCIATED WITH STRABISMUS

Strabismus is an important component of some of the syndromes; common ones are described below.

### Duane's Syndrome

#### Etiology

1. Duane's retraction syndrome is a congenital motility disorder characterized by limitation of abduction and/or adduction, narrowing of palpebral aperture and retraction of globe on an attempt for adduction.

2. It is caused by disturbances in the normal embryonic development.

3. Agenesis of the VIth cranial nerve nucleus and innervation of lateral rectus muscle by the inferior division of the IIIrd cranial nerve contribute to simultaneous contraction of lateral and medial rectus muscles.

4. The syndrome is familial and transmitted as autosomal dominant. It is often unilateral and involves left eye more frequently (80%).

5. The syndrome has three types:
   - Type I is the most common.
     - Besides classical clinical features of syndrome like limitation of abduction or adduction or both, retraction of the globe and narrowing palpebral fissure, A-V phenomenon of affected eye may be seen on an attempt for adduction or abduction.

- Exotropia is present in the primary position and face is usually turned toward affected side in unilateral cases.
- Type II syndrome presents exotropia due to marked limitation or absence of adduction but abduction may be slightly limited or normal.
  - An attempt on adduction causes narrowing of palpebral fissure and retraction of the globe.
  - In unilateral cases, face is turned away from the affected eye.
- Type III syndrome presents a combination of type I and type II.
  - The affected eye remains in primary position due to equal degree of limitation of both lateral and medial rectus muscles.
  - If adduction is more defective, the eye will diverge. An attempt for adduction results in narrowing of palpebral aperture and retraction of globe.
  - Other signs found in Duane's syndrome include optic nerve hypoplasia, morning glory syndrome, congenital ptosis, heterochromia with or without iris dysplasia and choroidal coloboma.
  - Duane's syndrome may be associated with other syndromes like Goldenhar and Klippel-Feil.

#### Diagnosis

Characteristic evidence of retraction of the globe and narrowing of palpebral aperture on an attempt for adduction help in diagnosis.

#### Treatment

1. If eyes are straight in the primary position, no treatment is indicated.

2. Surgery is indicated in cases with unacceptable abnormal head posture, upshoot or downshoot and enophthalmos.

3. Duane's syndrome with esotropia can be corrected by recession of medial rectus of the involved eye. Resection of lateral rectus

is not favored because it is likely to enhance the globe retraction.

4. Exotropic Duane's requires unilateral or bilateral lateral rectus recession.

5. A posterior fixation suture on the lateral rectus muscle can prevent upshoots and downshoots.

## Brown Syndrome

### Etiology

1. Brown or superior oblique sheath syndrome is characterized by restriction of elevation in adduction.

2. It may be congenital or acquired. The etiology of congenital form is not known. Defective development of muscle and its attachment limits the elevation.

3. Acquired Brown syndrome is caused by local trauma or inflammation in the region of trochlea.

### Signs

1. Elevation is limited in adduction.

2. In mild to moderate syndrome, there is no hypotropia in the primary position.

3. In severe cases, there is hypertropia in the primary position and a marked downshoot on adduction.

4. Head takes a compensatory posture with chin elevation and face turn to keep the affected eye in abduction.

5. Attempt for midline elevation causes divergence.

6. In adduction, the palpebral fissure widens with downshoot of the affected eye.

7. Eye intorts on upward gaze.

8. Fusion and stereopsis are present.

9. Forced duction test is positive.

### Differential Diagnosis

1. Inferior oblique palsy

2. Superior oblique muscle overaction

3. Duane's syndrome

4. Double elevator palsy.

### Diagnosis

1. Midline elevation differentiates the syndrome from inferior oblique palsy.

2. Downshoot of the affected eye in adduction differentiates it from superior oblique muscle overaction.

3. Forced duction test

4. CT and MRI may localize the etiology of the acquired Brown syndrome.

### Treatment

1. Mild-moderate grades of Brown syndrome do not need treatment.

2. Surgery is indicated in patients with hypotropia in primary gaze and unacceptable head posture. Guarded superior oblique tenotomy using a solid silicone band sewn to the cut ends of the muscle is effective. It does not need simultaneous weakening of inferior oblique muscle.

3. Inflammatory lesion near the trochlea can be managed by systemic administration of antibiotic and steroid or local injection of corticosteroids.

## Monocular Elevation Deficiency

### Etiology

1. Monocular elevation deficiency was known as double elevator palsy. It may be congenital or acquired.

2. Congenital deficiency may occur due to supranuclear defects, primary superior rectus paresis and inferior rectus restriction.

3. The acquired deficiency is due to CNS disorders, sarcoidosis and infectious disease.

### Signs

1. Eye is hypotropic.

2. Limitation of elevation in both adduction and abduction.

3. Abnormal head posture with chin elevation

4. Ptosis

10

5. Presence of Bell's phenomenon in supra-nuclear lesions
6. Acquired syndrome has an acute onset with diplopia in the primary position.

## Differential Diagnosis

Brown syndrome.

## Diagnosis

1. Bell's phenomenon is present only in supranuclear etiology and not other causes.
2. In supranuclear monocular elevation deficiency, saccades are absent above midline and but present below midline.
3. In primary superior rectus paresis, saccades are seen both above and below midline.
4. Upward saccades are normal in inferior rectus restriction but forced duction test is positive.

## Treatment

Treatment of monocular elevation deficiency is largely based on the result of forced duction test.
1. Restriction of inferior rectus (positive forced duction test) is managed by recession of the muscle.
2. Cases with negative forced duction test require transposition of split strips of medial and lateral muscles or full tendon of muscles near the insertion of the superior rectus muscle.

## Möbius Syndrome

### Etiology

1. Möbius syndrome is characterized by congenital facial diplegia, bilateral VIth cranial nerve palsies, and incomplete facial nerve palsy.
2. The etiology of the syndrome is not known.
3. However, an acute flexion of brain in the 4th week of embryonic life is incriminated. The event may contribute to hypoplasia of nuclei of VIth and VIIth cranial nerves.

## Signs

1. Bilateral VIth nerve palsies cause loss of lateral movement in both eyes, therefore patient turns head to look either way.
2. Bilateral lagophthalmos occurs due to facial palsies.
3. The patient has a mask-like face with open mouth.
4. The child is unable to smile and there is complete lack of facial movements during crying.
5. Cranial nerves from VIth to XIIth may be involved; however, VIIIth may be spared.
6. Cranial nerves IIIrd and IVth are rarely involved.
7. Speech is defective.
8. Skeletal deformities such as bilateral club-foot, brachydactyly and syndactyly may be present.

## Diagnosis

1. Classical clinical picture
2. CT or MRI shows calcification in the region of VI nerve nuclei.

## Treatment

Initially, the treatment is conservative and later cosmetic.

## Congenital Fibrosis Syndrome

### Etiology

1. Congenital fibrosis syndrome is a conge-nital disorder characterized by fibrosis of a single or all extraocular muscles resulting in limitation of their movements.
2. The etiology of the syndrome is unknown.
3. The syndrome may be inherited in an autosomal dominant or recessive manner.
4. Inflammation of orbit has also been suggested in some cases.

### Types

Congenital fibrosis syndrome may be divided into five types:
1. *General fibrosis:* It involves all extraocular muscles of both eyes including LPS. Marked

10

limitation of movements of both eyes with bilateral ptosis.

2. *Congenital unilateral fibrosis:* It involves all muscles of only one eye and also associated with ptosis and enophthalmos.
3. *Congenital fibrosis of the inferior rectus muscle:* It involves unilateral or bilateral inferior rectus muscle only.
4. *Strabismus fixus:* It usually involves medial rectus muscles resulting in severe esotropia.
5. *Vertical retraction syndrome:* It involves the superior rectus muscle resulting in inability to depress the eye.

### Diagnosis

1. Acquired fibrosis (thyroid ophthalmo-pathy) should be excluded.
2. Forced duction test confirms the restriction of movement.
3. Histopathology reveals replacement of extraocular muscle by fibrous tissue.

### Treatment

1. Surgery is possible in some cases.
2. Fibrosis of single muscle can be released by weakening procedure, however, rotation cannot be restored.

### 10.11 AMBLYOPIA

### Etiology

1. Amblyopia is an unexplained reduction of best corrected visual acuity usually in one eye and occasionally in both eyes.
2. It develops due to visual deprivation.
3. The neurophysiological mechanism of development of amblyopia is not clear.
4. It seems that cells of visual cortex become less responsive to inputs from the amblyopic eye.
5. Strabismus, anisometropia and visual deprivation are common causes.

### Classification

Amblyopia may be classified under the following categories:
1. *Strabismic amblyopia* is the most common and seen in cases with unilateral constant strabismus (Fig. 10.11) with poor vision. Amblyopia does not develop in alternate strabismus.
2. *Anisometropic amblyopia* is more common in unilateral hyperopic or astigmatic eye than myopic. It develops due to a large difference of refractive error between the two eyes that remains uncorrected. Besides anisometropia, aniseikonia is another amblyopic factor.
3. *Deprivation or amblyopia ex-anopsia* develops in early childhood due to opacities in media blocking visual stimulus. Common causes are cataract (congenital or traumatic) or corneal opacities.
4. *Bilateral anisometropic amblyopia* develops in children with uncorrected high hyperopia. The error causes marked blurring and prevents the development of binocular vision.
5. *Meridional amblyopia* is often caused by uncorrected astigmatism.
6. *Occlusion amblyopia* can develop in the fellow eye as a result of excessive patching or penalization use of atropine for a long-time.

### Symptoms

1. Most patients with amblyopia remain symptom-free and may be detected during routine eye check-up.
2. Occasionally, patient can report with decreased vision in one eye or in both eyes.

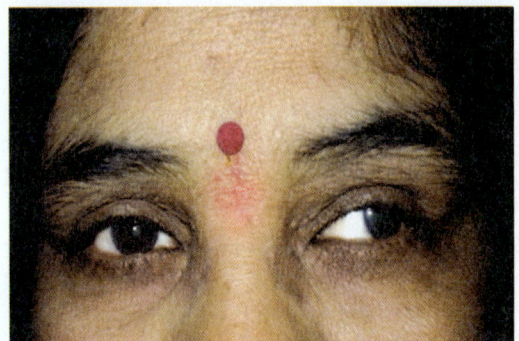

**Fig. 10.11:** Strabismic amblyopia LE

10

### Signs

1. Visual acuity (VA) is poor in one eye
2. VA is better if single letter charts are used than full line charts (crowding pheno-menon).
3. In amblyopia, central vision is decreased while peripheral visual field remains normal.
4. Amblyopic eye may have higher refractive error, and correction of error does not improve vision.
5. The eye is deviated (strabismic). It may or may not have associated anisometropia.
6. Opacities in the ocular media like corneal scar, congenital cataract, persistent hyperplastic primary vitreous (PHPV), etc may be found.
7. Relative afferent pupillary defect may be found in deep amblyopia.
8. Examination of the affected eye reveals no organic lesion accountable for poor vision.
9. In reduced illumination, the visual acuity of an amblyopic eye is relatively less reduced than in an eye with organic lesion.

### Diagnosis

1. History of ocular deviation in childhood, congenital cataract or squint surgery.
2. Refraction reveals anisometropia; the optical correction does not improve vision
3. Pin-hole test shows no improvement in vision.
4. Strabismus is manifest in some cases while in others cover-uncover and alternate cover tests should be performed.

### Treatment

1. Amblyogenic factors like refractive error, congenital cataract or complete ptosis must be treated at an early age to prevent visual deprivation.
2. Forced use of amblyopic eye by patching (2–6 hours/day, 6 weeks) of the normal eye is the mainstay of management.
3. Penalization of fellow eye is cosmetically more acceptable.

4. Strabismus surgery should be performed soon after visual improvement with patching.
5. The amblyopic eye in the past used to be stimulated with CAM stimulator, red filter or pleoptics treatment.
6. Treatment with levodopa may improve the vision in amblyopic eye.

### 10.12 BENIGN TUMORS OF CHILDHOOD

### Dermoid

1. Dermoid is the most common benign tumor of the orbit.
2. It may cause proptosis.
3. Histology may show hair, teeth, bone and other tissues.

### Lipodermoid

1. Lipodermoid is a solid tumor seen at the upper part of the lateral canthus (Fig. 10.12).

### Teratoma

1. Teratoma is a rare congenital tumor arising from multiple germinal layers.
2. Malignant teratomas need excision or exenteration of the orbit.

### Capillary Hemangioma

1. Capillary hemangioma is common. It involves the skin of the medial part of upper eyelid and produces strawberry discoloration.

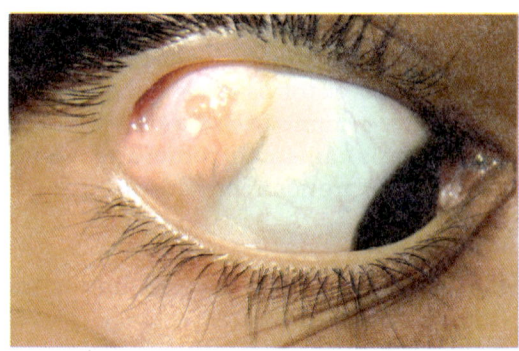

**Fig. 10.12:** Conjunctival dermoid

2. It may cause blue discoloration of lid.
3. The tumor may cause lid deformities.
4. Treatment of capillary hemangioma comprises an injection of a mixture of betamethasone (6 mg) and triamcinolone (10 mg).
5. Pulse-dye-laser may be used.
6. Small lesions can be excised.

### Glioma

1. Glioma of the optic nerve may or may not be associated with neurofibromatosis (25–60%).
2. It manifests in the first decade of life.
3. Glioma produces, unilateral axial proptosis.
4. Other manifestations include strabismus, papilledema and optic atrophy.
5. Chiasma may be involved.
6. A fusiform dilatation of the optic nerve is seen on CT scan.
7. A long follow up is often recommended.
8. Tumor threatening visual loss is dealt with surgical excision or radiotherapy.

### 10.13 MALIGNANT TUMORS OF CHILDHOOD

### Retinoblastoma

#### Etiology

1. Retinoblastoma is the most common intraocular malignant tumor of childhood.
2. Unilateral familial cases (about 60%) manifest during first year of life while bilateral (about 40%) between 1 year and 3 years.
3. Retinoblastoma is inherited as an autosomal dominant trait with high penetrance.
4. Children with hereditary retinoblastoma have one abnormal retinoblastoma gene in all their cells. The retinoblastoma gene is located within the q14 band of chromosome 13.
5. The retinoblastoma gene codes for a protein which dominantly suppresses tumor formation. In the absence of this antioncogenic protein, the retinal cell division may continue unchecked causing retinoblastoma.

6. About 60% of retinoblastoma cases arise from somatic nonhereditary mutations in retinal cells.
7. Most of the retinoblastoma are sporadic.
8. Retinoblastoma is usually of multicentric origin. It arises from the premature cells of photoreceptor.

#### Symptoms

1. Leukocoria cat's eye reflex (50%) and deviation of eye are common presentations.
2. Later, the child cries with pain.
3. Redness, watering, proptosis and loss of vision are other complaints.

#### Signs

The clinical course of retinoblastoma is divided into four stages:
1. *Stage of quiescence*
   - The amaurotic cat's eye reflex in a child's eye creates anxiety in parents (Fig. 10.13).
   - The pupil is dilated and does not react to light.
   - Ophthalmoscopy may present a cream colored growth protruding from the retina into the vitreous—endophytic retinoblastoma, or an exophytic retinoblastoma growing in the subretinal space and causing retinal detachment. The

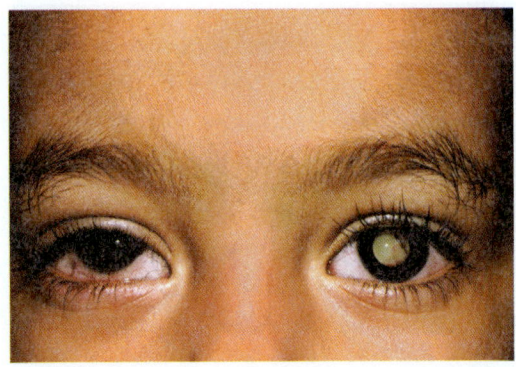

**Fig. 10.13:** Child showing leukocoria left eye (*Courtesy:* Dr Vikas Khetan, Consultant, Oncology, Sankara Nethralaya, Chennai)

10

endophytic retinoblastoma shows neovascularization on its surface.

2. *Stage of glaucoma*
   - IOP is increased due to tumor mass pushing the iris-lens diaphragm anteriorly and occluding the chamber angle.
   - IOP can also be increased due to blockage of the trabecular meshwork by tumor cells.
   - The eyeball becomes enlarged (buphthalmic).
   - Retinoblastoma cells in the anterior chamber can produce a pseudohypopyon with convex level.
   - Occasionally, the tumor presents a picture of anterior uveitis causing some clinical diagnostic problem.
   - Rubeosis iridis is often seen, it may be associated with hyphema.

3. *Stage of extraocular extension*
   - The growing retinoblastoma can cause rupture of the eyeball either at the limbus or near the optic disk resulting in extraocular extension (Fig. 10.14).
   - Orbital involvement can also occur through scleral emissaries and through optic nerve by direct extension.

4. *Stage of metastasis*
   - Metastasis in preauricular and cervical lymph nodes is common.

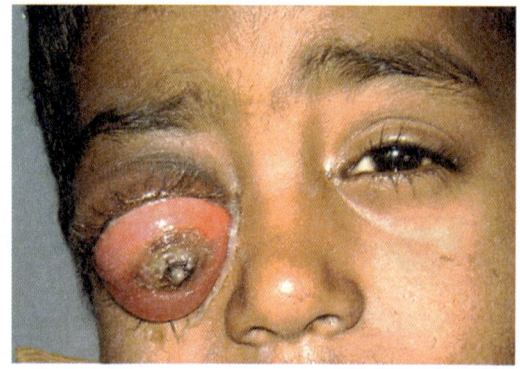

**Fig. 10.14:** Extraocular stage of retinoblastoma (*Courtesy:* Dr Vikas Khetan, Consultant, Oncology, Sankara Nethralaya, Chennai)

- Retinoblastoma may metastasize to brain, flat bones like, iliac crest and sternum.
- Blood-borne metastasis is uncommon.
- A combination of bilateral retinoblastoma with pineoblastoma is known as trilateral retinoblastoma.

### Differential Diagnosis

Endophytum retinoblastoma gives a white reflex in the pupil and must be differentiated from following conditions:

1. Congenital cataract
2. Acute iridocyclitis with vitreous exudation
3. Persistent hyperplastic primary vitreous
4. Toxocariasis
5. Retinopathy of prematurity
6. Retinal astrocytoma.

Exophytum retinoblastoma causes detachment of retina and should be differentiated from:

1. Retinal detachment
2. Coats' disease.

### Diagnosis

The child should be examined under general anesthesia. The examination should include:

1. Corneal diameter and IOP measurement.
2. Dilated fundus examination to locate tumor(s) and assess the extent of tumor.
3. Examination of the fellow eye for bilateral involvement.
4. CT for intraocular (Fig. 10.15) and intracranial calcification and enlargement of the optic foramen.
5. B-scan ultrasonography for mass lesion and calcification.
6. Histopathology for type of tumor
   - Differentiated (Flexner-Wintersteiner or Homer Wright rosettes)
   - Undifferentiated retinoblastoma (Fig. 10.16).

### Treatment

1. Genetic counseling may be provided to the parents of the child with retinoblastoma.

10

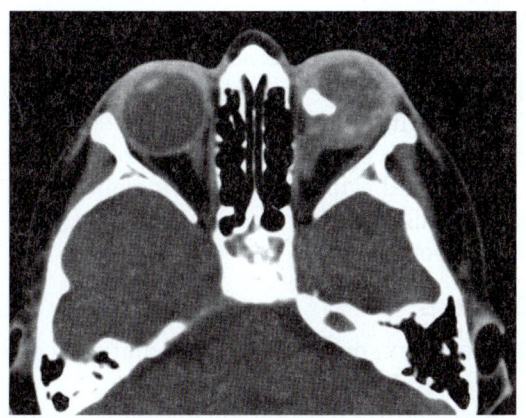

**Fig. 10.15:** CT of patient with retinoblastoma showing intraocular calcification left eye (*Courtesy:* Dr Vikas Khetan, Consultant, Oncology, Sankara Nethralaya, Chennai)

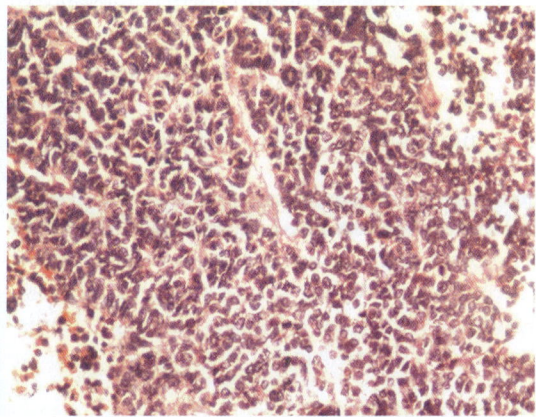

**Fig. 10.16:** Photomicrograph of retinoblastoma showing small round cells with hyperchromatic nuclei and scanty cytoplasm

2. Enucleation is indicated if retinoblastoma involves more than 50% of globe. Postoperatively radiation or chemotherapy may be needed in some patients.

3. In the third stage of large retinoblastoma, debulking is recommended followed by chemotherapy and radiation.

4. Chemoreduction of the tumor can be achieved by intravenous administration of chemotherapeutic drugs (carboplatin, vincristine, etoposide and cyclosporine every 3 weeks for 4–9 cycles).

5. Chemotherapy is preferred in children with metastasis.

6. A direct photocoagulation treatment is preferred for retinoblastoma smaller than 3 mm in apical height and less than 10 mm in basal diameter.

7. Children with bilateral retinoblastoma are treated with external beam radiation therapy (4,000–4,500 cGY over a period of 4–6 weeks). The therapy may cause radiation-induced cataract and optic neuropathy and osteosarcoma.

8. Medium size retinoblastoma (8 mm × 16 mm) can be managed by iodine-125 plaque radiotherapy.

## Rhabdomyosarcoma

### Etiology

1. Rhabdomyosarcoma is the most frequent primary orbital malignancy of childhood.

2. It takes origin from pluripotent mesenchymal elements and not from extraocular muscles as thought earlier.

### Symptoms

The child may complain of progressive bulging of eye with watering.

### Signs

1. A progressive proptosis develops unilaterally.

2. The growth often involves the superonasal quadrant.

3. Ptosis and strabismus are found.

4. The tumor can destroy the orbital bone.

### Diagnosis

1. CT and MRI can demonstrate the extent of the tumor.

2. An excisional biopsy confirms the diagnosis.

### Treatment

1. Small, encapsulated and localized tumor should be excised.

**10**

2. A combined local irradiation (a total of 4,500–6,000 cGy of irradiation is given in 6 weeks) with chemotherapy is effective. Radiation induced-cataract and retinitis are common complications.

## Metastatic Neuroblastoma

1. Neuroblastoma is a primary tumor that develops in the abdomen of children.
2. It often metastasizes to the orbit.
3. The metastatic neuroblastoma causes marked ecchymosis of lids and conjunctiva, proptosis and Horner's syndrome.

## 10.14 LEUKEMIA

Acute lymphoblastic leukemia is most common in childhood. Acute myelogenic and monocytic leukemias are less common.

### Symptoms

Prominent eye, swelling of conjunctiva and lids and decreased vision may occur.

### Signs

1. Eyes may be affected with progressive proptosis, ecchymosis and swelling of eyelids due to orbital infiltration (Fig. 10.17).
2. Retinal hemorrhages, Roth spots and optic nerve infiltration with edema and visual loss are often seen.

3. Localized collection of myeloid cells in the retina, called chloroma may be found.
4. Leukemic cells can infiltrate in the iris and cause iritis.
5. The angle of the anterior chamber may be infiltrated causing secondary glaucoma.
6. The child may become anemic or thrombocytopenic.

### Diagnosis

1. Blood examination for immature cells (Fig. 10.18)
2. Slit-lamp examination and IOP measurement
3. Dilated fundus examination.

### Treatment

1. Topical cycloplegic and corticosteroids can manage iritis.
2. Topical timolol to control secondary glaucoma.
3. Leukemia responds to radiation therapy.

## 10.15 PHACOMATOSES

The phacomatoses include neurofibromatosis (NF), Sturge-Weber syndrome, von Hippel-Lindau syndrome, tuberous sclerosis, Louis-Bar and Wyburn-Mason syndromes.

### Neurofibromatosis

Neurofibromatosis (NF) or von Recklinghausen disease is distinctly divided into two types: (1) NF1 and (2) NF2. They are described under

10

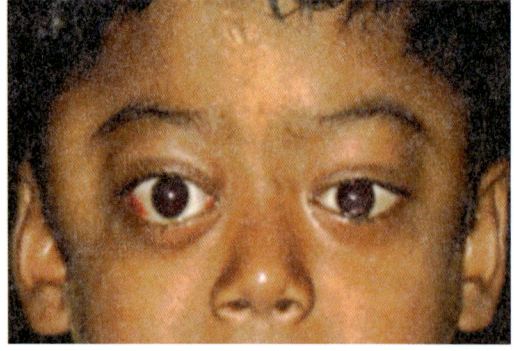

**Fig. 10.17:** Leukemia causing proptosis right eye (*Courtesy:* Shivcharanlal Chandrawanshi, Leucemia, Eye in Systemic Disorders. HV Nema, et al., editors, New Delhi, Wiley, India, 2015)

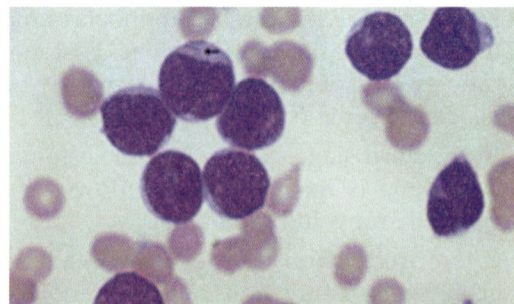

**Fig. 10.18:** Immature cells (*Courtesy:* Shivcharanlal Chandrawanshi, Leucemia, Eye in Systemic Disorders. HV Nema et al., editors, New Delhi, Wiley, India, 2015)

separate heads for better understanding of the disease.

## 1. Neurofibromatosis Type-1 (NF1)

### Etiology

1. NF1 is an autosomal dominant disease with 100% penetrance. It occurs in 1 out of every 3,000 births.
2. The gene for NF1 is located on the long arm of chromosome 17q11.2. It is thought to be a tumor suppressor gene.
3. NF1 occurs due to mutation of gene; although the cause of mutation is unknown.
4. It is suggested that the size of the NF1 gene is very large and therefore it is prone to high rate of mutation.

### Symptoms

Drooping of lid, ocular discomfort due to pulsating exophthalmos and decreased vision may occur.

### Signs

1. Plexiform neurofibroma of the upper lid is a characteristic sign causing ptosis (Fig. 10.19). It may be associated with secondary glaucoma.

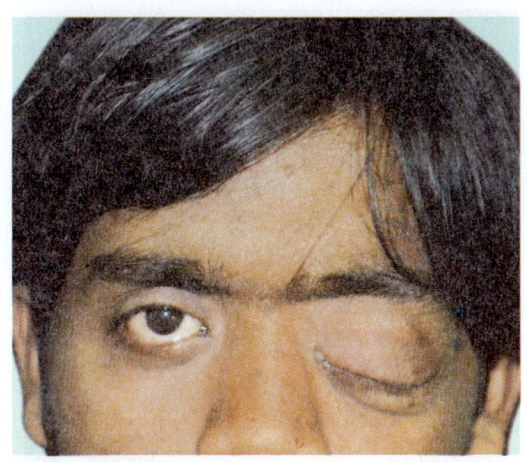

**Fig. 10.19:** Plexiform neurofibroma of the left eyelid causing ptosis (*Courtesy:* Prof. M Subramanyam, Visakhapatanam)

2. Lisch spots (hamartomas) on the iris are often present.
3. Other ocular features include pulsating proptosis, prominent corneal nerves, optic nerve glioma, uveal thickening and hamartomas of retina and choroid.
4. Systemic features include spheno-orbital encephalocele, absence of greater wing of sphenoid bone, vertebral deformities, isolated solitary neurofibromas, cardiovascular abnormalities, multiple *café au lait* spots and axillary or inguinal freckling.

### Diagnosis

1. Presence of six or more *café au lait* spots (5 mm diameter), two or more neurofibromas of any type or one plexiform neurofibroma, freckling in the axillary or inguinal regions, optic nerve glioma and two or more Lisch nodules are classical diagnostic features.
2. MRI of orbit and brain
3. DNA testing is helpful.

## 2. Neurofibromatosis Type-2 (NF2)

### Etiology

1. NF2 is also an autosomal dominant disease that is ten times less common than NF1. It occurs in 1 out of every 37,000 births.
2. The gene for NF2 is situated on chromosome 22q12.2. It is known as merlin or schwannomin (SCH).
3. The most important hallmark is the presence of bilateral vestibular schwannomas.

### Symptoms

Hearing loss, tinnitus and body imbalance are common.

### Signs

1. Presenile posterior subcapsular cortical cataract (57–80%) is common.
2. Pseudopapilledema, optic nerve head glioma, macular and paramacular epiretinal

**10**

membrane and hamartomas of the retina may be found.

3. Lagophthalmos may occur due to facial nerve palsy.
4. The eye becomes dry and corneal anesthesia may develop.
5. Bilateral vestibular schwannomas, spinal and intracranial meningiomas and subcutaneous spherical tumors on the trunk are also seen (Fig. 10.20).

### Diagnosis

1. Clinical evidence of neurofibroma, glioma, schwannoma, and presenile posterior subcapsular cataract.
2. CT scan or MRI (gadolinium contrast) shows bilateral VIIIth nerve masses.
3. DNA testing.

### Treatment

1. Treatment of solitary neurofibromas is total excision.
2. Children with plexiform neurofibroma should be treated well in time, lest they are likely to develop amblyopia.
3. Plexiform neurofibroma is vascular and diffusely intertwined with the normal tissues, therefore, its complete removal is associated with hemorrhage. The use of the $CO_2$ laser has been recommended for its excision.
4. Medical and surgical treatment is needed to control the increased IOP.

### Follow-up

Plexiform and diffuse tumors may show recurrence after incomplete excision.

## Sturge-Weber Syndrome

### Etiology

1. Sturge-Weber syndrome or encephalo-trigeminal angiomatosis, is a nonheritable neurocutaneous disorder with nevus flammeus.
2. A somatic mutation is implicated in its etiology. It has a prevalence of about 1 in 50,000 population.

### Symptoms

Congenital discoloration of one side of face, headache, hemianopsia, poor memory and fits may occur.

### Signs

1. Unilateral hemangioma of the face in the distribution of ophthalmic and maxillary nerves and upper eyelid (Fig. 10.21).
2. Glaucoma (30%) on the side of facial hemangioma is common and may cause optic atrophy.
3. Iris heterochromia is common.

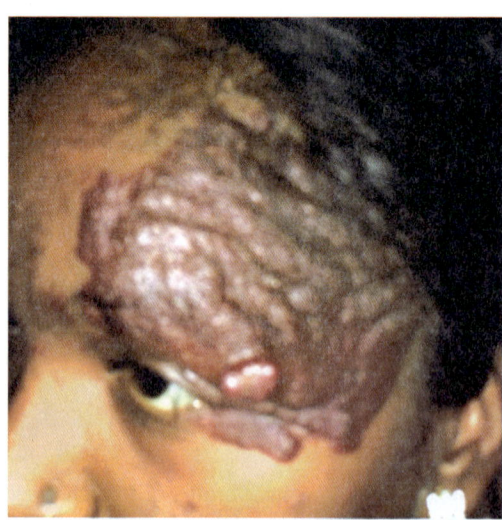

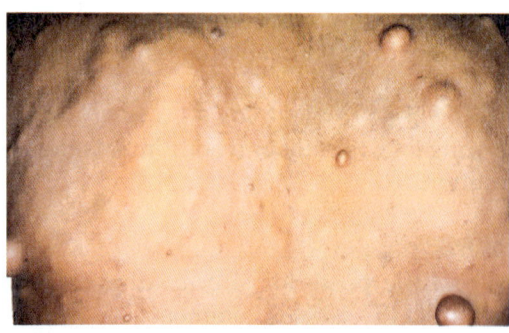

**Fig. 10.20:** Neurofibromatosis: Multiple neurofibromas on the back (*Courtesy:* Dr M Subramanyam, Visakhapatnam)

**Fig. 10.21:** Sturge-Weber syndrome: Angioma of the left face

10

4. Presence of diffuse choroidal hemangioma (70%) imparts a tomato catsup reflex to the fundus.
5. Serous retinal detachment may occur.
6. Systemic features include facial hemiatrophy, seizures, intracranial angioma, learning disability and mental retardation.

### Diagnosis

1. Clinical picture is characteristic
2. Dilated fundus examination can locate diffuse angioma and typical fundus reflex.
3. B-scan ultrasonography can demonstrate diffuse choroidal angioma and retinal detachment.
4. Skull X-ray shows intracranial calcification mostly in the occipitoparietal region showing typically a tram-track appearance.
5. CT scan and MRI highlight the extent of calcification with cortical atrophy and dilatation of lateral ventricle.

### Treatment

1. Control seizures by medical treatment.
2. A combined trabeculotomy-trabeculectomy approach may be tried for early onset glaucoma.
3. Choroidal hemangioma associated with retinal detachment can be treated with photocoagulation or transpupillary thermotherapy.

### Follow-up

Periodic measurements of IOP in operated or unoperated patients with glaucoma are necessary for proper control.

### von Hippel-Lindau Syndrome

### Etiology

1. von Hippel-Lindau syndrome (angiomatosis retinae) is inherited as an autosomal dominant trait with variable penetrance.
2. It is caused by mutation of the von Hippel-Lindau (VHL) tumor suppressor gene (80%) located on chromosome 3p25–26.

3. Syndrome manifests between 30 years and 40 years of life, more commonly in males and bilateral in 50% of patients.

### Symptoms

1. Headache, nausea, vomiting, dizziness, fits and tremors are common.
2. Hemangioma located in the periphery of retina remains undiagnosed for a long time in the absence of symptoms.

### Signs

1. Retinal capillary hemangioma with a dilated and prominent feeding artery and a draining vein is characteristic (Fig. 10.22).
2. It is small, round and red in color and may be single or multiple (33%).
3. Gray-white exudate rich in lipids surrounds the growth. Exudates may take the form of a macular star or circinate retinopathy.
4. There may be recurrent hemorrhages and massive exudative retinal detachment.
5. Epiretinal membrane and macular traction are not uncommon.
6. The final end stage of disease is marked by secondary glaucoma, perforation of eye and phthisis bulbi.

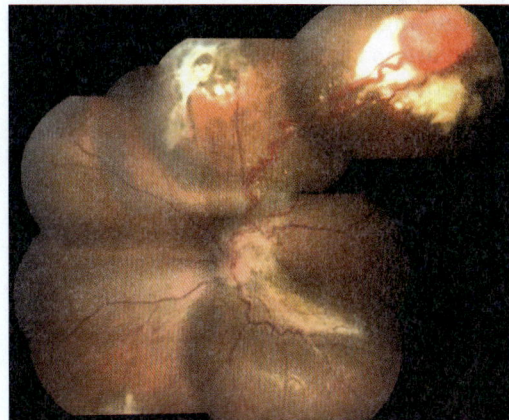

**Fig. 10.22:** Retinal angioma in von Hippel-Lindau disease (*Courtesy:* V Gupta, T Sharma. von Hippel-Lindau disease, Eye in Systemic Disorders. H V Nema et al., editors, New Delhi, Wiley, India, 2015)

10

7. Hemangioblastoma of the cerebellum is the most common CNS lesion (35–75%) causing raised intracranial pressure.
8. Disturbances of gait and posture, tremors, dysmetria, and speech defects may also be seen. Lesions of the spinal cord may lead to bladder dysfunction.
9. Carcinoma of kidney, pheochromocytoma of adrenal medulla and polycythemia may be associated with von Hippel-Lindau disease.

## Diagnosis

1. The clinical picture is characteristic (presence of angioma) and dilated fundus examination can diagnose majority of cases.
2. Fundus fluorescein angiography is very useful for detecting small hemangiomas which may be missed by the indirect ophthalmoscopy.
3. CT and MRI are advised to detect hemangioblastomas in the brain and other visceral organs.

## Treatment

1. All cases of von Hippel-Lindau disease should be treated as early as possible in order to retain or save the vision.
2. Photocoagulation is the treatment of choice for angiomas up to 1.5 mm in size.
3. Large angioma feeder vessels are treated with argon laser to reduce the blood flow.
4. If media are opaque, cryotherapy should be considered.
5. Retreatment is indicated after 4–6 weeks in those patients with incomplete regression.
6. Angiomas greater than 4 mm in size, plaque brachytherapy (ruthenium 106/rhodium 106 plaque) is the treatment of choice as these angiomas respond poorly to laser or cryotherapy.
7. Exudative retinal detachment or fibrotic membranes requires pars plana vitrectomy or scleral buckling.
8. Hemangioblastoma of cerebellum and carcinoma of kidney need surgical resection at an early stage.

## Follow-up

1. Periodic dilated fundus examinations should be performed as recurrences or formation of new angiomas are not rare.
2. Cerebellar hemangioblastoma and renal cell carcinoma are lethal.

## Tuberous Sclerosis

### Etiology

1. Tuberous sclerosis (Bourneville disease) is inherited as an autosomal dominant trait with variable penetrance although most cases are sporadic.
2. It is caused by mutations in the genes of tuberous sclerosis complex (TSC); TSC1 located on chromosome 9q34 and TSC2 on 16p13.
3. TSC1 encodes a protein, called hamartin and TSC2 encodes the protein tuberin; both proteins act at the golgi apparatus.

### Symptoms

Patient may complain of decreased vision.

### Signs

1. Mulberry-like astrocystic hamartomas of the retina and/or optic nerve are characteristic lesions.
2. They may be bilateral, multiple and undergo calcification.
3. Punched-out depigmented areas in the retina and choroid are found.
4. Coloboma of iris may be present.
5. Adenoma sebaceum (adenoma sebaceum is in fact an angiofibroma and there is no involvement of sebaceous glands) is seen in a butterfly distribution on cheeks (50–87%).
6. Ash-leaf spots of depigmentation (90%) and papules around and beneath nails are often seen.
7. CNS involvement may present seizures, cognitive impairment and behavioral abnormalities.

10

8. Cystic lesions in the lung and renal hamartoma may be found in some cases.

9. Rhabdomyoma and rhabdomyolipoma of the heart may cause fatal arrhythmias.

## Diagnosis

1. Astrocystic hamartoma of the retina or optic nerve and ash-leaf spots are diagnostic.

2. Cranial CT and MRI are advised for CNS lesions.

3. Molecular genetic tests should be carried out in suspected cases.

## Treatment

1. Control seizures by medical therapy (adrenocorticotropic hormone and vigabatrin).

2. Retinal hamartomas are benign and undergo calcification.

## Louis-Bar Syndrome

### Etiology

1. Louis-Bar syndrome is also known as ataxic telangiectasia.

2. It has an autosomal recessive trait.

3. The ataxia telangiectasia mutated (ATM) gene is located on chromosome 11q22–23.

### Symptoms

Difficulty in gait.

### Signs

1. Telangiectasia of bulbar conjunctiva and oculomotor apraxia with supranuclear gaze palsies may be found.

2. Strabismus and nystagmus may be seen.

3. Systemic features include progressive ataxia, immune deficiency and T-cell dysfunction, high incidence of malignancy especially leukemia and premature senility.

### Diagnosis

1. Clinical evidence

2. Molecular analysis.

### Treatment

No treatment is available.

## Wyburn-Mason Syndrome

### Etiology

1. Wyburn-Mason syndrome is also known as racemose angioma of the retina.

2. Etiology of the syndrome is not known and condition is nonheritable.

### Symptoms

Patient is symptom-free, occasionally the patient may complain of prominent eyes and fits.

### Signs

1. Retinal vessels are enormously dilated and tortuous.

2. Retinal vascular obstruction and hemor-rhage in the retina and vitreous may occur.

3. Racemose hemangioma may also involve the midbrain and pterygoid fossa.

4. Pulsatile vascular nevi are seen in the distribution of the trigeminal nerve.

### Diagnosis

1. Typical fundus picture

2. CT scan shows intracranial calcification.

### Treatment

No treatment is available.

10

# Neuro-ophthalmology

## 11.1 PAPILLEDEMA

Papilledema is defined as noninflammatory edema of the optic disk.

### Etiology

1. Papilledema is caused by intracranial tumors especially of midbrain, temporal and parietal lobes and cerebellum.
2. Inflammatory conditions like meningitis, encephalitis and brain abscess.
3. Subarachnoid hemorrhage, subdural and epidural hematoma and cerebrovenous sinus thrombosis.
4. Hydrocephalus and arteriovenous malformation
5. Systemic diseases like malignant hypertension, idiopathic intracranial hypertension, and blood dyscrasias can induce papilledema.
6. Ocular causes include orbital tumors or abscess, central retinal vein occlusion (CRVO) and ocular hypotonia.

### Symptoms

1. Patients may be symptom-free or may present transient episodes of blackouts, decrease in vision, headache associated with nausea, vomiting and diplopia.
2. Visual loss is due to macular edema/or optic atrophy.

### Signs

The clinical course of papilledema can be divided into four phases:

1. *Early phase*
   - It presents with hyperemia of the disk, blurring of the nasal disk margin, congestion of veins and absence of spontaneous venous pulsations.
   - Soon peripapillary folds *Paton lines,* tortuous and dilated retinal veins and flame-shaped hemorrhages may appear.
2. *Acute phase*
   - The optic cup is obliterated. The optic disk is edematous (1–3 disk diameter) with blurred margins (Fig. 11.1).
   - It is accompanied by peripapillary flame-shaped hemorrhages and cotton-wool

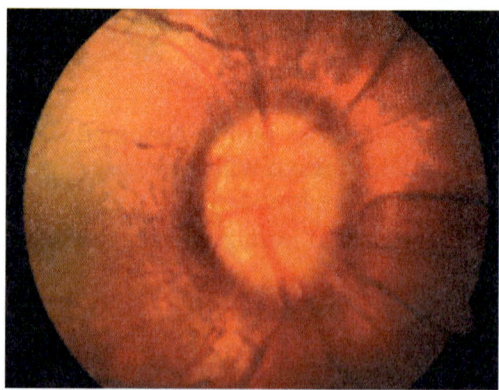

**Fig. 11.1:** Papilledema (*Courtesy:* Dr S Ambika, Director, Neuro-ophthalmology, Sankara Nethralaya, Chennai)

spots, exudates arranged in a radial manner or forming an incomplete macular star (Fig. 11.2).
- Pupillary reaction is normal.

3. *Chronic phase*
- In the chronic phase, retinal edema, hemorrhages and exudates start resolving. The disk appears as dome of a champagne cork with small refractile bodies like small drusen.
- Retinal vessels show sheathing and there occurs peripapillary gliosis.
- Pupils show sluggish reaction and an enlargement of blind spot may be found on perimetry.

4. *Atrophic phase*
- It is the end stage of papilledema characterized by grayish-white atrophic optic disk, narrowing of arteries and sheathing of vessels.
- Pupillary reaction is sluggish or lost depending on the amount of damage to optic nerve.
- There occurs loss of vision and concentric contraction of visual fields.

### Differential Diagnosis

1. Pseudopapillitis, seen in the following conditions:
   - High hyperopia (optic disk is small and the optic nerve fibers are heaped up)
   - Drusen of optic disk.

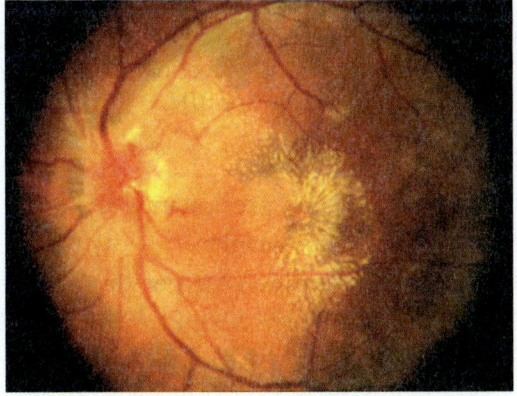

**Fig. 11.2:** Papilledema with incomplete macular star

2. Papillitis
3. Ischemic optic neuropathy
4. Diabetic papillopathy
5. Secondary optic nerve infiltration due to sarcoidosis, leukemia, etc.

### Diagnosis

1. Funduscopy shows edema of the disk
2. Systemic clinical examination may reveal etiology of papilledema
3. Visual field charting
4. Cerebrospinal fluid (CSF) analysis for ruling out inflammatory conditions
5. Computed tomography (CT) and magnetic resonance imaging (MRI) for intracranial tumors
6. Gadolinium MRI or magnetic resonance angiography (MRA) to look for vascular lesions.

### Treatment

1. The basic cause of papilledema should be treated.
2. Control of raised intracranial pressure (ICP) either medically or surgically may resolve papilledema.
3. Persistent papilledema leads to post-papilledematous optic atrophy and gross visual loss.

### 11.2 IDIOPATHIC INTRACRANIAL HYPERTENSION

### Etiology

1. The etiology of idiopathic intracranial hypertension (IIH) or pseudotumor cerebri is unknown.
2. The rise in intracranial pressure may be due to an impaired absorption of CSF.
3. Administration of contraceptives, systemic corticosteroids (or their rapid withdrawal), tetracyclines, cyclosporin A and high doses of vitamin A may precipitate the condition.
4. Obesity, weight gain and pregnancy are risk factors.

11

5. The incidence of IIH peaks in the third decade of life with a strong female preponderance (2:1).

## Symptoms

1. The most common presenting symptom is headache, worse in the morning, that aggravates by sneezing, coughing and straining.
2. Other symptoms include transient visual loss on change of posture, nausea, vomiting, diplopia, dizziness and pulsatile tinnitus.

## Signs

1. Bilateral papilledema is a cardinal sign of IIH seen in about 90% of patients (Fig. 11.3).

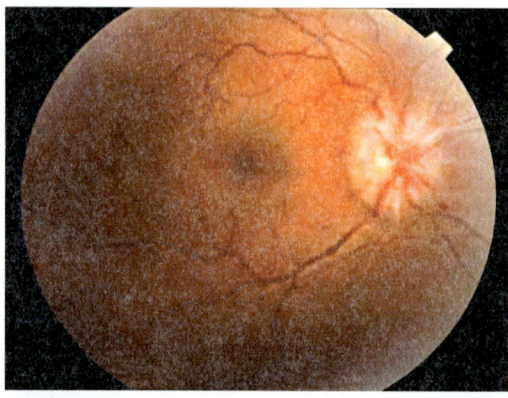
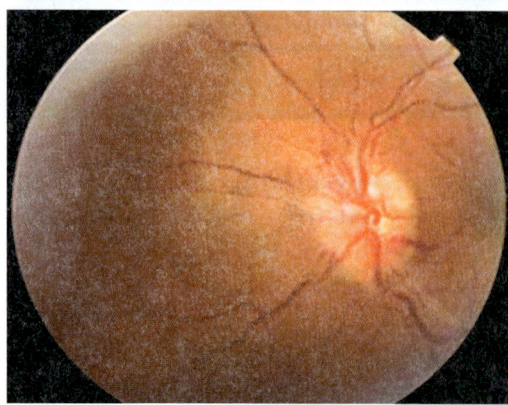

**Fig. 11.3:** Bilateral papilledema in IIH (*Courtesy:* Suneetha Lobo. Idiopathic intracranial hypertension. Eye in Systemic Disorders. HV Nema et al., editors, New Delhi, Wiley India, 2015)

2. Unilateral or bilateral VIth cranial nerve palsy is the next most frequent sign.
3. Chorioretinal folds, macular edema or exudates, subretinal peripapillary hemorrhages and neovascular membrane extending to the fovea are often seen.
4. ICP may remain elevated.
5. Optic atrophy develops in untreated patients.
6. Visual field defects and visual impairments are common.

## Differential Diagnosis

1. Cerebral venous thrombosis
2. Other causes of papilledema.

## Diagnosis

1. History of drug intake.
2. Dilated funduscopy shows presence of bilateral papilledema.
3. Periodic visual field charting should be done to know the progress of IIH.
4. Lumbar puncture (LP) demonstrating a CSF pressure of 250 mm of $H_2O$ is consistent with the diagnosis of IIH.
5. A normal cellular content, protein and glucose concentration in CSF suggests IIH.
6. CT may show slit-like cerebral ventricles due to enlarged brain volume.
7. Magnetic resonance venography is currently the study of choice.
8. Serial B-scan ultrasonography to measure the retrobulbar optic nerve sheath diameter is helpful in monitoring IIH.

## Treatment

1. Stop all medicines precipitating IIH.
2. Advice to reduce weight.
3. Oral acetazolamide (2 g per day) is the mainstay of medical therapy for lowering intracranial pressure.
4. Topiramate, an antiepileptic medicine may be used.

11

5. A short course of high dose intravenous corticosteroids may be useful in the acute phase of the disease.
6. Optic nerve sheath decompression (ONSD) or CSF diversion procedure (lumboperitoneal or ventriculoperitoneal shunt) is recommended in patients with progressive and severe visual loss.

## 11.3 ARTERITIC ANTERIOR ISCHEMIC OPTIC NEUROPATHY

### Etiology

1. The disease is less common than nonarteritic anterior ischemic optic neuropathy. It affects people above 60 years of age.
2. It may be accompanied with giant cell arteritis.

### Symptoms

1. Sudden, painless blindness associated with headache occurs in one eye, the other eye may soon be involved.
2. Pain during chewing, joint pains, fever, loss of appetite and weight loss are other symptoms.

### Signs

1. Visual loss is severe; vision is reduced to count fingers.
2. RAPD is present.
3. Temporal arteries are prominently dilated, tender and nonpulsatile.
4. Optic disk becomes swollen and pale with blurred margins (Fig. 11.4).
5. Retina shows hemorrhages, cotton-wool spots, edema and occasionally, CRAO.
6. In late stage, optic atrophy develops and optic disk may present cupping.
7. Abducens nerve palsy may be found.

### Differential Diagnosis

1. Nonarteritic ischemic optic neuropathy
2. Optic neuritis.

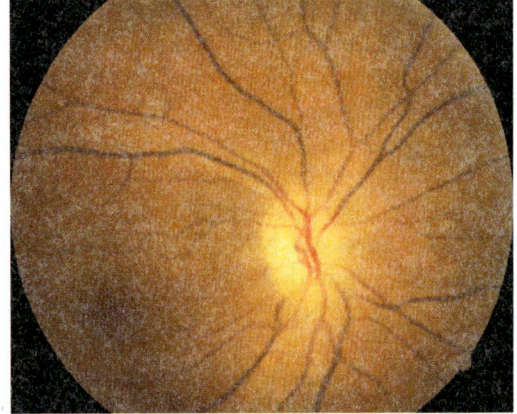

**Fig. 11.4:** Anterior ischemic optic neuropathy

### Diagnosis

1. Age of the patient
2. Dilated funduscopy presents a characteristic pallid disk swelling.
3. Raised erythrocyte sedimentation rate (70–100 mm/hour) and abnormally high C-reactive protein
4. Temporal artery biopsy often confirms the diagnosis.

### Treatment

1. Treatment must be started early to prevent the involvement of the fellow eye.
2. Intravenous methyl prednisolone followed by oral prednisolone should be administered. A maintenance dose of the drug is recommended for 3–12 months.

## 11.4 NONARTERITIC ANTERIOR ISCHEMIC OPTIC NEUROPATHY

### Etiology

1. Nonarteritic anterior ischemic optic neuropathy (NAION) is an idiopathic disease that affects patients between 40 years and 60 years of age.
2. Compromise in the optic nerve head microcirculation is implicated in its etiology.
3. Hypertension, diabetes, arteriosclerosis, hyperlipidemia, nocturnal hypotension,

**11**

sleep apnea, smoking, and migraine are known risk factors.

## Symptoms

1. Unilateral sudden loss of vision on awakening is a common symptom.
2. It may become bilateral.
3. In nonprogressive NAION after initial fall in vision, vision does not decline further.
4. In progressive NAION vision continues to decrease for about a month.

## Signs

1. Optic disk edema is diffuse or segmental.
2. Flame shape hemorrhages, cotton-wool exudates and telengiectasia of optic nerve are often seen.
3. A secondary optic atrophy develops following resolution of edema.
4. A small optic disk with absence of cup in the fellow eye is considered as a bad sign. Hence called "disk at risk."
5. Altitudinal visual field loss is usually seen (Fig. 11.5).

## Differential Diagnosis

1. Arteritic ischemic optic neuropathy

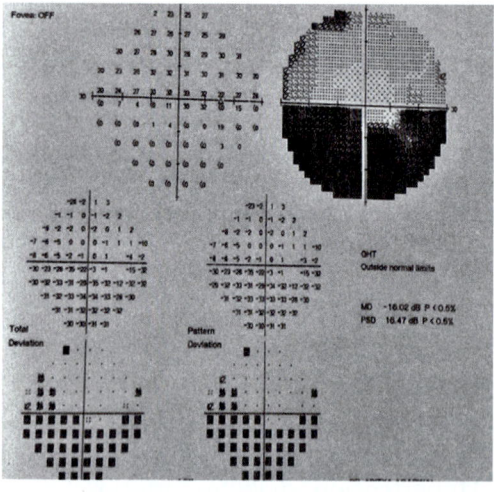

**Fig. 11.5:** Altitudinal visual field defect in NAION

2. Postoperative posterior ischemic optic neuropathy (following head and neck surgery, spinal surgery, open heart surgery, etc in high risk patients).

## Diagnosis

1. The diagnosis is mainly clinical.
2. Fellow eye examination should be done to look for "disk at risk"
3. FA shows segmental hypofluorescence of optic disk. Later on, luxury perfusion may be seen as hyperfluorescence of disk.

## Treatment

1. Avoid or treat risk factors. Antihypertensive drugs should be avoided at bedtime to prevent nocturnal hypotension.
2. Approximately, half of the patients improve over time.

## 11.5 OPTIC NEURITIS

Commonly optic neuritis represents an underlying demyelinating disorder. It may manifest as:

1. Papillitis
2. Retrobulbar neuritis.

## Etiology

1. The most common cause of optic neuritis is multiple sclerosis.
2. Other causes include herpes, poliomyelitis, tuberculosis, sarcoidosis, neurosyphilis, meningitis, sinusitis, orbital cellulitis, retinochoroiditis and autoimmune vascular disorders.
3. Many cases are idiopathic.

## Papillitis

### Symptoms

Unilateral loss of vision, depressed brightness and color defects are common.

## Signs

1. Pain on ocular movements
2. Pupillary reaction to light is sluggish and ill-sustained.
3. Optic disk is hyperemic, cup is filled and margin is blurred (Fig. 11.6).
4. Edema is seen in peripapillary area.
5. Retinal hemorrhages and exudates around the papilla are found.
6. Cells are seen in the vitreous.
7. Central or centrocecal scotoma is common.
8. Untreated cases of papillitis may pass on to postneuritic optic atrophy characterized dull gray disk, obliterated cup and blurred margins.

## Differential Diagnosis

Papilledema

## Acute retrobulbar Neuritis

### Symptoms

Patients may complain of sudden loss of vision, reduced perception of light intensity, defective color vision, pain in eye and headache.

### Signs

1. Upward and inward ocular movements are painful.

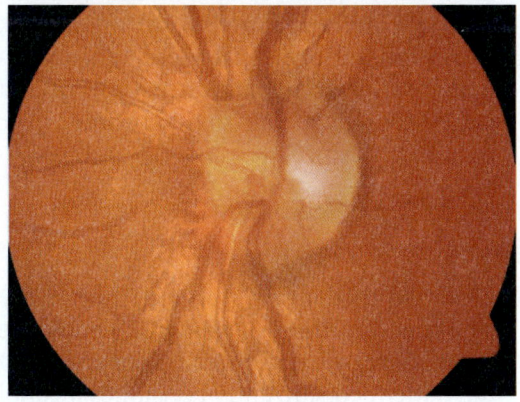

**Fig. 11.6:** Papillitis

2. Tenderness at the site of insertion of superior rectus muscle.
3. Ill-sustained pupillary reaction (*Marcus-Gunn pupil*).
4. The colored object appears faded.
5. The patient develops poor depth perception for moving objects.
6. Symptoms are aggravated if body temperature increases.
7. Funduscopy may show temporal pallor of the optic nerve head.
8. Common field defects are central or centrocecal scotomas.

## Differential Diagnosis

1. Cortical blindness
2. Papilledema
3. Ischemic optic neuropathy.

## Diagnosis

1. History of viral fever or previous multiple sclerosis (MS)
2. Pupillary reactions to light and dilated funduscopy
3. Color vision test
4. Visual field test
5. Serology for suspected etiology
6. MRI of brain and orbit may provide diagnostic clue.

## Treatment

1. Optic Neuritis Treatment Trial (ONTT) recommends the use of pulsed methyl prednisolone 1 g intravenous daily for 3 days followed by oral prednisolone 1 mg/kg body weight daily for 11 days, then oral prednisolone should be tapered. Initial oral corticosteroid therapy increases the risk of recurrence of optic neuritis.
2. In patients showing 2 or more MS lesions on MRI the treatment is with interferon β-1a, interferon β-1b or glatimer acetate.

11

## 11.6 LEBER HEREDITARY NEUROPATHY

### Etiology

1. Leber hereditary optic neuropathy (LHON) is transmitted in an atypical sex-linked manner, it affects predominantly the males.
2. Mothers transmit the disease to all offsprings by a mitochondrial DNA mutation, at position 11778.
3. Majority of sons (70%) and a few daughters (10%) manifest LHON.
4. The disease is commonly seen at the age of 20 years.

### Symptoms

Unilateral or bilateral decrease in vision is a common symptom. Patient may see a scotoma and notice defect in identifying colored objects.

### Signs

1. Acute form of the disease presents swelling of the optic disk and peripapillary nerve fiber layer.
2. Optic disk telangiectasia and arteriovenous shunts are found near the optic disk.
3. Telangiectatic vessels do not show leak on fundus flourescein angiography (FFA).
4. Centrocecal scotoma is a common field defect.
5. In chronic form of the disease, optic atrophy ensues (Fig. 11.7).
6. Cardiac conduction defects may be found in some patients on electrocardiogram.

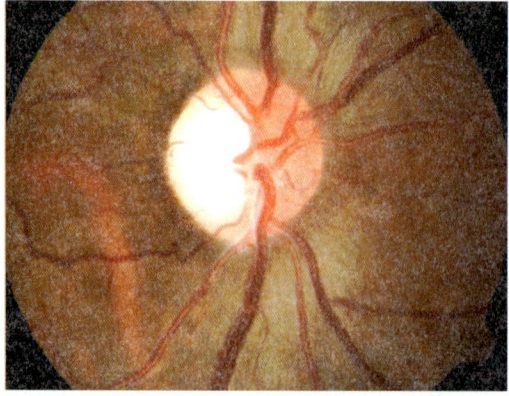

**Fig. 11.7:** Leber optic neuropathy

### Diagnosis

1. History of familial and hereditary character of LHON
2. Dilated funduscopy shows swelling of the disk and peripapillary telangiectasis.
3. Chronic cases reveal optic atrophy.
4. FFA shows absence of leakage of fluorescein from the telangiectatic vessels.
5. Visual field recording presents a central or centrocecal scotoma.
6. Molecular genetic testing can confirm the disease.

### Treatment

1. No treatment is effective
2. Cardiac conduction defects should be treated by a cardiologist.
3. Patient may be referred for genetic counseling.

## 11.7 TOXIC CHRONIC OPTIC NEUROPATHY (TOXIC AMBLYOPIA)

### Etiology

1. Toxic chronic optic neuropathy can cause painless loss of vision.
2. It is caused by a direct or indirect (through ganglion cells) effect of toxins on the retinal nerve fibers.
3. Tobacco, ethyl alcohol, methyl alcohol, cannabis, ethambutol, isonicotinic hydrazide, chloroquine, streptomycin, quinine, amiodarone, vigabatrin, sulfonamides, digitalis, chloramphenicol, chlorpropamide and tolbutamide are neurotoxic and capable of inducing toxic chronic optic neuropathy.

### Tobacco Optic Neuropathy

#### Etiology

1. Overindulgence in tobacco either by smoking, snuffing or chewing can cause toxic neuropathy. The toxicity increases if the patient concurrently consumes alcohol in a large amount and is malnourished.

11

2. Cyanide present in tobacco is toxic and damages the ganglion cells of retina.

## Symptoms

Decreased vision, impaired color vision, difficulty in reading and near work.

## Signs

1. Initially, signs may be minimal or undetectable but gradually decrease in vision manifests.
2. Pupillary reaction is ill sustained and later becomes sluggish.
3. Temporal pallor of the disk may be the only sign initially.
4. Color confusion occurs.
5. Centrocecal scotoma is seen on field charting.
6. The relative scotoma is bigger for red than white target.

## Diagnosis

1. History of abuse of tobacco and alcohol
2. Color vision defects
3. Sluggish pupillary reactions
4. Centrocecal scotoma
5. Poor nutritional status
6. Lower serum levels of vitamins $B_1$, $B_2$ and folate.

## Treatment

1. Complete abstinence from tobacco.
2. Large doses of vitamins $B_1$, $B_2$, $B_{12}$ and folate.
3. Systemic vasodilators were claimed to be beneficial.

## Methyl Alcohol Optic Neuropathy

### Etiology

1. Methyl alcohol optic neuropathy is caused by accidental or intentional drinking of methylated spirit.
2. The spirit causes metabolic acidosis.
3. Optic neuropathy occurs due to degeneration of the ganglion cells.

## Symptoms

1. Methyl alcohol toxicity may have an acute or chronic onset.
2. Symptoms of acute onset are vomiting, respiratory distress, abdominal pain, delirium and coma.
3. Bilateral loss of vision is a chronic mode of presentation.

## Signs

1. Semidilated pupil with sluggish/no reaction to light.
2. The fundus examination may show mild papilledema and attenuation of retinal vessels.
3. Later, optic atrophy develops.

## Diagnosis

1. History of consumption of methylated sprit.
2. Amsler chart testing shows depression of visual sensitivity around fixation point.
3. Centrocecal scotoma on visual field charting.

## Treatment

1. Gastric lavage and intravenous soda bicarbonate may save the life in acute stage.
2. Administration of folic acid and ethyl alcohol may help the patient.

## Quinine Optic Neuropathy

### Etiology

Toxic amblyopia can occur following use of quinine. It is used for treating malaria, arthritis and nocturnal cramps.

## Symptoms

The patient complains of near total blindness tinnitus and deafness.

## Signs

1. The pupils are dilated and fixed.
2. Funduscopy shows pallor of the optic disk, marked attenuation of retinal vessels and edema of retina.

11

3. Patients with retained vision may show constricted visual fields.

4. A complete optic atrophy can develop.

### Diagnosis

1. History of intake of quinine
2. Characteristic fundus picture
3. Constricted visual fields
4. Electroretinography (ERG) shows reduced bipolar cells and ganglion cells response. Electro-oculogram (EOG) is invariably abnormal.

### Treatment

1. Stop the use of quinine
2. Administration of multivitamins ($B_1$, $B_6$, $B_{12}$)
3. Hyperbaric oxygen, vasodilators and nutritional supplementation.

## Ethambutol Optic Neuropathy

### Etiology

1. Ethambutol is administered orally 15 mg/kg/day for the treatment of tuberculosis.
2. Toxicity of ethambutol is dose-related and more in alcoholic and diabetic patients.

### Symptoms

Decreased visual acuity and defective color vision are early symptoms.

### Signs

1. Pupillary reaction is sluggish and ill sustained.
2. Funduscopy reveals papilledema, optic neuritis and splinter hemorrhages.
3. Central or centrocecal scotoma is common.
4. Bitemporal hemianopia reflects early involvement of chiasm.
5. Later bilateral optic atrophy can develop (Fig. 11.8).

### Diagnosis

1. History of intake of ethambutol
2. Fundus picture shows disk edema.

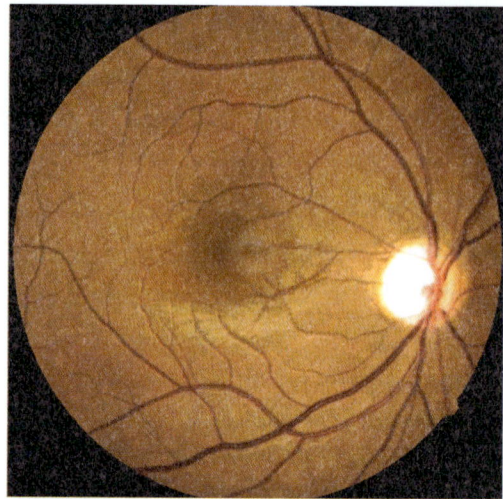
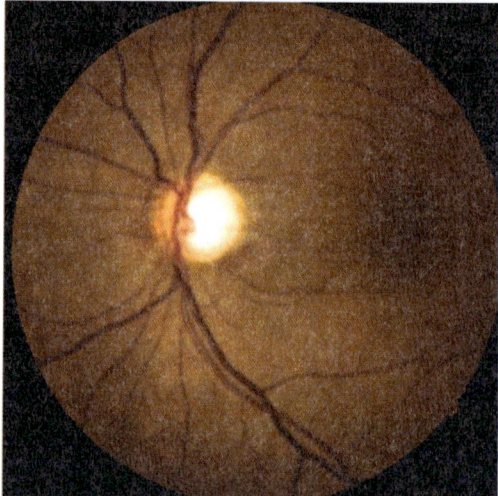

Fig. 11.8: Bilateral optic atrophy due to ethambutol

### Treatment

1. Withdraw the drug
2. Administration of vitamin B-complex, vitamin C and zinc may improve the vision.

## Chloroquine Optic Neuropathy

(*Refer* 8.15)

## Nutritional Optic Neuropathy

### Etiology

Malabsorption syndrome, chronic alcoholism, prolonged abstinence from food, general starvation and deficiency of essential vitamins B$_1$, B$_6$, B$_{12}$ and niacin in the diet can induce chronic optic neuropathy.

## Symptoms

Visual impairment is the main symptom. Nystagmus, strabismus and drooping of lids are other symptoms.

## Signs

1. Vitamin B$_1$ deficiency causes external ophthalmoplegia, retinal hemorrhages and optic neuropathy.
2. Niacin deficiency causes pellagra characterized by optic neuropathy, cystoid macular edema (CME), diarrhea, dermatitis and dementia.

## Treatment

A proper intake of food rich in essential vitamins should be given.

## 11.8 MIGRAINE

### Etiology

1. The etiology of migraine is not known. A family history is common.
2. Dopaminergic genes may be involved in the disorder.
3. Migraine is more common between 30 and 40 years of age and it shows a predilection for women especially those using contraceptives or are pregnant.
4. Psychic stress, insomnia, menopause, intake of nitrates, nitrites, glutamate, cheese, chocolate, wine and bright light may trigger an attack of migraine.

### Symptoms

1. Recurrent, severe, pulsating or boring unilateral headache is associated with nausea and vomiting.
2. Patients may complain of visual disturbances, photophobia, phonophobia and speech disturbances.

3. Some patients of migraine present an aura of symptoms.
4. Other symptoms include fatigue, mood changes, failure to concentrate, stiff neck, tingling, numbness, anorexia and intolerance to food odors.

### Types

1. *Migraine with typical aura (Classical migraine):* It is less common and seen in only 10%. A visual aura begins with flashes of light in a zigzag manner and covered nearly three-fourth of visual field. It is also known as scintillating scotoma. The aura is followed by severe hemicrania.
2. *Migraine without aura:* Migraine without aura is the most common type of migraine that lasts for 4–72 hours. It occurs without preceding aura. Typically, it is unilateral pulsating and of moderate to severe intensity.
3. *Acephalic migraine:* Acephalic migrane is also known as silent migraine or migraine with aura without headache. Some patients with advanced age may report scintillating scotoma but without headache. The visual symptoms remain for about 60 minutes.
4. *Familial hemiplegic migraine:* Familial hemiplegic migraine has an aura accompanied by motor weakness (hemiplegia).
5. *Retinal migraine:* Retinal migraine presents visual aura and unilateral headache which is fully recoverable.
6. *Basilar-type migraine:* Occasionally, symptoms of migraine mimic symptoms of vertebrobasilar artery insufficiency.
7. *Ophthalmoplegic migraine:* The onset of ophthalmoplegic migraine occurs in the first decade of life. The migraine causes paresis of the third cranial nerve which takes long time to recover or the recovery may not be complete.

### Diagnosis

1. Family history of migraine

**11**

2. The diagnosis of migraine is largely based on clinical features.
3. Exclude other causes of headache that can mimic or coexist with migraine by thorough ocular and central nervous system (CNS) examination.
4. CT and MRI of head can exclude secondary migraine.
5. Response to treatment is helpful in the diagnosis.

## Treatment

1. Avoid risk factors or manage them properly.
2. Prophylaxis: Propranolol (10–80 mg/day) and flunarizine (10–20 mg daily) may be taken for prophylaxis.
3. Rest, reassurance and avoidance of bright light may relieve headache.
4. Antiemetics may be used to manage nausea and aspirin or nonsteroidal anti-inflammatory drugs (NSAIDs) in low doses for persistent headache.
5. Specific medications include ergotamine 1 mg tablet 3–4 times a day, selective 5 HT agonists, sumatriptan 50–100 mg/day, rizatriptan 5–10 mg/day and zolmitriptan nasal spray.

## 11.9 CAROTID ARTERY INSUFFICIENCY

### Etiology

1. Carotid artery insufficiency (CAI) is caused by stenosis, thrombosis or embolism of carotid artery. Thrombosis is common in old age while embolism in young adults.
2. Thrombosis may occur due to giant cell arteritis, Takayasu's disease, herpes zoster, sarcoidosis, leukemia, thrombocythemia, polycythemia, oral contraceptive agents, pregnancy and antiphospholipid antibodies.
3. Hyperlipidemia, hypertension, hypotension, ischemic heart disease, smoking, obesity and diabetes mellitus are risk factors for CAI.

## Symptoms

1. Carotid insufficiency presents transient ischemic attacks (TIA) of loss of vision (*amaurosis fugax*), flashes of light, permanent monocular visual loss and contralateral homonymous hemianopia.
2. TIA occurs due to sudden, focal ischemia, lasting a few minutes.

## Signs

1. The monocular involvement is seen ipsilateral to affected internal carotid artery. Contralateral homonymous visual field defects and bitemporal visual field defects may occur in cases of bilateral carotid artery disease.
2. Bilateral simultaneous visual loss may result if the disease is bilateral.
3. Headache, mental confusion, seizure, vertigo, ataxia, dysarthria, dysphagia and hemiparesis may occur.
4. The carotid insufficiency may clinically manifest as central retinal artery occlusion (CRAO), branch retinal artery occlusion (BRAO), venous stasis retinopathy, ischemic optic neuropathy and ocular ischemic syndrome.
5. Dilated retinal veins (but not tortuous), pulsation of central retinal artery, hemorrhages in the mid-peripheral retina, neovascularization of iris and retina and cotton wool spots are found.
6. Mild anterior uveitis, iris atrophy, neovascular glaucoma and cataract may develop as complications of the disease.
7. Horner syndrome may occur in patients with occlusion of ICA.
8. Systemic features include contralateral hemiparesis, contralateral hemianesthesia, aphasia and weakness of tongue and face.

## Diagnosis

1. Complete ocular and neurological examinations including auscultation of cervical vessels.

2. Fundus examination allows direct visualization of the retinal circulation.

3. Duplex Doppler flow imaging is a noninvasive technique to assess the carotid and vertebral system.

4. CT scan and MRI can detect both acute and silent infarcts.

5. Contrast angiography though invasive, remains the gold standard to diagnose carotid stenosis.

6. MRA is preferred as it is noninvasive technique and can detect carotid artery dissection but not stenosis.

7. Echocardiography is useful in detecting cardiac valve and wall defects.

## Treatment

1. Medical therapy is aimed to prevent platelet aggregation by the use of thrombolytic drugs in acute stroke.

2. Surgical therapy includes angioplasty and endarterectomy.

3. Management of the risk factors like hypertension has a major role in decreasing the morbidity and mortality.

## 11.10 VERTEBROBASILAR INSUFFICIENCY

### Etiology

1. The vertebrobasilar arterial system supplies the entire brainstem, ocular motor system, the posterior visual sensory pathways and visual cortex.

2. The vertebrobasilar insufficiency is caused by thromboembolic diseases like atherosclerotic carotid disease, cardiac disease, atrial fibrillation, giant cell arteritis, systemic lupus erythematosus, migraine and hyperviscosity state.

### Symptoms

1. Visual signal acquistion (VSA) insufficiency usually presents ophthalmic symptoms first. They include transient loss of vision (approximately, 30% of TIA progress to cerebral infarction), flickering or flashing stars, photopsia, visual hallucinations of variable duration, achromatopsia and decreased vision.

2. Headache, diplopia and nystagmus are frequent.

3. Dizziness, vertigo, tinnitus and deafness are common.

4. Transient dysphagia, dysarthria and drop attacks may occur.

### Signs

1. Vestibular nystagmus is seen.

2. Both pupils are miotic.

3. Diplopia is caused by transient ischemia of the ocular motor nerves or their nuclei manifesting as strabismus, skew deviation, internuclear ophthalmoplegia, nystagmus and gaze paresis.

4. Cerebral blindness occurs with bilateral posterior cerebral arteries occlusion.

5. An isolated congruous homonymous visual field defect with macular sparing is the hallmark of the occlusive vascular lesion of occipital lobe.

6. Alexia without agraphia results from infarction of the left occipital lobe and disruption of the left ventral visual association between the cortex and the left angular gyrus.

7. Associative visual agnosia (left posterior cerebral artery occlusion), prosopagnosia (occlusion of the right posterior cerebral artery) and simultagnosia may develop in patients with bilateral superior occipital lobe strokes.

8. Ataxia, unstable gait, perioral numbness, hemisensory loss, hemiparesis and sudden falls to the ground (drop attacks) are common.

### Differential Diagnosis

Migraine.

### Diagnosis

1. History of TIA, sudden blackouts or giant cell arteritis with hard and tender temporal artery

11

2. Exclude papilledema on fundus examination
3. ESR, prothrombin time, platelets count and complete blood picture
4. Electrocardiography (ECG), echocardiography and 24 hours Holter monitoring for cardiac defects
5. Vertebral artery Duplex Doppler ultrasonography to study posterior cerebral blood flow
6. MRA is considered a better tool.

### Treatment

1. Control risk factors like smoking, hypertension, diabetes, hyperlipidemia, etc.
2. Patients are treated with aspirin and/or anticoagulants.

## 11.11 MYASTHENIA GRAVIS

### Etiology

1. Myasthenia gravis (MG) is an autoimmune disease of the neuromuscular junction.
2. It is caused by blockade of neuromuscular transmission at postsynaptic acetylcholine receptors (AChR) sites by immune complexes.
3. Susceptibility to MG has been shown to be associated with HLA-DQ8, HLA-B8, HLA-DRw3 and HLA-DQw2 polymorphisms.
4. The disease may be associated with thymoma, thyroid disorder, rheumatoid arthritis and systemic lupus erythematosus in some cases.
5. Certain drugs like aminoglycosides, ciprofloxacin, erythromycin and ampicillin, penicillamine, lithium, quinidine and neuromuscular blocking agents may induce myasthenia gravis.
6. MG has its onset in third decade of life with female preponderance (F:M::3:1). However, over 50 years it is more common in males.
7. The ocular myasthenia gravis is more common in men.

### Symptoms

1. Patients are symptom-free in the morning. Symptoms fluctuate in the day and are worst in the evening or when the patient is fatigued.
2. Drooping of lids and diplopia are common, however, they improve with rest.
3. Some cases may present with difficulty in swallowing and breathing.
4. Approximately, 20% of patients with MG manifest only ocular symptoms; but majority of ocular myasthenia patients develop generalized MG over a period of 3–4 years.

### Signs

1. Ptosis is bilateral. It becomes more prominent on either sustained upward gaze or on repeated eyelid closure.
2. Ptosis is mild or absent in the morning but becomes marked in the evening (Fig. 11.9).
3. Bilateral ptosis is usually asymmetrical.
4. Lid twitching may be seen (lid twitch sign of Cogan) or it can be elicited by asking the patient to change gaze from the downward position to the primary position.
5. Poor eye closure is a sign of orbicularis oculi muscle weakness.
6. The spectrum of extraocular muscle palsies stretches from isolated muscle

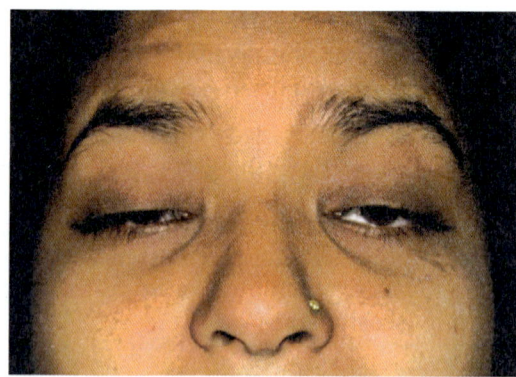

**Fig. 11.9:** A patient with myasthenia gravis showing bilateral ptosis in the evening (*Courtesy*: Rajnish Dubey and Amit Agrawal: Myasthenia gravis. Eye in Systemic Disorders, HV Nema et al., editors, New Delhi, Wiley India, 2015)

11

palsy (isolated medial rectus muscle palsy is most frequent) to total external ophthalmoplegia.

7. Weakness of convergence and upward gaze is often found.

8. Hypermetric or hypometric saccades may be seen.

9. Systemic features include weakness of jaw, neck, trunk and limb.

10. Dysphagia and dyspnea may be fatal.

## Differential Diagnosis

1. Graves' disease

2. Chronic progressive ophthalmoplegia

3. Myotonic dystrophy

4. Eaten-Lambert syndrome.

## Diagnosis

1. History of fluctuating ptosis and asymmetric external ophthalmoplegia with general weakness is virtually diagnostic of myasthenia.

2. Ask the patient to fix on a target in upward gaze for one minute, the degree of ptosis increases.

3. Absence of pupillary abnormalities

4. Apply ice-pack on closed eye for 2 minutes, an improvement in ptosis by 2 mm suggests MG.

5. Sleep test is based on improvement of MG symptoms following rest. It is used in children. Improvement in ptosis after 1 hour sleep for children or 30 minutes for adults is diagnostic of the disease.

6. Tensilon test: Edrophonium (2 mg/0.2 mL or 4 mg/0.4 mL, intravenously) results in improvement in ptosis and nystagmus. About 90% of patients with ocular myasthenia gravis (OMG) have a positive Tensilon test but it can cause syncopal attacks and respiratory arrest, therefore, it is less frequently used.

7. An elevated serum antiacetylcholine receptor antibody may confirm MG.

However, 20% of patients with general MG and 50% with OMG will be seronegative.

8. Antistriated muscle antibodies are positive in about 84% of patients with thymoma whose blood acetylcholine receptors antibodies are elevated.

9. CT chest is advised to rule out thymoma.

10. Thyroid function tests

11. Electromyography can differentiate between MG and Eaten-Lambert syndrome. Unlike MG, muscle strength increases in the latter after exercise.

12. Single fiber electromyography (SFEMG) of orbicularis oculi is the most-sensitive clinical test for detecting neuromuscular transmission defects.

## Treatment

1. Anticholinesterase drug, oral pyridostigmine bromide (Mestinon), the first line of treatment. The drug works better in systemic MG.

2. Oral prednisolone (60–80 mg/day) is prescribed in cholinesterase inhibitor non-responding cases with significant improvement. Side effects of long-term use of steroid should be prevented by tapering or stopping it.

3. Immunosuppressive cyclosporine (3–5 mg/kg/day) is an effective drug but it may cause hypertension and nephrotoxicity.

4. Azathioprine (1–2 mg/kg/day) is used in those patients who do not respond to either prednisolone or cyclosporine.

5. Diplopia may be relieved by applying a patch or Fresnel prism.

6. Plasmapheresis or plasma exchange is indicated for patients with sudden, severe and worsening of symptoms.

7. Ptosis surgery is considered for a stable ptosis that has failed to respond to the medical therapy.

8. Thymectomy is an accepted treatment for generalized MG.

11

## 11.12 CHRONIC PROGRESSIVE EXTERNAL OPHTHALMOPLEGIA

### Etiology

Chronic progressive external ophthalmoplegia (CPEO) is caused by mutation of mitochondrial DNA.

### Symptoms

Drooping of lids and inability to move eyes in any direction of gaze.

### Signs

1. Severe bilateral ptosis may be asymmetrical.
2. Initially the up-gaze is affected, later palsies of other directions of gaze develop.
3. Saccades are slow.
4. Gradually,the condition progresses to bilateral ocular immobility; both eyes appear frozen in the primary position.
5. Pupillary reactions remain normal.
6. Lagophthalmos and exposure keratitis occur due to orbicularis dysfunction.
7. Weakness of facial muscles and limb muscles may also manifest.

### Differential Diagnosis

1. MG
2. Oculopharangeal dystrophy (weakness of pharangeal muscle causing difficulty in swallowing)
3. Kearns-Sayre syndrome (besides CPEO, retinitis pigmentosa and heart block are also present).
4. Progressive supranuclear palsy (ophthalmoplegia, neck rigidity and gait instability, but there is absence of ptosis) may be present.

### Diagnosis

1. Clinical course of disease starts with ptosis and ends with complete immobility of eyes.
2. Absence of pupillary abnormality.

3. Exclude MG by absence of fluctuation of signs and ice-pack and rest tests.
4. Absence of RP and heart block rules out Kearns-Sayre syndrome.

### Treatment

1. Symptomatic relief may be provided to patients with CPEO as there is no cure.
2. Provide ptosis crutches or perform surgical ptosis correction.
3. Reading glasses generally help.
4. Exposure keratitis can be prevented by frequent use of preservative-free artificial tears or partial tarsorrhaphy.

## 11.13 INTERNUCLEAR OPHTHALMOPLEGIA

### Etiology

1. Internuclear ophthalmoplegia is caused by lesions of medial longitudinal fasciculi (MLF). It may be unilateral or bilateral.
2. MS is the most common cause of bilateral internuclear ophthalmoplegia.
3. Infarction of brainstem is the main cause of unilateral internuclear ophthalmoplegia seen in elderly people.
4. Tumors, hemangioma, hemorrhage, abscess, brainstem tuberculoma and Wernicke encephalopathy are other etiological factors.

### Symptoms

Diplopia, nystagmus, squint and decreased vision may occur.

### Signs

1. Unilateral internuclear ophthalmoplegia
   - Ipsilateral adduction saccades are slow.
   - Ipsilateral adduction is decreased and the contralateral abducting eye shows nystagmus and skew deviation.
   - In spite of adduction deficiency, convergence remains normal.

2. Bilateral internuclear ophthalmoplegia
   - Both eyes show loss of adduction.
   - Abducting eyes show nystagmus.
   - Upbeat nystagmus is found on elevation.
   - "Wall eyed bilateral internuclear ophthalmoplegia" can manifest if third nerve nucleus is also involved in the lesion of MLF resulting in a large angle divergent strabismus and loss of convergence.
   - Internuclear ophthalmoplegia is seen in "one-and-half syndrome" due to involvement of MLF and sixth nerve nucleus. "One-and-half syndrome" is characterized by ipsilateral adduction deficit, ipsilateral conjugate gaze paresis and retention of contralateral abduction.

### Differential Diagnosis

Myasthenia gravis.

### Diagnosis

1. A thorough examination of ocular movements; presence of slow adducting saccades have diagnostic value.
2. Exclude MG by history, ice-pack and sleep tests.
3. CT and MRI of brainstem.
4. If needed, MRA may be done.

### Treatment

1. Acute stroke should be treated on conservative lines.
2. Tumors may be dealt with surgery.

## 11.14 CAVERNOUS SINUS THROMBOSIS

### Etiology

1. The thrombosis of cavernous sinus is often caused by septic foci like facial furuncles, middle ear infection, erysipelas, paranasal sinusitis, inflammation of petrous bone and orbital osteomyelitis.
2. It may also occur in sarcoidosis, Behçet disease, hypercoagulability, following trauma, surgery and radiation.

### Symptoms

1. Symptoms include red eye, swelling of lids, drooping of upper lid, lacrimation, ocular pain, inability to open the eye(s) and proptosis.
2. Headache, nausea, vomiting, stupor, fever and tachycardia are general symptoms.

### Signs

1. Initially, ocular signs are unilateral, later they become bilateral.
2. Development of edema in the mastoid region (thrombosis of emissary veins) is an ominous sign for transfer of the symptoms to the other eye.
3. Contralateral VIth cranial nerve palsy is the earliest and the most consistent sign.
4. Bilateral orbital congestion, edema of lids, ptosis and proptosis are common (Fig. 11.10).
5. The paresis of the 3rd, 4th, 6th and ophthalmic division of the 5th cranial nerves may be seen.
6. Ophthalmoplegia and corneal anesthesia are not uncommon.
7. Pupils are dilated and fixed.
8. Optic nerve involvement decreases visual acuity markedly.
9. Horner syndrome, venous stasis retinopathy and facial numbness may be found in some cases.

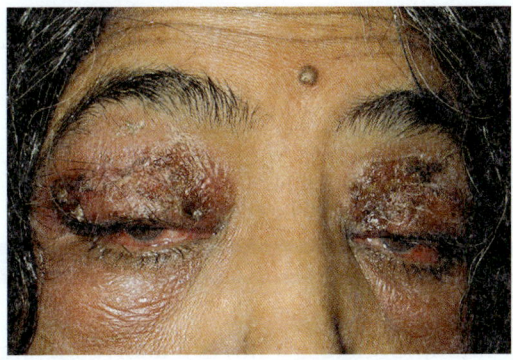

**Fig. 11.10:** Cavernous sinus thrombosis (*Courtesy:* Dr AK Grover, Ganga Ram Hospital, New Delhi)

11

## Differential Diagnosis

1. Orbital cellulitis
2. MG
3. Chronic progressive external ophthalmoplegia
4. Thyroid orbitopathy
5. Nasopharangeal carcinoma
6. Superior orbital fissure syndrome or orbital apex syndrome (painful ophthalmoplegia combined with optic nerve involvement) is attributed to inflammatory or neoplastic diseases of the superior orbital fissure.
7. Pituitary apoplexy (sudden headache, ophthalmoplegia and visual loss due to infarct or hemorrhage in a preexisting pituitary adenoma).

## Diagnosis

1. Mainly on the basis of clinical features.
2. History of infection of face or sinuses
3. Tenderness in the mastoid region
4. Unilateral signs become bilateral
5. Rule out nasopharyngeal carcinoma
6. CT or MRI of orbit and skull
7. Rarely, lumbar puncture is required.

## Treatment

1. The disease is controlled by high-doses of broad-spectrum antibiotics by intravenous route.
2. Systemic corticosteroids reduce inflammation and edema
3. Oral aspirin (325 mg/day)
4. Anticoagulants, heparin followed by warfarin, should be administered.

## 11.15 MULTIPLE SCLEROSIS

### Etiology

1. Multiple sclerosis (MS) is a demyelinating disease seen between the age of 25 and 40 years.

2. It affects females more often than males.
3. The etiology of MS is not known, however, there is an association of the disease with HLA-DR2 antigen.
4. Presence of multiple plaques in the white matter of brain on MRI suggests inflammatory event.

### Symptoms

1. Diplopia is the most frequent symptom, blurring of vision and nystagmus are other complaints.
2. Ataxia, tremors, vertigo, bladder or bowel disturbances, fatigue and depression may develop.

### Signs

1. Restriction in ocular motility and bilateral internuclear ophthalmoplegia are found.
2. Paresis of 6th cranial nerve is often followed by the 3rd nerve palsy.
3. Nystagmus is seen.
4. Incidence of optic neuritis is high (90%) in MS although it may show remission and recurrence.
5. Funduscopy shows retinal nerve fiber defects, vasculitis and sheathing of vessels.
6. Other findings include Bell's palsy, hemiparesis, paraplegia, paresthesia and electric-shock like sensation on flexion of neck.
7. Bitemporal or homonymous heminopic field defects are found.

### Diagnosis

1. Diagnosis of MS is mostly clinical.
2. History of two attacks separated by an interval of 1 month
3. Presence of bilateral internuclear ophthalmoplegia is highly suggestive of MS.
4. Examination of CSF shows raised IgG and IgG/albumin index.
5. FLAIR sequencing MRI demonstrates periventricular ovoid plaques (Fig. 11.11).

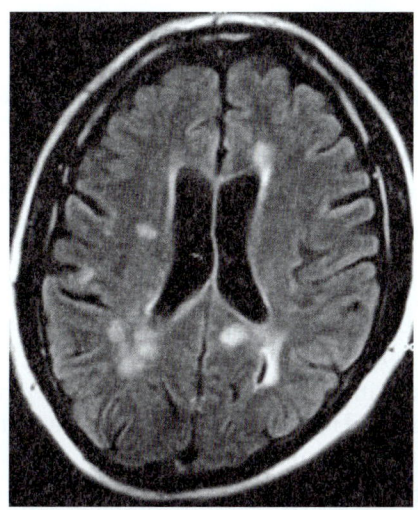

**Fig. 11.11:** Periventricular lesions in multiple sclerosis (*Courtesy:* Suneetha Lobo. Multiple sclerosis. Eye in Systemic Disorders. HV Nema et al., editors, New Delhi, Wiley India, 2015)

## Treatment

1. There is no rational treatment for MS, however, pulse steroid therapy is used in the acute stage.
2. Methotrexate in low doses is found beneficial in progressive MS.
3. Interferon-β1a (avonex) and interferon-β1b (betaseron) reduce the recurrence of attacks.

## 11.16 CEREBRAL BLINDNESS

### Etiology

1. Cerebral blindness or cortical blindness is caused by infarction of both occipital lobes due to embolism or thrombosis.
2. Emboli originate from cardiac valves or postpartum sepsis.
3. Systemic hypotension, secondaries in brain, head injury, encephalopathy and incontinentia pigmenti are risk factors.

### Symptoms

The patient has profound loss of vision in both eyes, visual hallucinations and denies blindness (*Anton syndrome*).

## Signs

1. The patient sees moving objects but not the stationary ones, known as *Riddoch phenomenon.*
2. In spite of blindness, pupils are normal and react briskly to light.
3. Funduscopy shows normal optic disk.
4. Marked visual field defect.

## Differential Diagnosis

1. Malingering (nonorganic visual loss)
2. Bilateral retrobulbar optic neuritis
3. Cone-rod dystrophy.

## Diagnosis

1. History of cardiac diseases like arrhythmia, valvular heart disease, etc.
2. Presence of blindness with normal pupil and optic disk.
3. Exclude malingering.
4. Complete cardiac checkup including ECG and echocardiography.
5. Brain MRI.

## Treatment

The patient needs hospitalization and should be treated under the care of cardiologist and neurologist. Visual prognosis mainly depends on the cause of blindness.

## 11.17 HORNER SYNDROME

### Etiology

1. Horner syndrome or sympathetic paresis is caused by the disorders of first to third-order sympathetic neurones. First-order or second-order Horner syndrome is preganglionic while the third-order is postganglionic.
2. Diseases of brainstem and spinal cord like tumor, stroke, demyelination and trauma may produce first-order neuron disorder.
3. The unilateral Horner syndrome associated with contralateral IVth cranial nerve palsy suggests lesion in the brainstem.

11

4. A lesion of second-order neuron may be due to pancoast tumor, mediastinal tumors, metastases from thyroid adenoma, neuroblastoma and lymphoma involving the brachial plexus at the apex of lung.

5. Lesions above the bifurcation of the carotid artery involve the third-order neuron. The lesions include carotid vascular insufficiency or carotid artery dissection, cervical trauma, nasopharyngeal carcinoma, cavernous sinus tumor, aneurysm or thrombosis, and migraine.

6. The unilateral Horner syndrome associated with contralateral VIth cranial nerve palsy indicates cavernous sinus lesion.

## Symptoms

Most patients remain asymptomatic, some may complain of drooping of lid, loss of sweating on one side of the face and pain in arm.

## Signs

1. Unilateral involvement is a rule and ptosis is mild.

2. Anhydrosis is present in first-order and second-order Horner syndrome but not in the third-order.

3. Reduced width of palpebral aperture (pseudoenophthalmos) is due to dysfunction of Muller's muscles.

4. Hyperemia of conjunctiva and heterochromia of iris are often present.

5. Miosis is common and the affected pupil shows a lag in dilatation in dark.

## Differential Diagnosis

Anisocoria.

## Diagnosis

1. Diagnosis is clinical in large number of cases.

2. Tests are needed for localization and for excluding life-threatening fatal diseases like internal carotid artery dissection, nephroblastoma or other neoplasms.

3. If a Horner pupil does not dilate equal to the size of the pupil in the fellow eye after 15 minutes of instillation of hydroxyamphetamine (1%) drops in both eyes, it suggests a third-order neuron disease. The test is sensitive and specific.

4. Instillation of cocaine (10%) in both eyes results in less dilatation of Horner pupil than normal pupil.

5. Instillation of apraclonidine (0.5–1%) shows that the Horner pupil dilates more than the normal pupil.

6. Internal carotid artery dissection can be excluded by the absence of visual loss, neck pain, foul taste and a negative MRA and CTA.

7. Duplex Doppler ultrasonography

8. CT scan for chest lesions

9. MRI of neck and brain lesions.

## Treatment

1. Patients with benign Horner syndrome do not need any treatment.

2. Ptosis surgery may be performed for cosmetic reason.

3. The underlying cause should be treated.

## 11.18 THIRD CRANIAL NERVE PALSY

### Etiology

1. The IIIrd cranial nerve (oculomotor nerve) palsy may occur either in isolation or in combination with other ocular motor nerves.

2. It may be partial or complete and pupil-sparing or not.

3. Common causes of IIIrd nerve palsy include, aneurysm, vascular occlusion, trauma, neoplasm and idiopathic in adults.

4. In children, the main cause is congenital followed by trauma.

5. Pupil-sparing IIIrd nerve palsy is the hallmark of vascular occlusion often seen

11

in diabetes. Initially, aneurysm (posterior communicating at the junction with the internal carotid artery) can also produce pupil-sparing IIIrd nerve palsy but after 3–5 days, the pupil dilates by compression from expanding aneurysm.

6. Subarachnoid hemorrhage from rupture of aneurysm causes sudden onset of painful IIIrd nerve palsy with meningeal irritation.

7. Meningioma, aneurysm, carotid-cavernous fistula and granuloma (Tolosa-Hunt syndrome) in the cavernous sinus may cause IIIrd nerve palsy with other cranial nerve palsies.

## Symptoms

Diplopia (horizontal or vertical), drooping of upper lid, blurring of vision, mild retrobulbar pain and outward deviation of eye.

## Signs

1. Ptosis, exotropia and hypotropia in the primary position are common presentations (Fig. 11.12).
2. Palsy of the superior division of IIIrd nerve presents ptosis and weakness or paralysis of superior rectus muscle resulting in an inability to elevate the eye.
3. Palsy of the inferior division of the IIIrd nerve presents internal ophthalmoplegia and palsies of medial rectus, inferior rectus and inferior oblique muscles.
4. Pupil is dilated and fixed and may show very poor reaction due to involvement of sphincter pupillae.

5. Ocular movements are restricted in adduction (Fig. 11.13) and depression.

## Differential Diagnosis

1. Chronic progressive external ophthalmoplegia.
2. MG
3. Idiopathic orbital inflammatory syndrome
4. Internal ophthalmoplegia
5. Giant cell arteritis.

## Diagnosis

1. History and age of the patient are helpful in excluding some diseases.
2. Blood pressure, fasting blood sugar, glycosylated hemoglobin, ESR, C-reactive protein and platelet count to exclude hypertension, diabetes and giant cell arteritis.
3. Refer the patient to neurologist to exclude meningitis and other CNS lesions.
4. CT and MRI to exclude neoplasm.
5. Gadolinium enhanced MRI is very sensitive.
6. Lumbar puncture should be performed, if imaging fails to show subarachinoid hemorrhage, for blood in CSF.

## Treatment

1. Treat the cause of the palsy.
2. Diplopia can be managed by prism or patching.

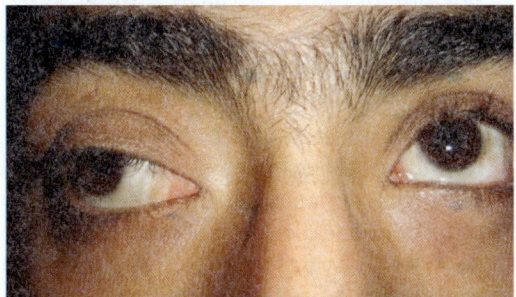

**Fig. 11.12:** Third cranial nerve palsy right eye showing ptosis and divergence

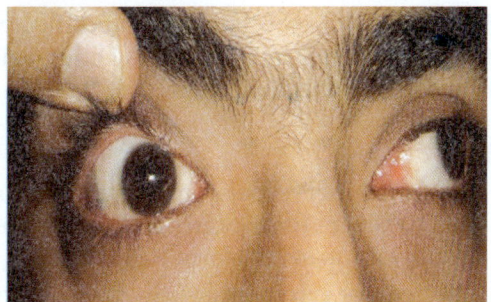

**Fig. 11.13:** Right third cranial nerve palsy showing restricted adduction on levoversion

11

3. After stabilization of the condition, cosmetic surgery for ptosis and squint may be performed.

### Follow-up

Aberrant regeneration of third nerve may occur.

1. Old palsies may show aberrant regeneration of the third nerve.
2. Aberrant regeneration of third nerve is found mostly in traumatic palsies and not in ischemic.
3. The regenerating third nerve fibers mixup with the original fibers supplying to extraocular muscles resulting in simultaneous movements of muscles supplied by different branches of the third nerve, for example, pupil shows constriction on adduction and ipsilateral retraction of upper eyelid on attempted infraduction.

### 11.19 FOURTH CRANIAL NERVE PALSY

### Etiology

1. Trauma is the most common cause of IVth cranial palsy in adults while in children, it is often congenital.
2. Other causes include vascular infarct, MS, neoplasm, aneurysm, hemorrhage, hydrocephalus and giant cell arteritis.
3. Cavernous sinus lesions give multiple nerve palsies due to their proximity.

### Symptoms

Diplopia, giddiness, brow pain and difficulty in reading as letters appear tilted. Diplopia is worse for near and downgaze.

### Signs

1. The fourth nerve palsy may manifest in mild to severe form. Signs and symptoms are obvious in severe form.
2. Affected eye is hypertropic in the primary position with head tilted on the opposite side to avoid diplopia.

3. Ipsilateral inferior oblique overaction (eye shoots up in adduction due to overaction of inferior oblique muscle), ipsilateral superior oblique underaction and contralateral superior oblique overaction can be elicited on version testing.
4. Torsional diplopia can be assessed and charted. Unilateral superior oblique palsy may present excyclotropia of about 7 to 8 degrees.
5. Hypertropia also increases on ipsilateral tilting of the head.
6. In congenital fourth nerve palsy, an asymmetry of face can be noticed because face on the side of head tilt is less developed.
7. Bilateral nerve palsy often manifests torsion more than 10 degrees, V-pattern esotropia, a chin-down posture and alternate hypertropia on head tilts on either side.

### Differential Diagnosis

1. MG
2. Idiopathic orbital inflammatory syndrome
3. Thyroid ophthalmopathy.

### Diagnosis

1. History may be taken to probe whether the palsy is recent or old (congenital).
2. Cover-uncover and Maddox rod tests can demonstrate hypertropia.
3. Bielschowsky head tilt test: Patient is asked to look at a distance in primary position of gaze. The head is tilted to the right and then to the left to compare the hypertropia. In superior oblique palsy hypertropia is more on same side head tilt.
4. Park's three-step test: In the first step try to find out the eye which is hypertropic in the primary position. In the second step determine the direction of horizontal gaze in which hypertropia is more as in superior oblique palsy it is more in opposite gaze. In the third step do Bielschowsky test.

11

5. The vertical fusion range is always more than 3 prism diopters (normal 1–3 prism diopters) suggesting a congenital fourth nerve palsy.

6. Fundus examination reveals relative displacement of optic nerve and fovea suggesting excyclotropia.

7. Double Maddox rod (one white and the other red) test is useful in the diagnosis of bilateral IVth nerve palsies.

8. Synoptophore test with vertical slides.

9. Hess screen test can confirm hypertropia.

10. Visual field charting shows displacement of blind spot.

11. Fasting blood sugar, glycosylated hemoglobin, C-reactive protein (CRP), ESR and platelets count tests are needed to rule out diabetes, inflammatory lesions and giant cell arteritis.

12. Axial and coronal CT scans for orbital lesions.

13. MRI brain for suspected CNS diseases.

## Treatment

1. Treat the cause

2. Annoying diplopia can be managed by patching or prisms

3. If diplopia or strabismus does not resolve in 9 months, surgical intervention should be done.

## 11.20 SIXTH CRANIAL NERVE PALSY

### Etiology

1. The causes of VIth cranial nerve palsy differ between adults and children.

2. Trauma, hypertension and diabetes are the main causes of VIth nerve palsy in adults or old patients.

3. Intracranial neoplasm, raised intracranial pressure, MS, giant cell arteritis, meningitis, neurosyphilis and mass lesions of the cavernous sinus are the other causes.

4. Viral infection, hydrocephalus, otitis media and trauma may cause VIth nerve palsy in children.

### Symptoms

Diplopia, headache, strabismus and inability to move the eye outward are common complaints.

### Signs

1. Eye is esotropic in the primary position (Fig. 11.14) and face is turned toward the side of palsy.

2. Diplopia (uncrossed) is horizontal and more for the distance than near.

3. Separation of images is wider in the direction of action of paretic muscle.

4. Paresis causes limitation of abduction while paralysis leads to complete loss of abduction and the eye does not move beyond the midline.

5. Funduscopy may reveal papilledema due to raised intracranial pressure.

6. Horner syndrome may be associated with VIth cranial nerve palsy in cavernous sinus lesion (carotid artery aneurysm).

### Differential Diagnosis

1. Thyroid ophthalmopathy

2. MG

3. Duane syndrome: In addition to limitation of abduction, variable degree of limitation of adduction and narrowing of palpebral

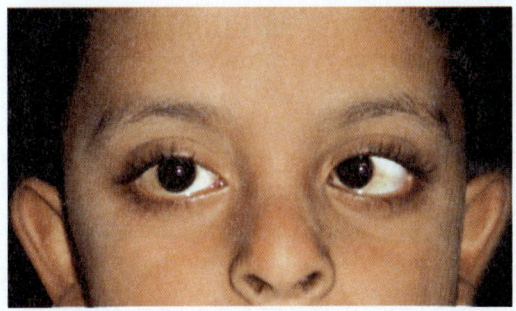

**Fig. 11.14:** Sixth cranial nerve palsy showing esotropia of left eye

11

aperture and retraction of globe may be found.

4. Möbius syndrome: Bilateral palsies of VIth and VIIth cranial nerves.

5. Convergence spasm: Both eyes are markedly converged associated with pupillary constriction and spasm of accommodation. The pupillary dilatation may relieve the condition.

### Diagnosis

1. History of trauma, hypertension and diabetes
2. Complete neurological examination
3. Relevant tests can exclude diabetes, thyroid disorder, myasthenia and giant cell arteritis.
4. Diplopia charting shows uncrossed diplopia
5. Ear examination to rule out otitis media
6. Funduscopy to look for papilledema or optic atrophy
7. MRI of brain
8. If MRI is negative in young patients (less than 45 years), lumbar puncture (LP) may be needed.

### Treatment

1. Manage diplopia by patching, prisms or injection of botulinum toxin in the medial rectus muscle.
2. Treat the underlying cause.

### 11.21 SEVENTH CRANIAL NERVE PALSY

### Etiology

1. The paresis of the VIIth cranial nerve can occur in supranuclear, nuclear and infranuclear lesions.
2. Sarcoidosis, basilar meningitis and Guillain-Barré syndrome may cause bilateral facial palsy.
3. Unilateral facial palsy occurs in Lyme disease, Melkersson-Rosenthal syndrome and Ramsay-Hunt syndrome.
4. Cortical lesions, pontine glioma, lesions of basal ganglion and cerebropontine tumors produce progressive facial nerve palsy with involvement of the Vth, VIth and VIIIth cranial nerves.
5. Exposure to cold, autoimmune disorders, viral infection (herpes) and trauma are other causes of the palsy.
6. Bell's palsy is considered as idiopathic.

### Symptoms

1. Sudden pain, lacrimation and inability to close eye properly
2. Loss of taste, impairment of hearing, nystagmus and vertigo.

### Signs

1. Supranuclear lesions produce upper motor neuron palsy predominantly involving the lower face.
2. Lagophthalmos (Fig. 11.15), decreased lacrimation and salivary secretion, and corneal and facial anesthesia may be present.
3. Weakness of facial muscles, and the corner of mouth is usually dropped.
4. Taste is decreased on the anterior two-thirds of tongue on the side of facial palsy.
5. Nuclear facial palsy presents facial monoplegia, VIth cranial nerve palsy, lateral gaze palsy, ataxia and Horner's syndrome.
6. Cerebellar signs may be seen.

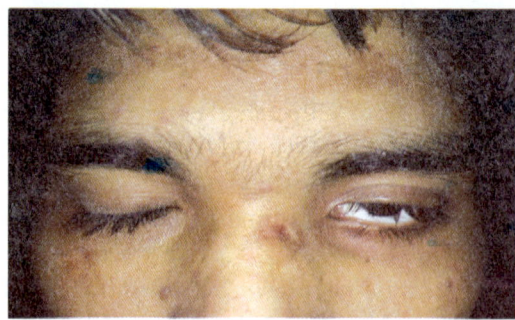

**Fig. 11.15:** Seventh cranial nerve palsy showing lagophthalmos left eye

## Diagnosis

1. History of trauma or stroke
2. Complete ocular examination including eliciting Bell's phenomenon.
3. Neurological examination to find whether the palsy is central or peripheral.
4. X-ray chest to rule out sarcoidosis
5. Multiple cranial nerve palsies warrant CT and MRI of brain.
6. If collagen disease is suspected ANA, RA, and ESR tests should be advised.
7. Occasionally, LP may be needed.
8. Bell's palsy in majority of cases is a diagnosis of exclusion.

## Treatment

1. Most cases of Bell's palsy (84%) show spontaneous recovery. However, systemic corticosteroids and a course of oral acyclovir are quite effective.
2. Cornea must be protected from exposure; use frequent preservative-free tear substitutes and lubricants.
3. Tape the lids or perform tarsorrhaphy
4. Injection of botulinum toxin is given to induce ptosis to cover the cornea
5. Correction of lagophthalmos with gold eyelid implants over tarsus.
6. Systemic diseases like sarcoidosis and Lyme disease may be treated by physician.

11

# CHAPTER

# 12

# Ocular Trauma

## 12.1 CORNEAL ABRASION

### Etiology

1. Corneal abrasions are caused by trivial trauma, corneal or conjunctival foreign body (FB), finger nail injury, plant and mascara brush.
2. Improper fitting contact lens often results in corneal abrasion.

### Symptoms

FB sensation, watering, photophobia and severe pain are common.

### Signs

1. Inspection of the cornea under slit-lamp can recognize abrasion.
2. The extent of epithelial defect is usually demarcated by fluorescein staining (Fig. 12.1).
3. Corneal haziness, mild peripheral pannus and diffuse central staining may be found in patients with contact lens over wear.
4. Anterior chamber reaction is absent.

### Differential Diagnosis

1. Recurrent erosions of cornea
2. Superficial punctate keratopathy.

### Diagnosis

1. Slit-lamp examination facilitates diagnosis of abrasion even in the absence of fluorescein staining

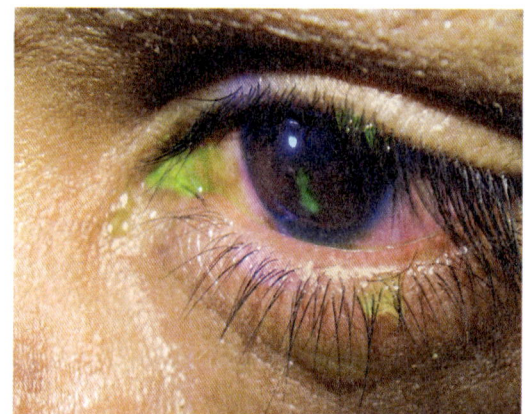

Fig. 12.1: Corneal abrasion

2. A linear abrasion indicates presence of a FB in the upper lid. Evert the lid to exclude it.
3. Staining with fluorescein reveals the size of abrasion.

### Treatment

1. Avoid wearing contact lens for the time being.
2. Old ill-fitting contact lens should be discarded.
3. Topical cyclopentolate (2%) and antibiotic ointment twice a day will heal the abrasion in most cases.
4. Patients with central corneal abrasion need patching.

## 12.2 CONJUNCTIVAL FOREIGN BODY

### Etiology

1. Minute particles of dust, sand, may be found on the conjunctiva in a windy climate.
2. Certain occupations like farmers, miners, carpenters and lathe workers are prone to get particles of husk, grain, coal, wood and metal in their eyes.

### Symptoms

1. Generally, tiny FBs are washed away by tear flow and do not cause any symptoms.
2. FB sensation, irritation, watering and redness are common if FB is retained.

### Signs

1. Sulcus subtarsalis and fornix are common sites for lodgment of FB in the conjunctiva.
2. A localized conjunctival hyperemia, edema or subconjunctival hemorrhage may be seen at the site of FB.
3. A FB in the upper lid may cause a vertical abrasion in the cornea.
4. FBs may be multiple following blast injuries.
5. Conjunctiva may show abrasion or laceration.
6. An embedded FB in the conjunctiva over a period can form a foreign body granuloma.
7. The FB may pierce the bulbar conjunctiva and lodge in the sclera (Fig. 12.2).
8. The nature of FB can be determined by the occupation of the patient.

### Diagnosis

1. A slit-lamp examination can help in finding the FB.
2. Double eversion of the upper lid is required to expose the FB retained in the upper fornix.
3. If conjunctiva is lacerated, scleral perforation must be ruled out.

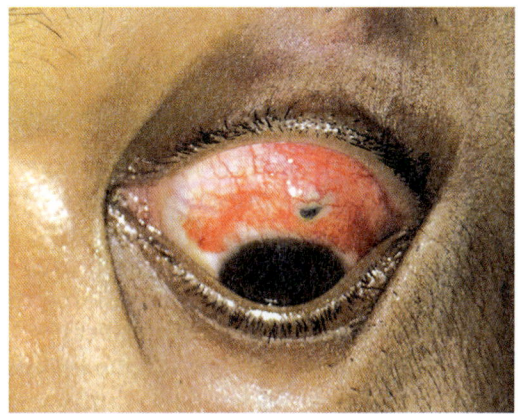

Fig. 12.2: Conjunctival FB partly embedded in sclera

### Treatment

1. Multiple superficial FBs are removed by a thorough irrigation with saline.
2. FB on the conjunctiva is often removed with a cotton bud.
3. Infected FB embedded in conjunctiva should be excised immediately.
4. FB granuloma needs excision.
5. Conjunctival irritation may be relieved by frequent use of preservative-free artificial tears.
6. Moxifloxacin eye drops (0.5%) or gatifloxacin eye drops (0.3%) are used 3–4 times a day for 1 week to avoid secondary infection.

## 12.3 CORNEAL FOREIGN BODY

### Etiology

1. Like conjunctiva, particles of coal, brick, stone and metal may be lodged onto or into the cornea during occupational work.
2. In certain industries, flying chips of iron, copper, zinc or steel may penetrate into the cornea (or enter into the eye).

### Symptoms

1. FB sensation, watering, photophobia, blepharospasm and pain are common.
2. Decreased vision may be noticed in some cases.

**12**

## Signs

1. A FB can be spotted on the cornea (Fig. 12.3) or limbus.
2. Iron FB is often surrounded by rust ring.
3. Presence of stromal infiltration suggests that FB has been present for more than 24 hours.
4. Flying metal pieces are often sterile (due to heat and velocity) that may pierce the cornea and may lie in its deep layers.
5. FBs of vegetable origin are usually infected and may cause microbial keratitis with varying degrees of anterior chamber reaction.
6. A severe uveitis with hypopyon and low intraocular pressure (IOP) suggests perforation of cornea with occult intraocular foreign body (IOFB).
7. Injury by a large piece of stone, brick, and glass usually causes corneal ulcer or perforation.

## Diagnosis

1. Slit-lamp examination of corneal surface and layers is the most important step in assessing the location, depth and nature of FB.
2. Retroillumination from iris and sclerotic scatter techniques are used to detect glass or plastic FBs.

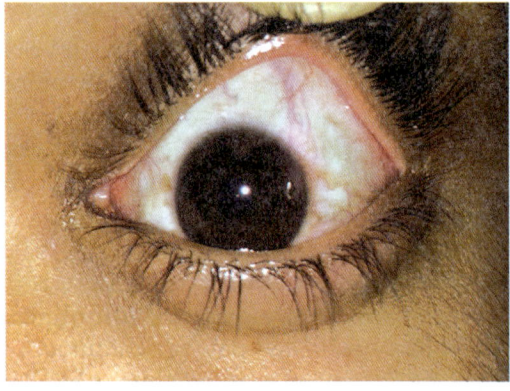

**Fig. 12.3:** FB on the cornea

3. Fluorescein staining may reveal the presence of a corneal abrasion caused by the FB.
4. If infection is suspected, corneal scrap should be sent for Gram-staining and culture.
5. Seidel test should be performed in suspected cases of ocular perforation.
6. Diagnosis of IOFB can be confirmed by dilated funduscopy, X-ray, B-scan ultrasonography and computed tomography (CT).

## Treatment

1. The wearing of safety goggles should be made mandatory for the workers who are engaged in grinding and lathe industries.
2. The corneal FB is removed with the help of FB spud or beveled edge of a 27-gauge needle after surface anesthesia.
3. Small, multiple superficial foreign bodies are removed by denuding the corneal epithelium with alcohol.
4. Iron FB lying in the deeper layer of the cornea is removed in the operation theater.
5. Rust-ring should be scraped by FB burr.
6. Treat the eye as corneal ulcer after the removal of FB.
7. In the presence of infection, fortified topical cefazolin (133 mg/mL) and vancomycin (25 mg/mL) and gentamicin (14 mg/mL) should be instituted.

## 12.4 LACERATION OF CORNEA

### Etiology

Corneal laceration is a partial or full-thickness injury of the cornea caused by sharp objects, flying metal fragment FBs, pellets, fireworks, blunt trauma, and automobile accidents.

### Symptoms

Symptoms include FB sensation, photophobia, watering, severe pain, blepharospasm and decrease in vision.

## Partial Thickness Corneal Laceration

### Signs

1. Trauma causes tear in layers of the cornea without any rupture.
2. IOP is usually normal and aqueous leak does not occur.
3. Hyphema may be present without air bubble in the anterior chamber.
4. Trauma can cause iridodialysis and dislocation of lens.

### Diagnosis

1. Slit-lamp examination can demonstrate the depth of laceration in the cornea.
2. Seidel sign is negative.

## Full-thickness Laceration

### Signs

1. A full-thickness laceration is also known as penetrating injury.
2. It results in a shallow or flat anterior chamber and an air bubble may be seen in the chamber.
3. The eye becomes soft; IOP is very low.
4. Pupil usually is irregular and may not react.
5. Hyphema is often found.
6. Undue pressure on the eye may result in iris prolapse.
7. Patients with corneal laceration are at a risk of developing retinal detachment and glaucoma as well as infection.

### Diagnosis

1. Seidel test (fluorescein test) is positive.
2. Slit-lamp examination is mandatory.
3. CT is indicated if IOFB is suspected.
4. Ultrasonography and optical coherence tomography (OCT) can provide information about dislocation of lens, IOFB and retinal detachment.

### Treatment

1. Use of protective glasses can prevent corneal laceration during high-risk occupation.
2. Administer tetanus toxoid and analgesic medication.
3. Corneal FBs should be removed.
4. Corneal tear should be repaired and dressed with atropine and antibiotic topically.
5. Patients with self-sealing corneal tear may be treated with soft bandage contact lens with frequent instillations of moxifloxacin eye drops (0.5%) and systemic carbonic anhydrase inhibitor 500 mg twice a day.

## 12.5 HYPHEMA

### Etiology

1. Hyphema is usually caused by a blunt or penetrating injury and may also occur postoperatively.
2. Spontaneous hyphema is usually small in amount (microscopic) and may be found in patients with neovascularization of iris, blood dyscrasia, sickle cell anemia, anterior chamber intraocular lens (IOL), ciliary body melanoma, leukemia and heterochromic iridocyclitis.
3. Hyphema may occur in patients who are on systemic nonsteroidal anti-inflammatory drug (NSAID) or warfarin therapy.
4. Hyphema occurs in two forms:
   1. Manifest and
   2. Microscopic (detectable only on slit-lamp examination).

### Symptoms

Blurring or loss of vision, watering, red eye and ocular discomfort may occur.

### Signs

1. The presence of blood in the anterior chamber may be very mild and can only be visible on slit-lamp examination, or massive filling the entire anterior chamber.

**12**

2. Recent hyphema presents a bright red blood in the anterior chamber covering the iris (Fig. 12.4).

3. The color of blood in the anterior chamber changes over time.

4. Old hyphema is characterized by black-clotted blood in the anterior chamber obscuring visibility of iris and pupil. It is known as black ball hyphema.

5. A massive hyphema becomes less due to settling of blood cells with passage of time.

6. Rebleeding is usually severe and occurs within 2–5 days of the trauma.

7. IOP is markedly reduced in penetrating injury but is usually raised in massive hyphema.

8. Sustained elevated IOP is an important predisposing factor for blood staining of the cornea.

### Diagnosis

1. History of trauma, eye operation, medication and family history of blood dyscrasia.

2. Slit-lamp examination to detect micro-hyphema hidden behind the corneoscleral ring and neovascularization of iris.

3. Gonioscopy can show the presence of new blood vessels in the angle.

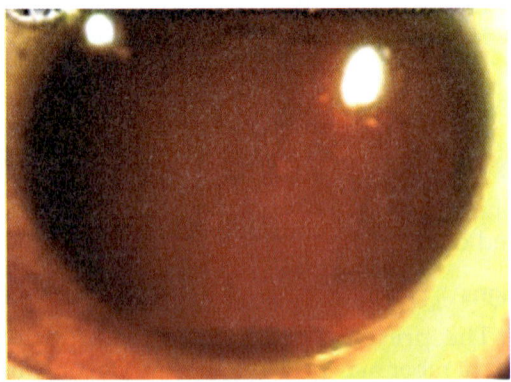

**Fig. 12.4:** Total hyphema (*Courtesy:* Prof. R Ramakrishnan, Aravind Eye Hospital, Tirunelveli)

4. Assess the type of injury; penetrating injury needs special attention and emergency treatment.

5. Blood examination for prothombin time and electrophoresis of hemoglobin (Hb) should be performed to rule out blood dyscrasia and sickle cell disease.

6. CT-scan is required for IOFB and orbital fracture.

7. Dilated funduscopy for retinal FB, retinal detachment and vitreous hemorrhage.

8. If fundus examination is not possible, B-scan ultrasonography is recommended.

9. Consider UBM for ciliary body lesion.

### Treatment

1. Stop immediately NSAID drugs and anti-coagulant therapy.

2. Patients with penetrating injury should be taken for emergency repair.

3. Microhyphema and postoperative hyphema are self-limiting and often do not need any treatment.

4. Use topical atropine (1%) twice a day and topical corticosteroids 2–3 times a day for a week and monitor IOP.

5. Put a shield over the eye and advice bed rest with elevated head end of the bed and no strenuous physical activities.

6. Use timolol (0.5%) twice a day for elevated IOP. If pressure is high, supplement with oral acetazolamide 500 mg bid.

7. In patients with sickle cell disease, acetazolamide should not be administered because it promotes sickling due to acidosis.

8. If IOP is not controlled by maximal medical therapy, a paracentesis should be considered for preventing blood staining of cornea.

9. Initially, the patient should be hospitalized but later should be seen daily or alternate days for amount of blood in anterior chamber, rebleed and IOP.

10. Argon laser photocoagulation may be used to stop bleeding from vessel in the angle of the anterior chamber.

## 12.6 IRIS TRAUMA

### Etiology

1. Iris can be traumatized in both blunt and penetrating injuries.
2. Metallic FBs can either be lodged in iris or create a hole in it.

### Symptoms

1. Blurring of vision or loss of vision, watering, photophobia and mild to severe pain in eye may occur.
2. Symptoms are more acute and severe in the penetrating injury of the eye than blunt.

### Signs

1. Blunt injury to iris may manifest as mild to moderate nongranulomatous uveitis with keratic precipitates (KPs), flare and cells in the aqueous.
2. The trauma causes dispersion of iris pigment on corneal endothelium, in the angle of the anterior chamber and on the anterior capsule of the lens in the form of Vossius ring.
3. Tear can develop in the sphincter pupillae or at the iris root causing iridodialysis. It can split the iris layer—iridoschisis.
4. The sphincter tear causes a tear drop-shaped pupil which may react segmentally. In severe trauma, the pupil is widely dilated and does not react.
5. Hyphema is common.
6. Goniosynechiae, angle recession and blood may be seen in the angle of the anterior chamber.
7. Anterior reflexion of the posterior surface may occur following iridodialysis.
8. The iris may be rolled backward (retroflexion).
9. Rarely, the iris may be completely torn from its root (aniridia).
10. Penetrating injury causes laceration of cornea, iris and lens and often iris presents in the wound.
11. Iris may plug the peripheral corneal wound.
12. The anterior chamber becomes flat or very shallow.
13. IOP is low.
14. Traumatic iritis and hyphema may produce posterior synechiae and occlusive pupillae, pupillary strands and later iris atrophy and secondary glaucoma.

### Diagnosis

1. Diagnosis is mostly on clinical evidence.
2. Slit-lamp examination is essential for detection of uveitis or hyphema.
3. Patients with penetrating injury needs special attention.
4. Suspected cases of IOFB should be subjected to B-scan ultrasonography, UBM and CT to localize it.

### Treatment

1. Mild uveitis is treated with topical cycloplegic [homatropine (2%) once a day], and prednisolone (1%) 3 times a day.
2. Massive hyphema should be treated aggressively.
3. Tear of the cornea, pupil and iridodialysis can be repaired surgically.
4. Elevated IOP is managed conservatively [timolol maleate (0.5%) and acetazolamide 500 mg twice daily].
5. Laser lysis of pupillary strands, adhesions and occlusive pupillae is recommended.

## 12.7 INJURY TO CILIARY BODY

### Etiology

Both blunt and penetrating injuries can damage the ciliary body.

12

## Symptoms

Glare, photophobia, diplopia and decreased vision are common.

## Signs

Trauma may cause iridodialysis and cyclodialysis.

## Iridodialysis

1. Iridodialysis is a disinsertion of the iris from its ciliary attachment. A black biconvex area is seen at the site of tear.
2. On ophthalmoscopy, red reflex and zonules are visible in the gap.
3. The pupil looks irregular due to inversion of the pupillary edge.
4. Anteflexion and retroflexion of iris may occur.

## Cyclodialysis

1. Cyclodialysis is a disinsertion of ciliary body from the scleral spur visible gonioscopically as a cleft.
2. Recession of the angle of the anterior chamber may occur due to tear between circular and longitudinal muscles.
3. The chamber angle recession is characterized by widening of ciliary band.
4. IOP is initially low but is raised if cleft is occluded.
5. Trauma can induce myopia following ciliary spasm and hyperopia can result from ciliary muscle paralysis (loss of accommodation).
6. Cyclodialysis may be accompanied by anisocoria, hyphema, and signs of traumatic uveitis and hypotony syndrome.
7. Cataract and maculopathy develop as complications.

### *Diagnosis*

1. Diagnosis of iridodialysis can be confirmed by ophthalmoscopic or plane mirror examination.

2. Slit-lamp examination should be carried out in all cases.
3. Gonioscopy is mandatory in the diagnosis of cyclodialysis.
4. UBM and anterior segment OCT are helpful in the diagnosis.

### *Treatment*

1. Traumatic uveitis is treated with topical cycloplegic and corticosteroids.
2. Iridodialysis can be repaired.
3. Elevated IOP is generally managed with the aqueous suppressants.
4. If hypotony is due to cyclodialysis cleft, atropine drops (1%) should be applied for approximation of the ciliary body to the sclera.
5. Persistent hypotony requires reattachment of the ciliary body to the sclera either by suturing or by laser photocoagulation.

## 12.8 TRAUMA TO THE LENS

### Etiology

1. Both blunt and penetrating injuries cause cataract and subluxation or dislocation of the lens.
2. Trauma may be inflicted by sharp toys in kindergarten, blunt trauma in sports, flying metal particles in industries and blast injuries in warfare.

### Symptoms

Watering, redness, photophobia, blepharospasm, uniocular diplopia and decreased vision or loss of vision may occur.

### Signs

1. Multiple iris pigments arranged in a circular manner (Vossius ring) on the anterior capsule of the lens may be found in blunt trauma.
2. Traumatic cataract develops due to rupture of posterior lens capsule and entry of aqueous humor in the lens causing a typical rosette-shaped cataract (Fig. 12.5).

**12**

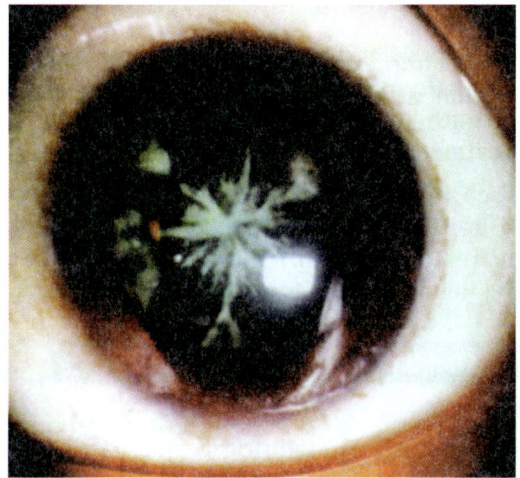

**Fig. 12.5:** Traumatic rosette-shaped cataract (*Courtesy:* HV Nema, Nitin Nema, Textbook of Ophthalmology, 6th ed, New Delhi, Jaypee-Highlights, 2012)

3. The cataract may remain stationary.
4. A concussion injury may cause a late rosette cataract.
5. Partial rupture of zonules causes subluxation of lens (Fig. 12.6).
6. Subluxated lens often gives diplopia. The AC is irregular, phacodonesis and segmental iridodonesis may be present.
7. Double images of the optic disk are seen through phakic and aphakic areas.
8. If the tear of zonules is complete, the lens is dislocated either into the vitreous or in the anterior chamber.

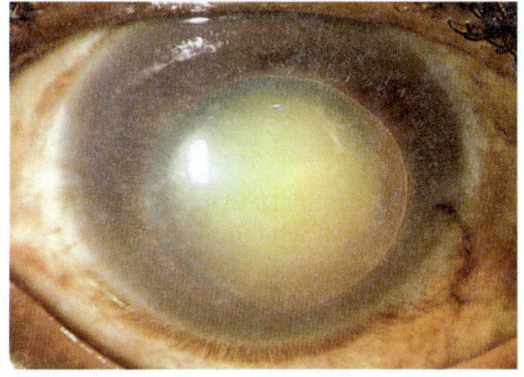

**Fig. 12.6:** Subluxated lens (*Courtesy:* Dr R Ramakrishnan, AEH, Tirunelveli)

9. The posterior dislocation of lens is marked by deep anterior chamber, iridodonesis and aphakia. It may be accompanied by vitreous in the anterior chamber, hyphema and elevated IOP.
10. A clear lens in the anterior chamber appears as an oil-globule and causes anterior uveitis and secondary glaucoma.
11. Rarely, lens may be found in the sub-conjunctival space due to rupture of the sclera.
12. An intraocular FB may be lodged in the lens that may not induce any reaction but only a localized opacity.

**Diagnosis**

1. Cataract is diagnosed clinically.
2. Posterior lens opacity, vitreous and small blood in the anterior chamber and sub-luxation of lens can be demonstrated on slit-lamp examination.
3. Ophthalmoscopy reveals both phakic and aphakic areas suggesting subluxation of lens.
4. B-scan ultrasonography is useful for diag-nosing poster capsule rupture, subluxation and dislocation of lens.

**Treatment**

1. Initially, inflammation caused by trauma and lens-induced uveitis should be treated with cycloplegic and corticosteroid.
2. Aqueous suppressants are used to control elevated IOP.
3. Traumatic cataract without dislocation is managed on general lines.
4. Phacoemulsification with IOL implantation is usually performed in patients with sub-luxated opaque lens with implantation of capsular tension ring.
5. A dislocated lens in the anterior chamber should be removed as early as possible followed by anterior vitrectomy and implantation of scleral fixated IOL.
6. A posteriorly dislocated lens in the vitreous may be removed by vitrectomy.

12

## 12.9 COMMOTIO RETINAE

### Etiology

1. Blunt trauma to the eye causes damage by three mechanisms: (1) coup, (2) countrecoup and (3) compression.
2. Countrecoup is the most common cause of commotio retinae. In countrecoup mechanism, damage occurs opposite to the site of direct impact through shock waves.
3. In commotio retinae shock waves produce whitening of retina as a result of fragmentation of photorecepter outer segments and intracellular edema.

### Symptoms

The patient may remain asymptomatic or suffer from decreased vision or acute loss of vision.

### Signs

1. Commotio retinae may develop either at the posterior pole (Berlin's edema) or peripheral retina. The lesion may arise soon after the impact or may be delayed.
2. The characteristic lesion is a gray-white cloudy opacification of retina at the posterior pole of the eye. Other parts of the retina remain normal.
3. A cherry-red spot may be seen in commotio retinae at the posterior pole.
4. Commotio retinae may be associated with retinal hemorrhages, uveitis, hyphema, serous macular detachment and choroidal rupture.
5. Gradually, the retinal whitening disappears and vision recovers.
6. Degeneration of photoreceptors results in a pigmentary disturbance in the retina.

### Differential Diagnosis

1. Retinal detachment
2. Branch retinal artery occlusion.

### Diagnosis

1. Slit-lamp examination
2. Dilated funduscopy.

### Treatment

Treatment is not needed because with disappearance of edema, central vision may be restored except in some cases where pigmentary changes involve the macula.

## 12.10 PURTSCHER RETINOPATHY

### Etiology

1. The pathophysiologic mechanism of Purtscher retinopathy is not known.
2. It is presumed to be caused by widespread infarcts in the peripapillary arterioles.
3. The typical Purtscher retinopathy is seen in patients with head trauma and chest compression without any direct eye injury.

### Symptoms

The patient may present with sudden decrease in vision, redness of eyes, swelling of lids, breathlessness and confusion.

### Signs

1. Ecchymosis of lids and subconjunctival hemorrhages are common.
2. Relative afferent pupillary defect (RAPD) is present.
3. Presence of bilateral multiple cotton wool spots (½–1 disk diameter in size) in the peripapillary area is a characteristic sign of the Purtscher's retinopathy.
4. Superficial and intraretinal hemorrhages are predominantly found at the posterior pole.
5. Generalized retinal and macular edema and areas of retinal whitening are found.
6. Optic disk edema is also seen.
7. Hard exudates, serous macular detachment and optic atrophy are the other features.
8. Systemic signs include cyanosis, cough, restlessness, skin hemorrhages, seizures, fracture of ribs and skull, and coma.

## Differential Diagnosis

Purtscher-like retinopathy may develop in the following conditions unassociated with the history of trauma.

1. Collagen diseases: Systemic lupus erythematosus (SLE), scleroderma, dermatomyositis and Sjögren syndrome
2. Acute pancreatitis
3. Chronic renal failure
4. Malignant hypertension.

## Diagnosis

1. In the absence of a history of trauma, a complete systemic examination and laboratory investigations are recommended.
2. A dilated fundus examination is mandatory.
3. Fundus fluorescein angiography (FFA) reveals retinal capillary nonperfusion in the area of retinal whitening and optic disk edema.
4. CT chest and skull can show the extent of damage.

## Treatment

1. Systemic condition of the patient should be managed on emergency basis.
2. Ocular treatment is not effective and most of the time the disease is self-limiting.

## 12.11 CHOROIDAL RUPTURE

### Etiology

1. Choroidal rupture (break in the choroid, Bruch's membrane and retinal pigment epithelium) is caused by blunt (countrecoup) trauma.
2. Presence of angioid streaks makes the eye more vulnerable for rupture.

### Symptoms

Decrease in vision is the main symptom.

### Signs

1. The rupture of the choroid develops as yellowish-white curved streak/s often concentric to optic disk.

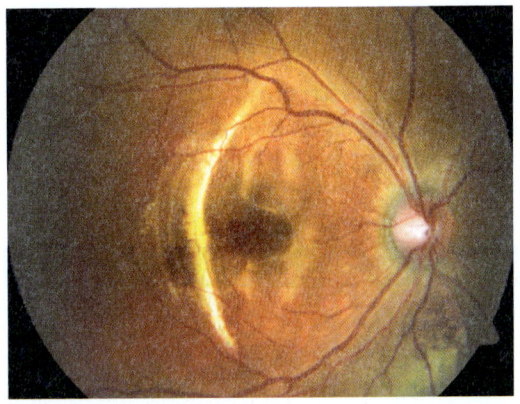

Fig. 12.7: Rupture of the choroid (*Courtesy:* Prof. Naresh Babu, AEH, Madurai)

2. The rupture of the choroid is usually found in the temporal (80%) fundus (Fig. 12.7).
3. Occasionally, the ruptures are multiple and appear radially oriented and can be on nasal side also.
4. The associated subchoroidal, intraretinal or vitreous hemorrhages may mask the details of choroidal rupture.
5. Pigments appear on the edges of the streak.
6. A rupture in the macular area (66%) causes loss of the central vision.
7. Later, choroidal neovascularization (CNV) appears during healing.
8. Central or paracentral scotoma is found on visual field charting.

### Differential Diagnosis

1. Angioid streaks
2. Lacquer cracks of high myopia.

### Diagnosis

1. Dilated fundus examination finds choroidal tears.
2. Slit-lamp biomicroscopy can reveal CNV.
3. FFA/indocyanine green angiography (ICGA) can confirm CNV.

### Treatment

1. Anti-vascular endothelial growth factor (anti-VEGF) drugs are used for the management of CNV.

**12**

2. Laser photocoagulation or photodynamic therapy may also be applied for CNV.
3. Pars plana vitrectomy with membrane extraction was in the past considered for subfoveal or juxtafoveal CNV if medical treatment failed.

## 12.12 CHORIORETINAL SCLOPETARIA

### Etiology

1. Chorioretinal sclopetaria is usually encountered in warfare.
2. It is caused by a high-velocity missile (BB bullet or shrapnel) injury to the orbit without hitting the eyeball.
3. Shock waves generated by the missile result in chorioretinal sclopetaria.
4. The ocular damage depends on the velocity and the size of the missile.

### Symptoms

Loss of vision is a prominent feature often associated with pain and watering.

### Signs

1. An area of chorioretinal rupture leaves bare white sclera; the ruptured tissue may undergo necrosis.
2. Extensive hemorrhages are found in retina, choroid and vitreous. It can also involve the macular area.
3. Fibrous bands develop following absorption of blood.
4. Other features include vitreous base detachment, retinal dialysis and IOFBs.

### Differential Diagnosis

1. Choroidal rupture
2. Avulsion of optic nerve: It results in loss of vision and manifests as retraction of the optic nerve head and vitreous hemorrhage.

### Diagnosis

1. A history of injury by a high velocity missile.

2. Dilated fundus examination shows rupture of retina and choroid with underlying bare sclera.
3. CT of orbit to rule out IOFB.
4. B-scan helps to localize IOFB.
5. UBM can locate FB.

### Treatment

1. No effective treatment is available for the chorioretinal sclopetaria.
2. Retinal dialysis and nonabsorbing vitreous hemorrhage are dealt surgically.
3. IOFB should be removed.

## 12.13 BLOWOUT FRACTURE OF THE ORBIT

### Etiology

1. The blunt trauma by a fist, cricket ball causes blowout fracture of the orbit.
2. There are two theories for mechanism of fracture:
   - The hydraulic theory suggests that shock wave generated by trauma shatters the weakest orbital bone.
   - The buckling theory advocates that a force at the inferior orbital rim causes fracture of the orbital floor.

### Symptoms

1. Symptoms are diplopia, pain, redness, watering, blurred vision and swelling of the eyelid.
2. Children may not complain of diplopia but keep their eye closed or may present with nausea, vomiting, bradycardia or syncope.

### Signs

1. Diplopia on the upward gaze
2. The upward ocular movement is restricted and painful. It indicates inferior rectus muscle entrapment. The eye looks enophthalmic. (Fig. 12.8).
3. Movements of horizontal muscles are also restricted.

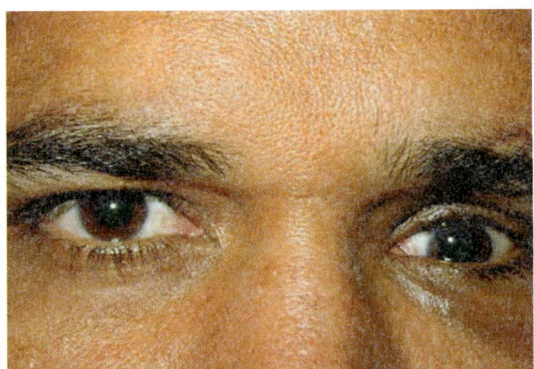

Fig. 12.8: Fracture floor of the left orbit (*Courtesy:* Dr AK Grover, Ganga Ram Hospital, New Delhi)

4. Some of the pediatric patients may develop trap-door fracture with restriction of ocular movements but without other external signs of fracture such a condition is known as "white-eyed blowout fracture".
5. Emphysema of the eyelid is seen in the fracture of the medial wall of the orbit
6. Periorbital ecchymosis or hemotoma may be found.
7. Unilateral hypesthesia of the face in the distribution of supraorbital and supra-trochlear nerves can be noticed.
8. Initial proptosis may be followed by enophthalmos.
9. Enophthalmos becomes marked after the orbital edema subsides. The prolapse of tissue in sinuses—maxillary or ethmoid can also cause enophthalmos.
10. A deformity of the inferior orbital margin may be palpable.
11. Traumatic retrobulbar hemorrhage and optic neuropathy may be found.
12. Other features include ptosis, traumatic iritis, hyphema, pupillary abnormalities, low/elevated IOP, retinochoroidal rupture, macular edema and rupture of the globe.

## Diagnosis

1. Recent history of trauma.

2. Clinical evidence of step-off deformity of lower orbital rim, hypesthesia of face and vertical diplopia.
3. The entrapment of the muscle can be confirmed on a forced duction test. Under topical anesthesia, the eye is grasped at the limbus and rotated in the deficient direction of gaze.
4. The diagnosis of a blowout fracture is confirmed by obtaining CT scan (Fig. 12.9); both axial and coronal views of the orbit.

## Treatment

1. Initially, all orbital fractures should be treated on conservative lines (analgesic, antibiotics and corticosteroids) for early resolution of lid and orbital swelling.
2. Instruct the patient for bed rest and not to blow the nose and use ice-packs on the affected eye.
   - Early surgical intervention is indicated in the following situations:
     - If muscle entrapment is associated with bradycardia and heart block.
     - White eye blowout orbital fracture
     - Early enophthalmos or hypoglobus.
   - Surgical correction is recommended within 2 weeks
     - Fracture is large.

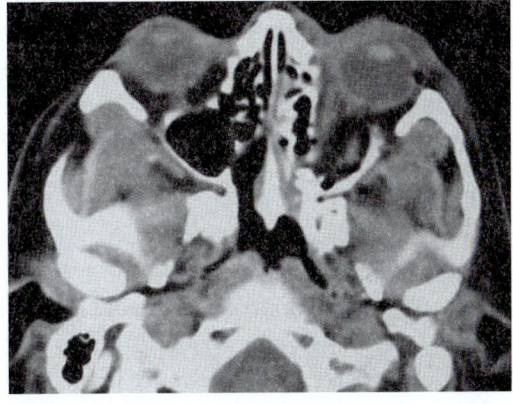

Fig. 12.9: CT showing fracture floor of the left orbit (*Courtesy:* Dr AK Grover, Ganga Ram Hospital, New Delhi)

12

- Diplopia persists for more than 10 days after the injury.
- Enophthalmos exceeds 2 mm.
- Infraorbital hypoesthesia is progressive.
  - Surgical approaches are:
    - Elevation of periorbita from the orbital floor
    - Release of entrapped inferior rectus muscle and orbital tissue, and placement of an implant.

## 12.14 RETROBULBAR HEMORRHAGE

### Etiology

1. The retrobulbar hemorrhage is caused by blunt trauma to eye, face and head injury and retrobulbar injection.
2. It is a common complication of sinus surgery, cosmetic surgery of eyelid and repair of orbital fracture.
3. Presence of orbital varix, lymphangioma and arteriovenous malformation can lead to hemorrhage.
4. Systemic disorders such as hypertension, blood dyscrasia, sickle cell disease, NSAID medication, and anticoagulant therapy are known risk factors.

### Symptoms

1. The common symptoms are pain, pressure on the eye and decreased vision.
2. Other symptoms include diplopia, swelling of lids and conjunctiva, inability to open the lids, red eye, bulging of eye, nausea and vomiting.

### Signs

1. A combination of ecchymosis of lid, hematoma of orbit and extensive subconjunctival hemorrhages presents an alarming picture.
2. Expanding proptosis is usually present.
3. Increased IOP, RAPD and ophthalmoplegia are other important signs.

4. Compressive optic neuropathy or pallor of the optic disk should be taken seriously.
5. Signs of retinal vascular occlusion may be present.

### Differential Diagnosis

1. Orbital fracture
2. Carotid-cavernous fistula
3. Orbital cellulitis.

### Diagnosis

1. History of trauma or intraocular surgery
2. Diagnosis of most cases of retrobulbar hemorrhage is clinical.
3. Detail eye examination including pupillary reflexes, IOP, dilated fundus examination for assessing the status of retina and optic nerve should be performed.
4. CT-scan can exclude the fracture of the orbit.

### Treatment

1. Use of anticoagulants and NSAIDs must be discontinued.
2. The main aim of treatment is to lower the intraorbital as well as IOP. It can be achieved by administration of intravenous mannitol and acetazolamide and topical timolol maleate.
3. If optic neuropathy is suspected, a course of intravenous methylprednisolone should be recommended to reduce soft tissue edema.
4. If medical therapy fails to reduce increased IOP and intraorbital pressure, lateral canthotomy with inferior cantholysis must be performed without further delay. The success of the procedure is evident by a decrease in IOP (there is a reliable correlation between IOP and intraorbital pressure).
5. If the lateral canthotomy and inferior cantholysis do not relieve the intraorbital pressure, an infrolateral anterior orbitotomy can decompress the orbit.

## 12.15 PENETRATING OCULAR INJURIES

### Etiology

1. The penetrating ocular injuries are caused by needle, knife, scissors, screw drivers and flying metallic FBs.
2. The incidence of penetrating injury is more common in young males than females; and especially in those who work in high-risk industries without wearing protective device.
3. The penetrating object may create a single wound at the site of entry and second at exit also.
4. The injury can produce an immediate or a delayed damage to the eye.

### Symptoms

Severe pain and loss of vision are common presentation. Children complain of nausea, vomiting and even abdominal pain.

### Signs

1. Cornea may suffer a minor cut or an extensive wound involving the limbus and sclera. The cut may be clean, linear or lacerated.
2. Small corneal shelving wound is usually sealed owing to swelling of margins and the anterior chamber depth is restored.
3. Large peripheral corneal wound may result in prolapse of iris (Fig. 12.10) and vitreous and need repair. There can be scleral tear with ciliary body prolapse or an occult scleral tear.
4. Anterior chamber may be flat, shallow or irregular and hyphema is often present
5. Presence of lens and vitreous in the wound is not rare.
6. IOP is very low; eye becomes soft.
7. Traumatic anterior uveitis is very common and infected cases may develop hypopyon.
8. FB or hole in the iris, aniridia and iridodialysis may be seen.

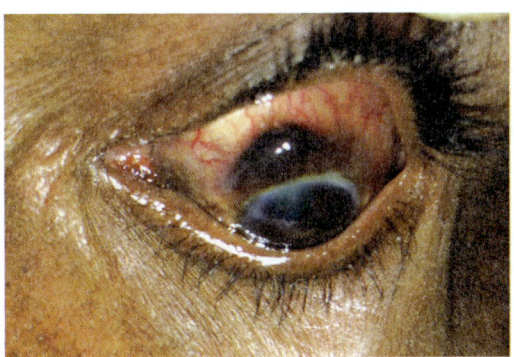

Fig. 12.10: A large traumatic wound with big iris prolapse

9. Pupil may be peaked due to prolapse and becomes irregular.
10. Ciliary body may be detached (cyclodialysis) and often bleeds.
11. The anterior capsule of the lens is usually ruptured and cataract develops. The lens may be subluxated, or dislocated in the vitreous.
12. Posterior vitreous detachment associated with vitreous hemorrhage and pigment dusting may occur. Later, fibrous proliferation in the vitreous may ensue.
13. Choroidal rupture, hemorrhages and secondary choroidal neovascularization may be visible.
14. Retinal hemorrhages, breaks and retinal detachment are often seen.
15. Optic neuropathy manifests with sudden loss of vision. Avulsion of optic nerve is rare.
16. Patient is likely to develop panophthalmitis if eye injury is caused by an organic matter and the eye has retained IOFB and remains untreated.

### Diagnosis

1. Clinical examination of the patient with penetrating injury should be done in the operation theater with minimal manipulation and utmost care.
2. Investigations like CT, B-scan ultrasonography should be done after repair of the wound.

**12**

## Treatment

1. A shelved wound of the cornea may heal quickly if treated.
2. Lacerated corneal wounds need repair and iris must be abscised and the wound should be sutured.
3. The scleral wound must be inspected after reflection of the conjunctiva and if iris, or vitreous, is present in the wound, they should be abscised and the sclera is sutured.
4. Subluxated lens must be removed followed by anterior vitrectomy.
5. Tetanus toxoid is administered in all the cases.
6. Topical, systemic and intravitreal anti-biotics are recommended in patients with high-risk of infection.
7. Severely injured eyes without any chance of restoration of sight should be enucleated.

## 12.16 TRAUMATIC OPTIC NEUROPATHY

### Etiology

1. Traumatic optic neuropathy is caused by direct trauma to orbit or indirect from injury to face and frontal part of skull.
2. The direct trauma may cause compression and laceration of optic nerve, hemorrhage in the optic nerve sheath or orbit and transection or avulsion of the nerve.
3. Indirect trauma is more common and occurs following fall from bicycle, auto-mobile accidents or hitting the head against the wall. The trauma may damage the nerve by deceleration injury by shearing of its blood supply or rotation of the globe.
4. Optic neuropathy may also be caused by fracture of the apex of the orbit, impinge-ment of optic canal and FB in the orbit.

### Symptoms

Pain, decreased vision or loss of vision, difficulty in recognizing colors, diplopia and field defects are common symptoms.

### Signs

1. Edema, ecchymosis of lid, ptosis and prop-tosis may be seen.
2. Pupil is dilated with RAPD.
3. Ocular mobility is restricted due to injury to extraocular muscles.
4. Orbital hematoma is not rare.
5. The optic disk appears normal or congested (Fig. 12.11) and later mild pallor develops.
6. Avulsion of the optic nerve head is rare may occur in war.
7. Vitreous hemorrhage can mask the fundus view.
8. Other signs of ocular trauma may be present.
9. There may be associated clinical features of intracranial injury.

### Differential Diagnosis

Preexisting optic neuropathy.

### Diagnosis

1. History of direct or indirect ocular trauma or head injury and visual status before trauma.
2. Visual acuity and color vision testing
3. Fundus examination
4. CT-scans of orbit and skull through optic canal for FB, fracture and bony impinge-ment on the nerve.
5. B-scan ultrasonography can reveal avulsion of the optic nerve head.

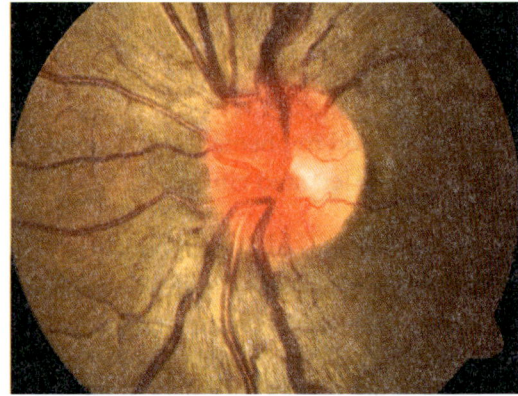

Fig. 12.11: Traumatic optic neuropathy

12

## Treatment

1. In spite of controversy, intravenous prednisolone (30 mg) therapy is recommended for 3 days followed by oral therapy. If visual improvement does not occur in 2–3 days, it should be stopped.
2. Orbital hematoma if compressing the optic nerve should be drained.
3. Optic nerve sheath fenestration may relieve the pressure from hematoma of the nerve sheath.
4. Early decompression is necessary in patients with impingement of optic canal.
5. Orbital FB causing compressive optic neuropathy must be removed.
6. There is no treatment for avulsion of optic nerve head.

## 12.17 INTRAOCULAR FOREIGN BODIES

### Etiology

1. Intraocular foreign bodies (IOFBs) are often seen in workers engaged in stone cutting, lathe, iron foundry, etc.
2. Chips of iron, copper, lead, stone, glass etc. may be found in the eye.
3. The chip may penetrate the eye especially when it strikes the eye with a high velocity.

### Symptoms

Severe pain, watering or decreased vision are common. Occasionally, patients remain symptom-free.

### Signs

1. The mode of entry of FB in the eye is either from cornea or sclera. Iris is not injured when FB enters from the center of the cornea.
2. FB entering through the peripheral part of the cornea creates a hole in the iris.
3. In case FB gets entry from the posterior sclera it passes through choroid and retina and found in the vitreous.

4. The IOFB is likely to damage the eye in four ways:
   - Mechanical
   - Infection
   - Chemical disintegration of IOFB
   - Inflammation in the sound eye (sympathetic ophthalmitis).
5. FB can be found in any intraocular structure of the eye as well as in the orbit.
   - The mechanical effects of the IOFB:
     - FB may be lodged in the iris or perforate it leaving behind a hole.
     - FB may be found in the lens, or forms an opaque track.
     - Initially, the IOFB remains suspended in the vitreous gel but with liquefaction of vitreous it sinks in the vitreous cavity. An opaque tract may be left in the vitreous by a fast moving FB.
     - Retinal FB may be associated with hemorrhages and exudation and tends to undergo encapsulation.
     - IOFB may be lodged on the choroid or sclera.
     - Occasionally, a high speed FB may cause double perforation of the eye and lodge in the orbital tissue (Fig. 12.12).

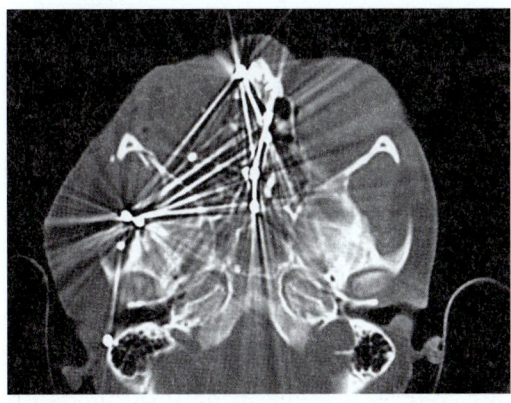

**Fig. 12.12:** CT showing bullets in the orbit (*Courtesy:* Dr AK Grover, Ganga Ram Hospital, New Delhi)

**12**

- Intraocular infection
  - Nonmetallic FBs such as stone, pieces of wood, thorns or vegetables often produce a proliferative reaction and form granuloma. They usually get contaminated with bacteria and fungi and cause severe ocular infection.
  - Infection manifests either as endophthalmitis or panophthalmitis and causes blindness.
- Chemical disintegration of IOFB
  - Depending on the composition, FBs are capable of inducing chemical reactions.
  - Iron and copper FBs induce characteristic siderosis bulbi and chalcosis, respectively.
  - Gold, platinum, glass and porcelain are considered inert.

## Siderosis Bulbi

1. The retained iron IOFB undergoes an electrolytic dissociation and causes brownish discoloration and degeneration of intraocular tissues, a condition known as siderosis bulbi.
2. Early sign of siderosis bulbi is development of brown oval patches on the anterior lens capsule followed by cataract formation.
3. The iris becomes brownish-red and pupil is dilated owing to degeneration of sphincter pupillae.
4. Iron pigments are found in the trabeculum with increased IOP.
5. Pigmentary degeneration of retina and optic atrophy are important manifestations of siderosis bulbi.

## Chalcosis

1. Pure copper IOFB causes a violent reaction while the copper alloy (brass) gives a mild reaction.
2. The deposition of copper in the periphery of the cornea gives Kayser-Fleischer ring.

3. Sunflower cataract with golden-green petals is formed due to deposition of copper under the lens capsule.
4. The copper deposition at the posterior pole is seen as a golden-green plaque.
5. Copper alloy FBs do not produce cell degeneration.

## Diagnosis and Localization of IOFB

1. History-taking is important; the surgeon can know the nature of the IOFB by inquiring the type of job the patient was engaged at the time of accident. Whether the FB was metallic or nonmetallic should be ascertained to facilitate treatment. Did it enter the eye like a missile or gently?
2. Slit-lamp examination should be conducted to find the corneal or scleral wound of entry, hole in the iris.
3. Gonioscopy is necessary to localize the IOFB in the chamber angle.
4. Presence of iris hole and opaque tract through the lens and vitreous have great diagnostic value.
5. Dilated fundus examination may detect the FB in the posterior segment of the eye. The presence of a retinal perforation indicates the FB may be in the posterior sclera or the orbit.
6. A plain X-ray of the orbit may reveal the presence of a FB.
7. CT-scan is the most preferred modality for localization of an IOFB.
8. MRI is contraindicated in metallic IOFB. However, it is preferred in organic IOFBs.
9. Both metallic and nonmetallic IOFBs can be diagnosed with the help of ultrasonography. It can also diagnose associated detachment and incarceration of retina and vitreous.
10. UBM is helpful in localization of IOFB in the anterior segment of the eye.

## Treatment

1. Although removal of an IOFB is almost always preferred, the removal is deferred

if it is likely to destroy the remaining vision in the injured eye. Inert FB may not further damage the eye.

2. FB lying in the anterior chamber can be removed under direct vision by making an incision at the limbus. If it is magnetic, a hand-held magnet may be used.

3. FB embedded in the iris is removed by iridectomy.

4. If lens with FB is opaque, it should be extracted.

5. Magnetic FB in the vitreous and retina can be removed either through the anterior route or the posterior route with the help of magnet.

6. Nonmagnetic FB from the posterior segment is removed by bimanual vitrectomy and with the help of intravitreal forceps.

7. A FB greater than 2 mm in size destroys the eye.

## 12.18 SYMPATHETIC OPHTHALMITIS

### Etiology

1. The etiology of sympathetic uveitis is not clear.

2. It is considered to be an autoimmune disease wherein uveal pigment acts as an allergen.

3. The uveal protein acts as antigen due to virus infection.

4. The incidence of sympathetic ophthalmitis is higher in children and in patients with penetrating injury in the danger zone (ciliary body) and retained FB.

### Symptoms

1. The development of watering and photophobia in a normal eye following injury to the contralateral eye hearlds the onset of sympathetic ophthalmia.

2. Symptoms like pain, photophobia and redness are aggravated in the injured eye.

### Signs

1. A granulomatous anterior uveitis sets in the uninjured eye marked by the presence of ciliary flush, mutton-fat keratic precipitates, flare, nodular infiltrations in the iris, and synechiae. The granulomatous uveitis in the exciting eye is flared up and its condition worsens.

2. A full blown case of sympathetic ophthalmitis presents severe uveitis. Marked exudation in the pupillary area, heavy posterior synechae and elevated IOP are found.

3. Eye becomes tender.

4. Multiple vitreous opacities, perivasculitis and papilledema are seen.

5. Fundus has a sunset glow due to pigmentary disturbances.

6. The exciting eye remains irritable.

7. Exacerbations and remissions are frequent

8. Systemic features include headache, tinnitus, vitiligo and alopecia.

### Diagnosis

1. History of injury in one eye.

2. Clinical evidence of severe uveitis in the uninjured eye.

3. FFA shows multiple foci of leakage and retinal detachment.

4. ICGA may reveal dark spots in the choroid; an evidence of active disease.

5. B-scan ultrasonography can reveal the presence of choroidal thickening and retinal detachment.

6. Histopathology of the enucleated eye often shows thickening of choroid and Dalen-Fuchs nodules.

### Prophylaxis

1. The incidence of sympathetic ophthalmitis has significantly decreased in recent years due to early repair of the wound and administration of corticosteroids.

2. Enucleation of injured eye with poor prognosis within first 2 weeks is an established prophylactic measure.

12

## Treatment

1. All cases of penetrating ocular injury should be considered as emergency and the injured eye must be repaired as early as possible.
2. Topical atropine sulphate (1% drops, 3 times a day), moxifloxacin eye drops (0.5%, 6 times daily) and prednisolone drops (1%, hourly) are instilled.
3. A systemic course of antibiotics and corticosteroids is administered for a considerable period with monitoring of IOP.
4. If systemic corticosteroids fail to improve the condition, antimetabolite therapy is indicated. Cyclosporine is preferred.
5. If the patient does not have any vision in the injured eye and ciliary injection persists in spite of treatment, the eye should be enucleated to prevent sympathetic ophthalmia.

## 12.19 CHEMICAL BURN

### Etiology

1. Strong alkali and acid usually produce serious chemical injuries to the eye.
2. Detergents, disinfectants, drain cleaners, fertilizers and pesticides can cause ocular burns.
3. Cyanoacrylate can also damage the eye due to its quick hardening after coming in contact with the eye mainly due to moisture.

### Alkali Burns

1. Alkali burn may be caused by caustic potash, ammonia, and mortar.
2. Alkali burn is more common and more severe than acid burn. However, initially, it appears less alarming because of its delayed effect.
3. Alkali damages the eye due to: (i) deep penetration in tissue (ii) sudden increase in the pH of tissue, (iii) destruction of cell membrane by saponification of fat (iv) destruction of limbal stem cells and (v) causing ischemia.

### Acid Burns

1. Sulfuric acid, nitric acid, glacial acetic acid, acid used in inverter batteries etc. cause serious ocular burns.
2. Acids do not penetrate deeply because they coagulate surface proteins that acts as a barrier. However, they are capable of inciting a severe inflammatory reaction causing destruction of the corneal stroma.

### Symptoms

Marked photophobia, lacrimation, blephrospasm, intense pain and loss of vision are common symptoms.

### Signs

1. Ocular signs of chemical burn show great variation depending on the duration of exposure to alkali or acid.
2. Mild degree of burn presents papillary conjunctivitis, conjunctival chemosis and SPK. There is no limbal ischemia and corneal damage.
3. *Moderate degree of burn* shows considerable damage to conjunctiva and cornea. There may be a total corneal erosion, superficial stromal destruction, superficial neovascularization of the cornea, mild anterior chamber reaction and visual impairment. It is accompanied with segmental limbal ischemia.
4. *Severe degree of burn* causes chemosis and blanching of the conjunctiva, opaque cornea and marked limbal ischemia. Cornea becomes necrotic and undergoes ulceration and perforation. Burn destroys limbal stem cells leading to conjunctivalization of the cornea associated with vascularization. It may cause severe reaction in the anterior chamber resulting in uveitis, cataract and secondary glaucoma. Hypotony can develop as a result of ciliary body injury.
5. Severe chemical burns are likely to cause complications like secondary glaucoma, nonhealing corneal ulcer, dry eye disease,

12

pseudopterygium and symblepharon (Fig. 12.13).

## Diagnosis

1. History may reveal the type of chemical agent, time of accident and the first-aid treatment received.
2. Slit-lamp examination is necessary to assess the extent of burn.

## Treatment

1. Immediate irrigation by normal saline regains its near neutral pH (7–7.4).
2. Particles of chemical material are removed with a swab stick or forceps after topical anesthesia.
3. Surgical debridement may be necessary for removal of embedded particles.
4. Topical atropine drops (1%, 3 times/day), moxifloxacin eye drops [0.5%, (4 times/day] and prednisolone acetate drops (1%, 8–10 times/day) are administered.
5. Systemic prednisolone (60 mg/day) is added if anterior uveitis persists.
6. Use of preservative-free artificial gel (6–8 times in a day) enhances epithelial healing.
7. Use of therapeutic soft contact lenses may help in epithelial healing.

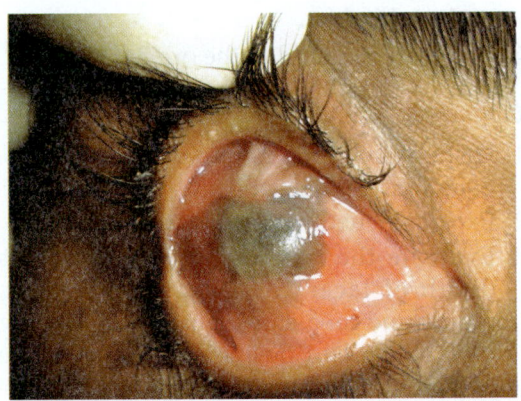

**Fig. 12.13:** Severe chemical burn with extensive symblepharon (*Courtesy:* Dr AK Grover, Ganga Ram Hospital, New Delhi)

8. Oral tetracyclines (500 mg bid) prevent polymorphonuclear-induced collagenolysis and corneal melting.
9. Intravenous or oral ascorbic acid (2 g per day) is given to promote collagen synthesis. It has been reported that it may prevent corneal melting in severe alkali burns.
10. After sweeping a glass rod in fornices, a conformer may be used.

### Surgical Measures

1. Tarsorrhaphy is performed.
2. An amniotic membrane graft may be transplanted.
3. Stem cells transplants may be helpful in restoring the corneal epithelium.
4. Extensive burn of the cornea may need penetrating keratoplasty (PK). However, it has a poor prognosis.
5. Keratoprosthesis can be tried in failed PK cases.

### Prognosis

The prognostic classification of Roper-Hall is shown in Table 12.1. It is mainly based on corneal transparency and ischemia of limbus.

## 12.20 INJURY TO OCULAR ADNEXA

### Etiology

1. Injury to ocular adnexa is caused by blunt or sharp objects.
2. Dog bite injuries are common in children.
3. Trauma may involve eyelids, lacrimal canaliculi, medial palpebral ligament, lacrimal gland, orbital fat and orbital bones.

### Symptoms

Pain, watering, swelling of lids and bleeding may occur.

### Signs

Signs depend on involvement of individual structure of the ocular adnexa.

**12**

**Table 12.1** Classification of ocular chemical burns and their prognosis

| Grade | Conjunctiva/cornea | Iris | Limbal ischemia | Prognosis |
|---|---|---|---|---|
| I | Some epithelial damage | Details clearly seen | No ischemia | Very good |
| II | Large epithelial damage, cornea hazy | Seen | Less than one-third ischemia | Good |
| III | Total epithelial loss, stromal haze | Blurring iris details | One-third to half ischemia | Guarded |
| IV | Opaque cornea | Not seen | Greater than half ischemia | Poor |

### Eyelids

1. Eyelid injury may vary from minor skin abrasion to complete tear.
2. Ecchymosis or hematoma of lid and ptosis are common after blunt trauma (Fig. 12.14).
3. Superficial laceration of eyelid margin with or without gaping wound may be seen.
4. Partial or full-thickness tear of the eyelid is not rare.
5. Injury to the lateral portion of eyelid may implicate the lateral canthal ligament and lacrimal gland.
6. Laceration of the medial part of the eyelid often damages lacrimal punctum and canalicui.
7. Injury to the medial canthal ligament causes its laxity or displacement resulting in rounding of the medial canthus.

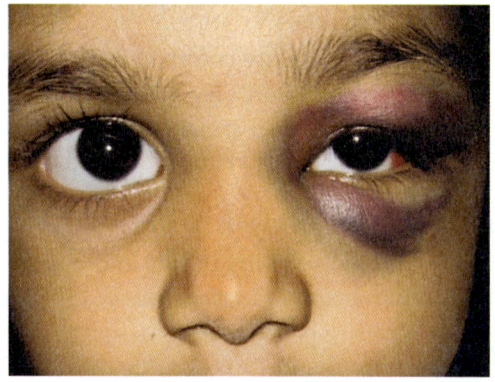

**Fig. 12.14:** Traumatic orbital ecchymosis, ptosis and subconjunctival hemorrhage

8. Laceration of eyelid is common in road traffic accidents.

### Conjunctiva

1. Subconjunctival hemorrhage and ecchymosis are common.
2. Tear and infection can occur.

### Orbit

1. Trauma can cause fracture of medial and lateral walls, floor of the orbit and apex.
2. Initially, the fracture produces proptosis followed by enophthalmos or hypo-ophthalmos.
3. Periorbital hematoma and restriction of ocular motility are important signs.
4. Fracture of apex of the orbit is rare.
5. Damage to orbital septum leads to prolapse of the orbital fat.
6. A FB can be found in the orbit.

### Diagnosis

1. History about the nature of injury: Blunt, penetrating, FB or dog bite.
2. Exclude penetrating injury to eyeball.
3. Evaluate the type of lid injury such as depth of laceration, degree of ptosis, puncta and canaliculi damage by syringing or probing, and position and appearance of medial and lateral canthal ligaments.
4. Dilated funduscopy to exclude retinal detachment, optic neuropathy and IOFB
5. CT scan to exclude IOFB or orbital FB.

## Treatment

1. Administer tetanus toxoid.
2. Patient with contaminated laceration of the lid should be given systemic broad spectrum antibiotics.
3. The superficial wound of the eyelid is thoroughly cleaned and FBs are removed. The wound is sutured under local anesthesia.
4. The tear of lid margin requires careful plastic repair to avoid postoperative notching.
5. The canalicular laceration is repaired with the help of a silicone tube. The tube is intubated from punctum to bridge the lacerated parts of canaliculi and threaded down to nasolacrimal duct opening in the nose.
6. Deep laceration with extensive tissue loss of eyelid needs major reconstructive surgery.
7. The wound should be dressed with antibiotic ointment and a protective shield is applied.

## 12.21 SHAKEN BABY SYNDROME

### Etiology

1. Shaken baby syndrome or child abuse occurs due to acceleration-deacceleration forces of violent shaking of the child by caregiver causing grave neurotrauma.
2. Although external signs of trauma may not be visible, the child may sustain internal injuries.
3. The age of the child is usually between 1 year and 3 years.

### Symptoms

Irritability, feeding difficulty, vomiting, lack of interest, lethargy, change in mental status and seizures are common.

### Signs

1. The anterior segment of the eye appears normal except RAPD or widely dilated nonreactive pupils.

2. Extensive superficial and intra- and subretinal hemorrhages are associated with subarachnoid and subdural hemorrhages.
3. Vitreous hemorrhage and hemorrhage in the sheath of the optic nerve may occur.
4. Hemorrhagic macular cyst, macular schisis, papilledema and optic nerve avulsion (rare) may be found.
5. Nystagmus, disconjugate eye movements, esotropia or exotropia, cranial nerve palsy and cortical blindness may develop.
6. Chronic cases of child abuse may present chorioretinal scars, pigmentary disturbances, retinitis proliferans, retinal detachment, macular degeneration and optic atrophy.
7. Multiple fractures of humeral shaft, skull, clavicles and ribs are found. The most common fracture is diaphyseal fracture.

### Differential Diagnosis

1. Birth trauma
2. Accidental fall
3. Blood dyscrasia.

### Diagnosis

1. Multiple and unexplained fractures in a child should arouse a suspicion of the abuse.
2. Social history of the family and frequent changes in the statement of the caregiver may help in the diagnosis.
3. Dilated fundus examination.
4. Blood examination to rule out bleeding disorders.
5. CT-scan for bone fractures
6. MRI to assess soft tissue damage.

### Treatment

1. Child is referred to pediatrician and neuro-surgeon for opinion, treatment and care.
2. Ocular treatment is mostly supportive.
3. If vitreous hemorrhage persists, vitrectomy is performed.

12

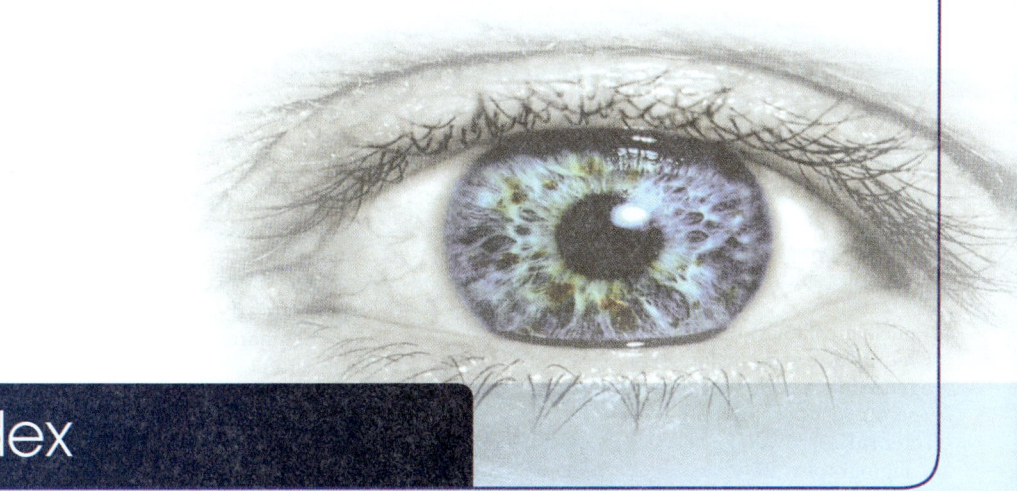

# Index